MANUAL OF
PAEDIATRICS

AN INTEGRATED APPROACH

Leon Polnay BSc MB BS FRCP FRCPCH DCH
Professor of Community Paediatrics
University of Nottingham
Queen's Medical Centre
Nottingham

Mandy Hampshire BMediSci BM BS MRCGP MEd DM
Senior Lecturer in Primary Care
Division of Primary Care
University of Nottingham
Nottingham

Monica Lakhanpaul MB BS DM MRCP MRCPCH
Senior Lecturer in Child Health
University of Leicester
Consultant Paediatrician
Specialist Community Child Health Services
Leicester

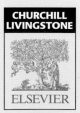

CHURCHILL LIVINGSTONE

ELSEVIER

Edinburgh London New York Oxford Philadelphia St Louis Sydney
Toronto 2007

CHURCHILL LIVINGSTONE
ELSEVIER

First published 2006

ISBN 10: 0-443-07494-1
ISBN 13: 987-0-443-07494-3

British Library Cataloguing in Publication Data
A catalogue record for this book is available from the British Library

Library of Congress Cataloging in Publication Data
A catalog record for this book is available from the Library of Congress

Notice

Knowledge and best practice in this field are constantly changing. As new research and experience broaden our knowledge, changes in practice, treatment and drug therapy may become necessary or appropriate. Readers are advised to check the most current information provided (i) on procedures featured or (ii) by the manufacturer of each product to be administered, to verify the recommended dose or formula, the method and duration of administration, and contraindications. It is the responsibility of the practitioner, relying on their own experience and knowledge of the patient, to make diagnoses, to determine dosages and the best treatment for each individual patient, and to take all appropriate safety precautions. To the fullest extent of the law, neither the Publisher nor the Editors assume any liability for any injury and/or damage to persons or property arising out or related to any use of the material contained in this book.

The Publisher

Printed in China

PREFACE

This book has been written with the intention of providing a concise reference source for both family doctors and paediatricians. We recognise the need for joined up clinical pathways between primary and secondary care. They are based upon published guidelines, where available, and our own clinical practice. We hope that the standardised format will provide an easily accessed format for readers. The contents cover the information that clinicians will need at their finger tips starting with the problem as it presents, e.g. problems with vision and working towards specific diagnoses. More detailed discussion can be found in the companion textbook, *Community Paediatrics,* or in the references quoted at the end of each section. We have had to make choices on the limited number of topics that we could cover in a handbook. We have focused on common clinical problems and have excluded tertiary care issues. The sections of the book are intended to reflect good clinical practice with headings such as 'who to talk to' and 'key points for parents' underlying the need for communication and discussion with both colleagues and parents.

This book comes with two warnings: firstly that information becomes obsolete and secondly that in the real clinical world pathways are a lot more complex and tortuous than our writing might suggest.

We are grateful to the contributors for helping us to complete this project and for remaining our friends in spite of our editorial demands.

We would like to thank Dr Jane Ravenscroft, Dr Yin Ng, Dr Pradip Thakkar and Mr David Spicer for critically reviewing some of the chapters.

Finally we would like to thank our families for their tolerance and support during this work.

Leon Polnay, Mandy Hampshire, Monica Lakhanpaul
Nottingham and Leicester
September 2005

CONTRIBUTORS

Maria Atkinson MB ChB MRCPCH
Paediatric Specialist Registrar
Queen's Medical Centre
University Hospital
Nottingham

David W. Bond MB ChB MRCP(UK) FRCPCH
Consultant Paediatrician
Kings Mill Hospital
Sutton-in-Ashfield
Nottinghamshire

Sandra Buck MB ChB DCH MRCPCH
Associate Specialist in Paediatrics
1 Bridgeway Centre
The Meadows
Nottingham

Liz Didcock BM BS BMedSci DTM&H FRCPCH
Consultant Paediatrician
RHR Medical Centre
Nottingham

Rosemary Dove MB ChB DCCH DRCOG
Associate Specialist in Community Paediatrics
Sherwood Rise Health Centre
Nottingham

Richard Gregson BM BCh MA DPhil FRCS(Ed) FRCOpth
Consultant Paediatric Ophthalmologist
Department of Ophthalmology
Queen's Medical Centre University Hospital NHS Trust
Nottingham

Catherine Griffin MB BCh MRCPCH
Associate Specialist in Paediatrics Integrated
Children's Services
Huntingdonshire PCT

Mandy Hampshire BMedSci BM BS MRCGP M Ed DM
Senior Lecturer in Primary Care
Division of Primary Care
University of Nottingham
Nottingham

Helen Heussler MB BS FRACP
Staff Specialist and Senior Lecturer University of Queensland
Mater Children's Hospital
South Brisbane 4101
Queensland
Australia

Liz Hutchinson MSc RGN RSCN DN cert
Clinical Nurse Specialist
Nottingham Children and Young People's Rheumatology Service
Queen's Medical Centre University Hospital NHS Trust
Nottingham

Derek Johnston MD FRCP FRCPCH DCH
Consultant Paediatrician/Paediatric Endocrinologist
Children's Department
Queen's Medical Centre University Hospital NHS Trust
Nottingham

Monica Lakhanpaul MB BS DM MRCP MRCPCH
Senior Lecturer in Child Health
University of Leicester
Consultant Paediatrician
Specialist Community Child Health Services
Leicester

Sam Majumdar BM BS BMedSci (Hon) BDS (Hon) FDS RCPS FRCS
Specialist Registrar
Otolaryngology and Head and Neck Surgery
Sheffield Children's Hospital
North Trent Deanery
Sheffield

Liz Marder BM BS BMedSci MRCP(UK) FRCPCH
Consultant Paediatrician
Child Development Centre
City Hospital Campus
Hucknall Road
Nottingham

Elaine Marlow MB BS MSc
Associate Specialist in Paediatric Audiology/Community
Paediatrics
United Lincolnshire Health Care Trust
Grantham Hospital
Lincolnshire

Dilip Nathan BM BS BMedSci MRCP MRCPCH
Consultant (Community Paediatrics)
Radford Health Centre
Nottingham

Janet Polnay BScHons MB BS MA
Formerly Associate Specialist in Paediatrics and Named Doctor
for Child Protection
Nottingham City Hospital NHS Trust
Nottingham

Leon Polnay BSc MB BS FRCP FRCPCH DCH
Professor of Community Paediatrics
University of Nottingham
Queen's Medical Centre
Nottingham

Satyapal Rangaraj MRCP (UK) MRCPCH DCH
Consultant Paediatric Rheumatologist
Queen's Medical Centre University Hospital NHS Trust
Nottingham

Venkat Reddy MRCP (UK) FRCPCH
Consultant Paediatrician
Peterborough District Hospital
Peterborough

Vikas Sharma MBBS BSc (Hons) FRCOphth
Specialist Registrar in Ophthalmology
King's College NHS Trust
Denmark Hill
London

Shailinder Jit Singh MS DNB MCh FRCSI FRCS (Eng) FRCS (Paed Surg)
Consultant Paediatric Surgeon
Queen's Medical Centre University Hospital NHS Trust
Nottingham

Fiona Straw BM BS BMedSci MRCP MRCPCH DFFP
Consultant Paediatrician
Beeston Health Centre
Nottingham

Helen E. Venning BMed Sci BM BS FRCP FRCPCH
Consultant Paediatric Rheumatologist
Queen's Medical Centre University Hospital NHS Trust
Nottingham

Michelle V. Vincent MBBS MRCSEd
Specialist Registrar, Department of Paediatric Surgery
Queen's Medical Centre University Hospital NHS Trust
Nottingham

Lisa Waddell BScHons Nutr RD PhD DipADP
Community Paediatric Dietitian
Nottingham Community Nutrition and Dietetic Service
Nottingham City PCT

Louise Wells MBBS BScHons MMedSci MRCP FRCPCH
Consultant Paediatrician
Queen's Medical Centre University Hospital NHS Trust
Nottingham

William Whitehouse MB BS BSc DCH FRCP FRCPCH
Clinical Senior Lecturer (Paediatric Neurology)
Academic Division of Child Health
Queen's Medical Centre University Hospital NHS Trust
Nottingham

Jane Williams MB BS DCH FRCPCH
Consultant Paediatrician, Community Child Health
Queen's Medical Centre University Hospital NHS Trust
Nottingham

Antonia Wolff BSc MB DCH MRCP FRCPCH
Consultant (Community Paediatrics)
Child Development Centre
City Hospital Campus
Nottingham

CONTENTS

SECTION SIX: CHILD HEALTH PROMOTION PROGRAMME

SECTION SEVEN: SOCIAL PAEDIATRICS

GLOSSARY OF ACRONYMS

Within this text, eponymous names for syndromes appear in the plural (e.g. Down's syndrome, Turner's syndrome). Although there has been considerable (and continuing) debate on this issue, since this book is principally directed at a readership for whom the plural style is more common, this terminology has been adopted throughout.

ACBS	Advisory Committee on Borderline Substances
ACPC	Area Child Protection Committee
AD	autosomal dominant
ADHD	attention deficit hyperactivity disorder
ADI	Autistic Diagnostic Interview [questionnaire]
AED	antiepileptic drug
AFP	alphafetoprotein
ALP	alkaline phosphatase
ALT	alanine transaminase
ANA	antinuclear antibody
AR	autosomal recessive
ASD	atrioseptal defect; autistic spectrum disorder
AST	aspartate transaminase
BESD	behaviour, emotional and social difficulty
BMI	body mass index
BRE	benign Rolandic epilepsy
BSER	brain stem evoked responses
BSL	British sign language
BXO	balanitis xerotica obliterans
Ca	calcium
CAE	childhood absence epilepsy

CAMHS	Child and Adolescent Mental Health Services
CDGP	constitutional delay of growth and puberty
CDH	congenital dislocation of the hip
CFS	chronic fatigue syndrome
CMPH	cow's milk protein hypersensitivity
CMV	cytomegalovirus
CP	cerebral palsy
CPAP	continuous positive airways pressure
CPK	creatine phosphokinase
CPR	child protection register
Cr	creatine
CRP	C-reactive protein
CSA	child sexual abuse; Child Support Agency; Children's Services Authority
CSF	cerebrospinal fluid
CXR	chest x-ray
DCD	developmental coordination disorder
DDH	developmental dysplasia of the hip
DfES	Department for Education and Skills
DISCO	Diagnostic Interview for Social and Communication Disorders [questionnaire]
DLA	disability living allowance
DNA	did not attend
DQ	developmental quotient
DSH	deliberate self-harm
E&U	urea and electrolytes
EAS	expiratory apnoea syncope
EBV	Epstein–Barr virus
ECG	electrocardiogram

EEG	electroencephalogram
ENT	ear, nose and throat
EPA	eicosapentanoic acid
ESR	erythrocyte sedimentation rate
ETN	erythema toxicum neonatorum
EU	European Union
EUA	examination under anaesthetic
EWO	Education Welfare Officer
FBC	full blood count
FISH	fluorescent in situ hybridisation
FSH	follicle stimulating hormone
FTT	failure to thrive
GH	growth hormone
GI	gastrointestinal
GnRH	gonadotrophin releasing hormone
GOR	gastro-oesophageal reflux
GTCS	generalised tonic–clonic seizure
Hb	haemoglobin
HCG	human chorionic gonadotrophin
HI	hearing impairment
HKD	hyperkinetic disorder
HNIG	human normal immunoglobulin
HPV	human papillomavirus
HSCR	Hirschsprung's disease
HSP	Henoch–Schönlein purpura
HUS	haemolytic uraemic syndrome
IBD	inflammatory bowel disease
ICPC	initial child protection conference
IEP	individual education plan

IGE	idiopathic generalised epilepsies
IQ	intelligence quotient
JCA	juvenile chronic arthritis
JIA	juvenile idiopathic arthritis
JME	juvenile myoclonic epilepsy
KFS	Klinefelter's syndrome
LBW	low birth weight
LD	learning difficulties
LEA	local education authority
LFT	liver function test(s)
LH	luteinising hormone
LRNI	lower reference nutrient intake
LSCB	Local Safeguarding Children Board
MCH	mean corpuscular haemoglobin
MCHC	mean corpuscular haemoglobin concentration
MCV	mean corpuscular volume
MEND	mind, exercise, nutrition and diet [programme]
MLD	moderate learning difficulty
MRI	magnetic resonance imaging
MSI	multisensory impairment
NAPC	National Autism Plan for Children
NARES	non-allergic rhinitis with eosinophilia
NICE	National Institute for Health and Clinical Excellence
NMS	neurally mediated syncope
NS	Noonan's syndrome
NSAIDs	non-steroidal anti-inflammatory drugs
NSF	National Service Framework
NT	nuchal translucency
OAE	otoacoustic emissions

OCP	oral contraceptive pill
OSAS	obstructive sleep apnoea syndrome
PCR	polymerase chain reaction
PH	physical disability
Pi	protease inhibitor
PKU	phenylketonuria
PMLD	profound and multiple learning difficulty
PTSD	post-traumatic stress disorder
PUO	pyrexia of unknown origin
PWS	Prader–Willi syndrome
RAP	recurrent abdominal pain
RAPD	relative afferent pupil defect
RAS	reflex asystolic syncope
RAST	radioallergosorbent test
RCT	randomised controlled trial
RF	rheumatoid factor
RNI	reference nutrient intake
RP	retinitis pigmentosa
SAT	standard assessment task
SBI	serious bacterial illness
SD	standard deviation
SGA	small for gestational age
SIDS	sudden infant death syndrome
SLCN	speech, language and communication needs
SLD	severe learning difficulty
SLE	systemic lupus erythematosus
SPA	suprapubic aspiration
SPF	sun protection factor
SpLD	specific learning difficulty

STC	slow transit constipation
STI	sexually transmitted infection
SUFE	slipped upper femoral epiphysis
TBC	transurethral bladder catheterisation
TFT	thyroid function test
TCR	target centile range
TIBC	total iron binding capacity
T-LOC	transient loss of consciousness
TM	tympanic membrane
TORCH	toxoplasmosis, other agents, rubella, cytomegalovirus, herpes simplex
TR	target range
TS	Turner's syndrome
TSH	thyroid stimulating hormone
URTI	upper respiratory tract infections
USS	ultrasound Scan
UTI	urinary tract infection
UV	ultraviolet
VI	visual impairment
VLBW	very low birth weight
VSD	ventriculoseptal defect
VZIG	varicella zoster immunoglobulin
YOT	Youth Offending Team

ACKNOWLEDGEMENTS

The editor and authors are grateful to the publishers for permission to reproduce illustrations from the following titles:

From Cohen BA (1999) Paediatric dermatology, 2nd edn. Philadelphia: Mosby
  Figures 39.1–39.6, 40.4, 40.6–40.8.

From White GM, Cox NH (2000) Diseases of the skin: a colour atlas and text. London: Mosby
  Figures 40.1–40.3, 40.5, 41.1, 41.2.

Permission has also been granted from other sources to reproduce the following illustrations:

• *From* the Down's Syndrome Medical Interest Group (DSMIG) 1998 – Figure 10.1.

• *From* Anne Stewart, from presentation to RIPM Symposium 2004 (unpublished) – Figure 15.1.

• *From* Didcock E, Waddell L, 2004 The Nottingham Integrated Care Pathway for the management of weight and growth faltering in young children (unpublished) – Figure 30.1.

CHILD HEALTH CONSULTATIONS

GENERAL NOTES ON CHILD HEALTH CONSULTATIONS

GENERAL

Appointment letters can contain details of travel directions, access, parking, cancellation and DNA policies, who they will see and what will happen.

All paediatric consultations should take place in a child-friendly environment – this will enhance cooperation.

Younger and older children may be frightened of a visit to see a doctor, especially when there are difficult social histories.

Interpreters may be needed for some children and chaperones for older children seen on their own.

The ability to attend may be limited by poverty, poor organisation, competing priorities or child protection issues – DNAs need careful assessment.

'Results' obtained in one environment may not be generalisable to all and caution needs to be exercised in interpreting findings from a single consultation. Whether problems are pervasive or occur in only one setting may be an important piece of information.

Interruptions can disturb the flow and effectiveness of a consultation.

90% of patients are expected to be seen within 30 minutes of their appointment time.

Ask to see Red Book (personal child health record) and make a note of the consultation and advice at the end of the consultation.

PRESENTATION

Presenting symptoms in paediatrics are often a proxy for other problems, e.g. tummy ache or headaches may indicate problems at school or difficult home relationships.

ASSESSMENT

Remember to relate findings to age and gestation.

Quality of performance may be as important as pass/fail criteria when looking at development.

History

Children are the subject rather than the object of consultations – they can usually give much of the history themselves rather than being left bored or excluded while you talk with the parent.

Parents' concerns are usually justified and should always be taken seriously, even when initial observations appear to contradict their beliefs.

It is often helpful to see parents on their own at an initial consultation to discuss sensitive family issues or concerns about progress at school. Hearing a catalogue of criticisms can be a devastating experience for a child.

A genogram (Fig. 1.1) – who lives in the household, and a professionogram (Fig. 1.2) – who is involved with the child and family, are both essential information.

History should follow the same format used in adults with additional information in the following areas:

- Birth history
- Developmental history
- Immunisations
- Family and social history.

The range of 'normal' with respect to feeding patterns and bowel habits, particularly in infants, varies considerably. It is useful to ask parents what is 'normal' and how it has changed.

It is also useful to ask parents and children what is worrying them the most. This will often elucidate parental and child worries not picked up in the rest of the history.

In very young children most of the history will be taken from the parent or carer. A history from the child, however limited this may be, should be sought when they have sufficient understanding. In an older child a joint history should be taken from the child and parent. (In some circumstances it may also be useful to see the child and parents individually.)

Examination

Children are entitled to the same level of privacy as adults and even very young children can feel shy or embarrassed at being undressed.

Explanation about what you are doing and what you are about to do is helpful.

Observation usually gives excellent information on development, relationships and interaction with parents.

Examining a young child is a challenge and as much information as possible should be gained from observation prior to starting the examination. Observation of the child playing or interacting with others, especially parents, is very important. As much information as

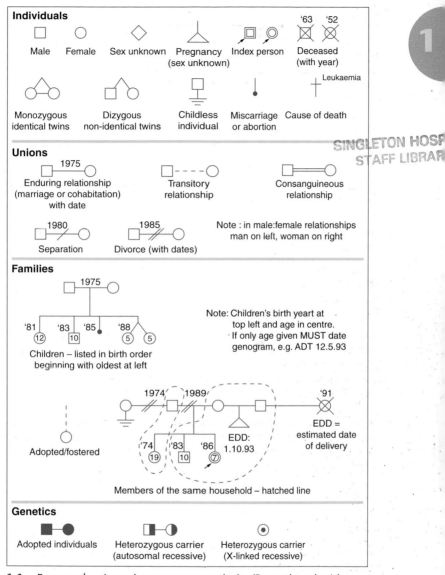

Fig. 1.1 Proposed universal genogram symbols. (Reproduced with permission from Tandy 1993, unpublished.)

possible should be gathered before touching the child. Younger children are often happier on a parent's lap and should be examined there. Try to get down to their level and explain what you are doing as you go along. The examination may need to occur in an opportunistic

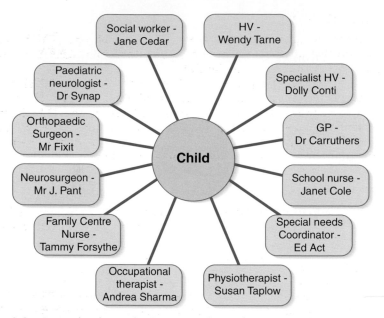

Fig. 1.2 Example of a professionogram for a 4½-year-old child with spina bifida transferring to school.

fashion rather than in any particular order. An overall view of the child's health is necessary, including an assessment of their cleanliness. Leave any unpleasant parts (e.g. ENT examination) until the end.

Diagnostic tests
Explain tests to children.
Topically applied local anaesthetic creams help greatly when blood tests are needed.

> **ALERTS**
>
> ⚠ Children who are labelled 'uncooperative' may be more than just unwilling – they may be frightened, shy, tired or unable to complete the task.

WHO TO TALK TO
Important information may often be available from others, e.g. the family doctor or class teacher. Always request permission to ask for or to pass on information or concerns that arise from the consultation.

WHEN TO REFER

Consultation involves obtaining further professional advice. This might not involve another practitioner seeing the child. *Referral* requires another practitioner to see the child.

Guidelines and referral pathways will be established locally for many common presenting problems. This publication attempts to provide generic guidance applicable to most settings in the UK. Clinical presentations are often complex and may involve multiple rather than single problems. Individual clinical judgement is always required, backed up by advice from more experienced colleagues.

THERAPY

Therapy needs to be explained to the parent and child. This includes medicines and how and when to administer them. Advice on safe storage is often needed.

FOLLOW-UP

Ensure there is enough time to get results of investigations or reports from others. Appointments on different days of the week mean that schoolchildren do not always miss the same lesson. For older children, especially those working for examinations, appointments outside of school hours will be very welcome.

KEY POINTS FOR PARENTS AND CHILDREN

It is good practice and is now a requirement to copy letters to parents. Children should not be excluded from this process. Language will need to be modified to reflect children's developmental levels and parents' literacy.

HEALTH PROMOTION

Every consultation is an opportunity for health promotion.

ADDITIONAL POINTS

Remember ask and advise about benefits – this is frequently forgotten.

See also

Chapter 6, Consent and confidentiality.

CHILD-FRIENDLY FACILITIES

DEFINITION

Key dimensions of good patient care include access, waiting times, information, choice, safety, and having a clean, comfortable and friendly environment. The Children's NSF makes specific reference to the importance of physical facilities in the provision of high-quality, child-centred care.

RESEARCH EVIDENCE

One observational study found that most baby clinics held in general practices were child friendly.

More practices could have had notice boards with information on child health issues and toilet facilities suitable for young children.

Most frequent problems identified by parents include poor access for prams, lack of provision of toys, cleanliness, inconvenient clinic times, lack of nappy changing facilities and lack of privacy for discussion with health visitors.

ACCESS

Appointment times need to be flexible, e.g. allowing different members of the family to be seen consecutively, fit in with school hours and allow ill children to be seen urgently.

Quick appointments and confidentiality are important to teenagers.

Short waiting times in clinic are less stressful for families with young children.

Easy access for prams and children with disabilities.

RECEPTION

Staff should be welcoming, consider the needs of the family and respect confidentiality.

Clear signposting.

WAITING ROOM

Play area with suitable, safe toys and activities for young and older children.
Space for prams.
Nappy changing facilities.
Toilet facilities appropriate for young children, e.g. with potty.
Provision of room for mothers to breast feed in private.
Health promotion information, e.g. notice board and leaflets.
Décor child centred if used predominantly by children, e.g. cartoon characters on walls and mobiles.

CONSULTATION AND TREATMENT ROOMS

Warm (22°C if young babies to be examined).
Privacy and avoidance of unintended interruptions.
Space for prams and children to play.
Toys and play materials.
Screened couch offering privacy for examination.
Appropriate equipment, e.g. height measure, scales, growth charts.
Consider need for chaperone for examinations.
Wash-hand basin.
Consider contents of low cupboards that toddlers might open.
Safe storage of sharps and medicines.
Siting of sharps disposal boxes.

> **ALERTS**
>
> ⚠ Safety, especially for young children. For example, storage of sharps and medicines, nappy changing facilities, doors, stairs, stacked furniture, electrical equipment.

HEALTH PROMOTION

Leaflets on relevant child health issues, notice boards in waiting rooms, appropriate information for teenagers.

KEY POINTS FOR PARENTS

Help the experience to be as convenient and stress free as possible.

ADDITIONAL POINTS

Availability of interpreters when needed.

SOURCES

Boyle G, Gillam S (1993) Parents' views of child health surveillance. Health Education Journal 52: 42–44

Department of Health (2004) National Service Framework for Children, Young People & Maternity Services. London: Department of Health

Department of Health – Estates and Facilities Management. Online. Available at www.dh.gov.uk/Policy and Guidance/Organisation Policy/Estates and Facilities Management.

Hampshire A, Blair M, Crown N, Avery A, Williams I (2002) Assessing the quality of child health surveillance in primary care. What are the problems? Child: Care, Health and Development 28: 239–249

Sutton J, Jagger C, Smith L (1995) Parents' views of health surveillance. Archives of Disease in Childhood 73: 57–61

See also

Chapter 1, General notes on child health consultations; Chapter 3, Equipment; Chapter 6, Consent and confidentiality.

3

EQUIPMENT

Community paediatricians and general practitioners working in surgeries, clinics, schools, family centres and in the home need a portable 'kit'. The following is a guide, though individual doctors will develop their own preferences.

TYPES OF EQUIPMENT

Technical equipment
- Paediatric stethoscope
- Head circumference tape measure (Lasso-o tape)
- Otoscope (spare batteries); fibreoptic models give best illumination
- Ophthalmoscope
- Thermometer
- Torch
- Magnifying glass
- Patella hammer
- Sphygmomanometer (paediatric cuff)
- Peak flow meter

Support equipment
- Notepaper and envelopes
- Pathology and x-ray request forms
- Range of bottles, swabs, syringes and needles
- Disposal toothbrush/card used for containing skin scrapings for mycology
- List of important telephone numbers, e.g. child protection register
- Dictating machine and spare tape
- Growth charts:
  - height, weight and head circumference: nine-centile standard charts for general population
  - separate charts for Down's syndrome
  - preterm babies to 1 year of age
  - body mass index
  - head circumference charts (over 2 years)
- Peak flow charts

- Attention deficit disorder rating scales, i.e. Connors, Wells, etc.
- *British National Formulary For Children*
- *Medicines for Children/Pocket Medicines for Children* (Royal College of Paediatrics and Child Health)
- *Immunisation Against Infectious Diseases* – 'The Green Book' (The Stationery Office)
- Height and weight conversion charts and/or pocket calculator (to imperial measurements)
- Star charts
- Small diaries for parents and children to keep records or for use in behaviour modification programmes/stickers for reward programmes
- Some key diagrams for explanations to parents and children, e.g. middle ear, constipation
- Frequently used health education materials, information on ADHD, constipation, autism, useful websites – e.g.

Contact a Family (www.cafamily.org.uk), providing information and support for parents caring for a child with a disability

- Access to national (e.g. NICE, SIGN, RCPCH) guidelines and local guidelines

Developmental equipment
- Books, e.g. first picture books
- Symbolic toys, e.g. small male and female dolls, chair, spoon, cup, fork, dog, cat, car
- Crayons and paper, plus ready-drawn shapes to copy
- Ten coloured 1-inch cubes to test block building, copying designs, matching colours, coordination
- Beads for threading
- Blunt scissors for testing fine motor skills
- Small jar with screw lid to test fine motor skills
- Access to standardised tests for those trained to use them, e.g. Griffiths, Denver, Schedule of Growing Skills

Bigger pieces of equipment for use in clinics
- Scales – modern, self-zeroing and properly maintained.
- Within the EU, directive 90/384/EEC demands particular specification for clinical weighing scales
- Height – Leicester height measure, minimeters and wall-mounted magnimeters are recommended by *Health For All Children* for accurate height measurement
- Formboards, posting box and bigger toys

1

SOURCES OF EQUIPMENT, MEDICINES AND FORMS

Growth charts and weight and height equipment
Child Growth Foundation
2 Mayfield Avenue
London W4 1PW
Tel: 020 8995 0257/8994; fax: 020 8995 9075
Email: cgflondon@aol.com

Developmental testing equipment
NFER-Nelson
The Chiswick Centre
414 Chiswick High Road
London W4 5TF
Tel: 020 8996 8444

Personal Child Health Record and Growth Charts
Harlow Printing Ltd
Maxwell House
South Shields
Tyne and Wear NE33 4PU

Harlow Healthcare: Online resource (www.healthforallchildren.co.uk) for purchase
of growth monitoring equipment and charts and information on the UK Child
Health Promotion Programme.

Medicines for Children
Royal College of Paediatrics and Child Health
50 Hallam Street
London W1W 6DE
Tel: 020 7307 5600
www.rcpch.ac.uk/publications/bnfc.html

Immunisation against infectious disease
If paper versions are unavailable, information should be downloaded from
the Department of Health website (www.dh.gov.uk) as updates are
incorporated as 'draft'. Search 'Immunisation' to locate the latest
version.

4

COLLECTING SPECIMENS

URINE SAMPLES

A confirmed urinary tract infection (UTI) in a young child (<2 years) may lead to the initiation of invasive radiological investigations. It is therefore important that care is taken when collecting urine specimens to ensure that a positive result indicates a UTI and not a contaminated sample. Unfortunately, some commonly used methods of urine collection are associated with contamination and therefore the method of collection should be taken into account when interpreting culture results. Ideally, two specimens should be taken prior to starting antibiotic therapy. Urinalysis sticks can be used to look for the presence of leucocytes and nitrites that are suggestive but not diagnostic of a UTI.

There are six main methods used to collect urine samples. The method used will depend on the age of the child and the speed with which a urine sample is required.

1. *Midstream urine sample*: This should be used in any child old enough to cooperate.
2. *Suprapubic aspiration (SPA)*: This is the most invasive method and is rarely used in children >18 months but the least likely to be contaminated. The procedure should be carried out under sterile conditions with the child held in a frogs' leg position, ideally, 45 minutes after a feed. A sterile container should be available as often the child will micturate while the bladder is being palpated or during the procedure. A 23-G needle is inserted in the midline vertically immediately above the symphysis pubis. The needle should be aspirated as it is advanced (not more than 2.5 cm).
3. *Transurethral bladder catheterisation (TBC)*: Again this is an invasive procedure but allows a clean specimen to be collected. There is a small risk of introducing infection during catheterisation. A sterile technique should be used with a fine nasogastric tube.
4. *Urine collection bag*: The bag is placed over the perineum, which should be clean. It should be removed as soon as urine is passed to avoid contamination. This method is non-invasive but is associated with a high false-positive rate due to contamination. However, a sterile culture from a bag specimen makes a UTI very unlikely.

5. *Clean catch*: This method requires patience and the parents should be encouraged to participate. After cleaning the area, the parents are given a sterile container and asked to catch the middle portion of the stream. This method is superior to a bag specimen.
6. *Urine collection pads*: The pad is placed in the nappy and urine is removed using a syringe and needle. This is a non-invasive method but associated with a high level of contamination.

If the sample cannot be sent to the laboratory immediately, it should be stored in the fridge.

TAKING BLOOD

Venesection

Various measures can be used to make this as pleasant an experience as possible for the child and family. Ideally, a play therapist should be present to distract the child while the procedure is undertaken. This can be very effective if the child is positioned so they are not aware when the blood is being taken. This technique works best when combined with topical anaesthetic cream to numb the skin. Apart from emergency situations, topical anaesthetics should always be offered. In practice it tends not to be used on infants <6 months of age although there is no reason why this should be the case.

Two preparations are available:

1. *Emla* (licensed for children >1 year): This is applied under an occlusive dressing and takes 45 minutes to be effective. The skin can become irritated if it is left on for more than 2 hours. Analgesia lasts for 1 hour. It can be associated with vasoconstriction which can make the procedure more difficult.
2. *Ametop gel* (licensed for children >1 month): Again this is applied under an occlusive dressing. Analgesia is achieved after 30 minutes and lasts for 4–6 hours.

The veins over the back of the hand, the flexor surface of the elbow and on the feet are the best in children. The distribution of subcutaneous fat in infants makes them a challenging group from which to take blood. If there are no visible veins the best approach is to insert the needle over an area where you would expect to find a vein. A 21- or 23-G butterfly needle ± syringe is introduced into the vein after cleaning the area. In small babies blood does not tend to flow freely and so a butterfly needle is often most effective, allowing the blood to drop directly into the collecting bottle which will be sent to the laboratory.

Capillary samples

These methods are less traumatic and quicker than taking blood from a vein. They are useful if venous access is a problem.

In older children capillary samples can be taken from a finger prick. This method is not ideal for taking large amounts of blood but can be useful for investigations such as a full blood count. It can also be used for urea and electrolytes; however, squeezing the finger can result in a falsely high reading for the potassium level due to haemolysis. The area should be covered with Vaseline cream to encourage the blood to form a globule that can be deposited directly into the collecting bottle. The skin is penetrated using a small lancet. The same method can be used in babies using the lateral and medial aspects of the heel.

STOOL SPECIMENS

The parents are provided with a container in which to place the stool specimen when collected. A 'spatula' is usually part of the lid and the parents can use this to scoop a small specimen of stool into the container. For most investigations there is no problem if the specimen is kept in a fridge; however, if the stool is to be examined for ova or parasites, it must be sent straight to the laboratories, i.e. get a 'hot specimen'.

5

CLINICAL RECORDS

Trusts are responsible for maintaining a comprehensive system for completion, use, storage and retrieval of medical records. They must be kept confidential, bound and securely stored so that loss of documents and traces are minimised. Employees are also responsible for following Trust guidelines.

The following reports have informed this process:

- *Setting the Record Straight: A Study of Hospital Medical Records* (Audit Commission Report 1995, updated 1999)
- *The Caldicott Report* (1997) (about weaknesses in the way parts of the NHS handled confidential patient data)
- *For the Record – Managing Records in NHS Trusts and Health Authorities* (Health Service Circular 1999/053)
- *Controls Assurance* (part of Department of Health; ceased August 2004)
- *Information for Health: An Information Strategy for the Modern NHS* (Health Service Circular 1998/168)
- *The Freedom of Information Act 2000*
- *The Data Protection Act 1998*
- *Clinical Negligence Scheme for Trusts* (NHS Trusts and certain other bodies providing services under the National Health Service Act 1977 may make provision for meeting liabilities to third parties in connection with personal injury arising out of negligence in the carrying out of the bodies' functions)

CONFIDENTIALITY AND DATA PROTECTION

Personal identifying information includes the clinical record, information held on computer, clinic appointment sheets, audiotapes, correspondence, telephone messages, etc.

Black ink is required.

Do not leave personal identifying information unattended.

Lock away all personal identifying information when not in use.

Only discuss patients for the purpose of carrying out care.

Only access information you have a right to access.

Only give access to those who have access rights.

Do not disclose your password to anyone else.

TRANSPORTING RECORDS

Only do this when necessary.
Always transport in the boot of your car.
Remove from car boot as soon as possible.
Do not leave in car boot overnight.
Only take personal identifying information home if it is justifiable, and ensure that it is secure.

RECORD KEEPING

Clinical records have many functions. They:

- provide continuity when different clinicians see a child
- serve to communicate from doctor to colleague and to other healthcare workers
- give a picture of care and treatment given
- fulfil a medicolegal function and are needed for clinical audit, research, resource allocation, and service planning.

Fulfilling these functions requires attention to detail:

- Each entry should outline treatment plans, medication prescribed, follow-up and referrals to other practitioners.
- Note advice and information given, and outcomes.
- Abbreviations should be limited to agreed local protocols.
- Mistakes should be countersigned and a line drawn through.
- Notes must be legible, accurate and contemporaneous.
- All entries should be signed and dated, and the doctor's name written in capitals on each page.
- The patient's full name, date of birth and identification number must be recorded clearly on every sheet of paper in the record.
- Records should not include meaningless phrases, irrelevant speculation, offensive subjective statements or irrelevant personal opinions regarding the patient.

Good clinical records ensure continuity of care. Letters are necessary to communicate with colleagues involved in the care of the child about your plans and to inform parents of actions and findings.
When signing notes, add General Medical Council (GMC) registration number.

ADDITIONAL POINTS

Keeping good clinical records is part of good medical practice, as advised by The General Medical Council, and supported by clinical governance.
Clinical governance is the framework through which NHS Trusts are accountable for continuously improving the quality of services and safeguarding high standards of care by creating an environment in which excellence in clinical care will flourish.

SOURCES

Trusts have their own standards for data and clinical records, as do individual
professional bodies, such as the Royal College of Physicians.

General Medical Council (1998, updated 2001) Good medical practice –
protecting patients, guiding doctors. London: GMC

See also

Chapter 6, Consent and confidentiality.

CONSENT AND CONFIDENTIALITY

UK GUIDANCE

From the age of 16 and 17 years, children can give their own consent for medical examination or treatment.

Under the age of 16, children who, in the doctor's opinion, fully understand what is involved in the examination or procedure can also give valid consent. Ideally, parents should be involved and the doctor should ask the young person's permission. If this is withheld, their request for confidentiality should be respected.

Parents cannot overrule valid consent given by a competent young person.

Where a child (age 16, 17 or younger) who is competent refuses treatment, those with parental responsibility can override the young person's wishes where there is a risk of the child suffering grave and irreversible mental or physical harm.

The Court can overrule refusal to consent by both the parents and the child in the same circumstances.

For children not included in either of the two above groups consent must be obtained from someone holding parental responsibility unless there is an emergency and they cannot be contacted. This includes all children who lack capacity to give consent. The power to give consent must be exercised with the child or young person's best interest as paramount.

CONFIDENTIALITY

The duty of confidentiality owed to a person under 16 is as great as that owed to any other person. (BMA et al 1993)

This is a general principle which cannot be applied in all circumstances, e.g. disclosure of child abuse.

There is a duty to protect patient information, to keep medical records securely and to disclose medical information on a 'need to know' basis. It is good practice to tell parents and children what will be contained in a letter. Copying clinical letters to patients is also good practice and is now a requirement. Care should be taken with the inclusion of information about third parties.

WHO TO TALK TO

NHS Trusts will generally have local procedures to ensure valid consent before disclosing medical records.

They will also have access to legal advice where there are difficult decisions to be made on consent or confidentiality.

SOURCES

British Medical Association, General Medical Services Committee, Health Education Authority (1993) Confidentiality and people under 16. British Medical Association, London

Department of Health (2001) Reference guide to consent for examination and treatment. London: Department of Health

Department of Health (2003) Confidentiality: NHS code of practice. London: Department of Health

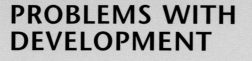
PROBLEMS WITH DEVELOPMENT

7

LEARNING DISABILITY AND DEVELOPMENTAL DELAY

DEFINITION

Learning difficulties (LD) and developmental delay are defined by scores of IQ and DQ on standardised tests (Table 7.1).

EPIDEMIOLOGY AND AETIOLOGY

Epidemiology

Severe learning difficulty (SLD): 0.3–0.4% by age 3 years. Diagnosed earlier and with a more constant rate in the population, until fall-off with earlier death.

Mild learning difficulty (MLD): 1.5% by age 7 years. Usually diagnosed between 3 and 7 years of age, but may be later.

Boy 1.5:1.0 girl.

Aetiology

This is outlined in Table 7.2.

PRESCHOOL CHILD WITH MILD OR SEVERE DEVELOPMENTAL DELAY

PRESENTATION

Babies with chromosomal defects, multiple congenital abnormalities and syndromes, or problems resulting from intrauterine infection, are likely

Table 7.1 IQ scores compared with population norms

IQ	Range
Normal*	85–115
Borderline disability	71–84
Mild disability (MLD)	50–70
Severe disability (SLD)	<50
Profound disability	<20
* 90% of the population.	

Table 7.2 Aetiology of learning disabilities and developmental delay

	SLD (%)	MLD (%)
Identified probable cause	80	45
Unknown	20	55
Prenatal (genetic defects, syndromes, intrauterine problems)	55	23
Perinatal (birth problems)	15	18
Postnatal (brain injury, autism)	12	4

After Hagberg & Kyllerman (1983).
Foetal alcohol exposure is an important cause of MLD in 8%.
Family clustering is common in MLD unknowns.
MLD is influenced by psychosocial factors including understimulation.
Parents may well have MLDs themselves.

to be identified by staff on the neonatal unit and referred directly to the child development team.

Others may present to the primary care team with concerns about:

- feeding and growth
- level of arousal (irritable or lethargic)
- handling (floppy or stiff)
- lack of normal developmental progress.

ASSESSMENT

History
Pregnancy and birth history, neonatal problems
Detailed family history and family tree
Medical history – illness (seizures)
Social circumstances
Feeding and growth pattern
Developmental history
Behaviour problems

Examination
Alertness of child.
Is the child ill?
Hand function.
Current developmental skills – levels in each field.
General and neurological examination, with particular attention to:

- muscle tone and reflexes
- dysmorphic features (hands, face, ears, feet)
- heart for murmurs
- palate for cleft

- abdomen for hepatosplenomegaly
- skin for neurocutaneous stigmata
- spine (other skeletal abnormalities)
- length/height, weight, and head circumference, and plot on charts.

Vision and hearing assessments are very important.
Likely to need specialist assessment, brain stem evoked responses (BSERs) and ophthalmologist.

Diagnostic tests
FBC, ferritin.
? lead, depending on FBC.
Chromosomes, including fragile X.
Fluorescence in situ hybridisation (FISH) – 22q11 deletion if heart, palate and learning problems (velocardiofacial syndrome).
Thyroid function, creatinine kinase.
Urine screen for metabolic disorders, including amino acids, organic acids and mucopolysaccharides.
Neuroimaging if head circumference is big or small for age.
EEG if history of seizures.

DIFFERENTIAL DIAGNOSIS
Developmental delay without LD (a child with a chronic illness may have developmental delay).
Understimulation and neglect.
Hearing or vision impairment.
Familial developmental patterns, e.g. late walkers.
Children with specific developmental disorders.
Severe physical disability in a child with normal cognitive skills.

ALERTS
Accurate and comprehensive vision and hearing tests are essential.
Parents may have learning difficulties – may not be able to read or keep appointments; may not appreciate any problem.
Statutory duty to give information about relevant voluntary agencies, e.g. MENCAP, Contact a Family, etc.
Benefits – Disability Living Allowance.
Respite care.
Refer to preschool education service and educational psychologist as soon as it is clear that the child will have ongoing educational difficulties – (need parental consent).

WHO TO TALK TO
Health visitor
Disability paediatrician – child development team

Preschool teacher team/educational psychologist
Community paediatrician
Clinical geneticist
Local speech and language therapist
Social worker or family centre
Occupational therapist – home modifications

WHEN TO REFER

To paediatrician – child with severe delay, i.e. <50 DQ in any developmental field.
If further specialist investigations, including neuroimaging, are likely to yield a diagnosis.
Suspect chronic disease, poor growth.
Abnormal head growth.
Dysmorphic features.

THERAPY

Child with SLD

Will need multidisciplinary intervention programme as early as possible, i.e. whole child development team including physiotherapy, occupational therapy, speech and language therapy, teacher, social worker and psychologist.

Child with MLD

Health visitor and community nursery nurse – support of normal stimulation and behaviour management, access to other support services including playgroup and nursery.
Local speech and language therapist – promotion of communication skills.
Local physiotherapist/orthotist – gait and motor programme.
Local preschool teacher team/portage – play and cognitive skills, communication, fine motor skills.
Behaviour is often a problem and may need specialist help – psychologist.

FOLLOW-UP

Regular follow-up is essential to monitor developmental progress and growth, and to review diagnosis, plus effective liaison with other agencies, e.g. education and social services, voluntary sector.
Minimum 6-monthly in preschool period; possibly 3-monthly for a child with SLD or medical problems.
Referral to the education team as soon as it is clear that the child will have ongoing special educational needs.

HEALTH PROMOTION

Dental health.
Regular vision and hearing checks.

Immunisation.

Maternal nutrition, avoidance of alcohol, drugs and smoking; immunisation (e.g. rubella) may prevent learning difficulties in a child.

Screening for hypothyroidism and PKU in neonatal period.

SCHOOL-AGE CHILD WITH LEARNING DIFFICULTIES

2

PRESENTATION

Most children with SLD will present in the preschool period and therefore come into mainstream or special schooling with a comprehensive intervention programme in place.

Children with MLD are often not identified until cognitive abilities are challenged by the school.

May present with teacher or parent concerns about lack of normal academic progress; may also present with secondary behaviour problems.

Likely to have problems with attention control, fine motor skills and social skills as part of their learning difficulties.

Teacher or parent may query ADHD, developmental coordination disorder (dyspraxia), dyslexia or autistic spectrum disorder.

Children with overall low IQ can also have these diagnoses if they have relatively severe problems or disordered development in the relevant specific areas compared with their other cognitive skills and 'mental age equivalent'.

ASSESSMENT

As for preschool child.

WHO TO TALK TO

School nurse

Class teacher

School special needs coordinator

Local educational psychologist

Community paediatrician

Child and adolescent psychiatry team

Connexions (career guidance for 14–19 year olds) for older child

Resource library

WHEN TO REFER

Child with SLD if they have not had thorough investigations in the past 5 years and are not under paediatric review (a child in a special school is likely to be having annual medical reviews with the school paediatrician).

Child with MLD if there is absence of progress or loss of skills.

Indications for further investigation, e.g. dysmorphic features or neuro-cutaneous stigmata.

THERAPY

Speech and language therapist may contribute advice to a programme to develop communication skills but these are likely to be delivered mainly in a school context by education staff.

Physiotherapist/occupational therapist may advise on motor programme and equipment but motor skills will develop in line with the child's cognitive development and the main intervention will be through education staff.

Behaviour problems are common and a psychologist may be helpful.

FOLLOW-UP

Children with SLD often need medical review for associated problems, e.g. seizures, constipation.

Children with MLD do not need regular medical follow-up, but need a point of access if there are medical concerns or support is required. The latter is often needed at transition to secondary school or college.

HEALTH PROMOTION

Young people with learning difficulties are very vulnerable, and the following should be addressed:

- sexual health issues
- consent to sex and contraception
- leisure opportunities
- alcohol and drugs
- social inclusion and employment.

SUPPORT ORGANISATIONS

Connexions – www.connexions.gov.uk.

SOURCES

Hagberg B, Kyllerman M (1983) Epidemiology of mental retardation – a Swedish survey. Brain and Development 5: 441–449

HYPOTONIA AND GROSS MOTOR DELAY

8

DEFINITION

Wide range of normal motor development. There will be an average age of attainment of a motor milestone and an upper limit of normal, i.e. 98% children have attained by this age.

Upper age limit for sitting = 10 months; for walking = 18 months.

PRESENTATION

Baby or toddler with hypotonia and gross motor delay.

ASSESSMENT

Is the baby ill?
Are there neurological signs?
Is this a problem of the central or the peripheral nervous system?
Are there other organ problems?
Is this a syndrome?

History

Pregnancy and birth.
Neonatal problems.
Medical history, particularly feeding, growth, constipation and respiratory problems.
Development problems.
Family history.

Examination

Dysmorphic features?
Active and alert?
General physical examination:

- Bladder, bowel
- Hepatosplenomegaly?
- Hips and spine
- Skin for neurocutaneous markers, e.g. in neurofibromatosis.

Vision and hearing.
Neurological examination:

- Is the baby weak? Gower's manoeuvre in a child over 3 years.
- Tone, power and tendon reflexes.

Length/height, weight and head circumference, and plot on charts.

Diagnostic tests
Creatinine kinase if not walking by 18 months.
Neuroimaging of brain and spinal cord, particularly if abnormal head size
    or abnormal neurological signs other than mildly hypotonic.
Consider metabolic and genetic studies.

DIFFERENTIAL DIAGNOSIS
Normal variant, may be familial
Understimulation and neglect
Brain problem – cerebral palsy or learning disability
Peripheral nerve disorders
Muscle disorders
General disease
Metabolic disease
Syndrome

ALERTS
Baby walkers inhibit normal motor development.
Dislocated hips can cause delayed motor development.
Check creatinine kinase in non-walkers at 18 months.
Bottom shufflers can have an underlying abnormality.

WHO TO TALK TO
Health visitor.
Community paediatrician.
Paediatric physiotherapist.
Paediatric occupational therapist.

WHEN TO REFER
Abnormal head size
Not active/alert
Dysmorphic
Failure to thrive
Very floppy with absent tendon reflexes
Respiratory problems
Any indication of muscle weakness

Delayed motor milestones as above, *i.e. child not sitting by 10 months, not walking by 18 months*

THERAPY

Advise re normal stimulation and opportunities for motor development. Encourage crawling, discourage supported walking.
Health visitor support to encourage normal development.
Paediatric physiotherapy to promote motor development.

FOLLOW-UP

In a child with no identified pathology, review 3 monthly, until running and walking upstairs without support (indicates no weakness).
Child with an underlying disorder is likely to need the multidisciplinary child development team.

9

MOVEMENT AND DEXTERITY

DEFINITION

Delayed development of motor skills, i.e. late motor milestones
Development is normally distributed in the population.
Generally, development assessment tools use the 50th centile to indicate the age around which most children will achieve this skill.
Where there is a wide range of normal, the 98th centile is more discriminating.

	50th centile	98th centile
Sitting unsupported	7 months	10 months
Walking	13 months	18 months

Early motor milestones (3–18 months)
- Holds a rattle placed in hand – 3 months
- Reaches for an object and gets it – 5 months
- Transfers object from hand to hand – 7 months
- Pincer grip (tip of index finger and tip of thumb) – 12 months
- Stops mouthing and casting – 18 months

Subsequent motor milestones (2–7 years)
- At 2 years – runs and jumps and climbs stairs (two feet per step); with pencil, draws lines and dots.
- At 3 years – stands on one leg, pedals a trike, climbs stairs (one foot on each step); with pencil, copies a circle.
- At 4 years – hops, walks on tiptoe; with pencil, copies a cross.
- At 5 years – hops on the spot; with pencil, copies a square, writes name.
- At 6 years – skips; copies a triangle, writes small words (e.g. cat, mum).
- At 7 years – rides a bike, ties shoelaces; writes sentences and starts to join up writing.

DEVELOPMENTAL COORDINATION DISORDER (DCD)

DEFINITION
Child's motor coordination is significantly below that expected for their age and intelligence, and there is no diagnosable neurological disorder such as cerebral palsy or muscular dystrophy.

PRESENTATION
Baby or toddler with hypotonia and gross motor delay.
Nursery age child with delayed motor skills.
Schoolchild with motor coordination difficulties.

ASSESSMENT
Is the child ill?
Is this specifically motor delay or global developmental delay?
Is there muscle weakness?
Are there neurological signs?
Is this a problem of the central or the peripheral nervous system?
Does the child have a syndrome?

History
Pregnancy and birth.
Preterm birth/neonatal problems.
Medical history, particularly feeding, growth, constipation and respiratory problems.
Family history of motor problems.
Developmental history in all fields.
Detailed history of motor development.
Feeding, dressing, ball and pencil skills in older child.

Examination
Alertness and activity level.
Social responsiveness.
Dysmorphic features.
Skin for neurocutaneous markers.
General physical examination:

- Chest shape
- Hepatosplenomegaly?
- Bladder/bowel
- Hips and spine.

Neurological examination:

- Tone, power, tendon reflexes
- Motor coordination in older child, mirror movements
- Gower's manoeuvre in a child over 3 years.

Length/height, weight and head circumference, and plot on charts.

Diagnostic tests

Creatinine kinase if not walking by 18 months.
Chromosomes including fragile X if global delay or dysmorphic.
Standardised tests of motor coordination, e.g. Movement ABC.

DIFFERENTIAL DIAGNOSIS

Global developmental delay due to:

- understimulation/neglect
- learning disability.

Normal variant, may be familial.
Cerebral palsy
Muscle disorder, e.g. Duchenne muscular dystrophy
Peripheral nerve problem, e.g. hereditary motor and sensory neuropathy
Progressive ataxia
Various syndromes, e.g. neurofibromatosis
Systemic illness or metabolic disease.

ALERTS

Hand dominance under 12 months suggests hemiplegia.
Baby walkers inhibit normal motor development.
Late walkers may have dislocated hips.
Creatinine kinase in all non-walkers at 18 months.
Bottom shufflers can have underlying abnormality.

WHO TO TALK TO

Health visitor.
Community paediatrician.
Paediatric physiotherapist.
Paediatric occupational therapist.
Teacher.

WHEN TO REFER

Global developmental delay

Lethargy, poor feeding, failure to thrive – urgent referral.
Dysmorphic, small stature – needs further genetic/metabolic studies.

Abnormal head size.
Asymmetry.
Abnormal muscle tone/reflexes.
Muscle weakness:

- very floppy baby with diminished tendon reflexes
- child over 3 years with positive Gower's manoeuvre.

Motor milestones severely delayed, e.g. not sitting by 12 months, not walking at 2 years.
Loss of previously acquired skills.

DCD
Lack of school progress despite extra help.
Socially isolated.
Behaviour problems.
Secondary somatic symptoms, e.g. headache, abdominal pain.
Other overlapping specific developmental problems, e.g. autistic spectrum disorder, ADHD.

THERAPY
Advise re normal stimulation and opportunities for motor development.
Encourage crawling, discourage supported walking.
Health visitor support to encourage normal development.
Paediatric physiotherapy to promote motor development.
Paediatric occupational therapist.

FOLLOW-UP
In a child with no identified pathology and mild delay – 3-monthly monitoring until running and walking upstairs without support.
Others – 6-monthly review to monitor for progressive disorders and support educational and social problems.

KEY POINTS FOR PARENTS
Motor development is highly variable in normal children.
Encourage physical activity of any kind, especially swimming.
Children with motor coordination difficulties may prefer non-team sports.
Make dressing as easy as possible – Velcro fastenings, elastic waistbands.
DCD is a developmental disorder and children improve as they mature.
Keeping up their confidence, self-esteem and willingness to try is crucial.
Children with DCD often have other specific developmental disorders.

SUPPORT ORGANISATIONS

The Dyspraxia Foundation
  Tel: 01462 454986
  Email: admin@dyspraxiafoundation.org.uk
  www.dyspraxiafoundation.org.uk
Muscular Dystrophy Campaign
  Tel: 020 7720 8055
  Email: info@muscular-dystrophy.org
  www.muscular-dystrophy.org

10

DOWN'S SYNDROME

DEFINITION

Down's syndrome is characterised by typical facial, other physical features, and learning disability. It is associated with an increased incidence of a number of medical problems.

EPIDEMIOLOGY AND AETIOLOGY

The natural prevalence is around 1:600 live births. Prenatal screening and termination of some affected foetuses, together with demographic changes, make the current birth prevalence in the UK 1:1000.

95% of cases are caused by an additional chromosome 21 (trisomy 21); minority caused by translocation or mosaicism.

PRESENTATION

Many diagnoses are now antenatal. Despite this, almost half of all diagnoses are made in the neonatal period. Usually suspected because of facial features, floppiness or associated medical problems (Box 10.1).

Occasionally, diagnosis is made later, usually presenting with developmental delay.

MANAGEMENT IN THE NEONATAL PERIOD

Karyotype to confirm diagnosis.

Examination as for all newborns, but specifically look for cataracts, gastrointestinal anomalies and congenital heart disease (50% of all babies born with Down's syndrome will have congenital heart disease).

ECG and CXR or echocardiogram and referral for paediatric cardiology opinion.

Ensure all babies are included in neonatal hearing screening programme, and have Guthrie screen for hypothyroidism.

Explanation to parents of diagnosis, associated medical problems, likely developmental prognosis, and available resources, including contact with support organisations.

BOX 10.1 Specific medical problems that occur more frequently in people with Down's syndrome

Cardiac
- Congenital malformation
- Cor pulmonale
- Acquired valvular dysfunction

Orthopaedic
- Cervical spine instability
- Hip subluxation/dislocation
- Patellar instability
- Scoliosis
- Metatarsus varus
- Pes planus

ENT
- Conductive hearing loss
- Sensorineural hearing loss
- Upper airway obstruction
- Chronic catarrh

Ophthalmic
- Refractive errors
- Blepharitis
- Nasolacrimal obstruction
- Cataracts
- Glaucoma
- Nystagmus
- Squint
- Keratoconus

Gastrointestinal
- Congenital malformations
- Feeding difficulties
- Gastro-oesophageal reflux
- Hirschsprung's disease
- Coeliac disease

Endocrine
- Growth retardation
- Hypothyroidism
- Hyperthyroidism
- Diabetes

Immunological
- Immunodeficiency
- Autoimmune diseases, e.g. arthropathy, vitiligo, alopecia

Haematological
- Transient neonatal myeloproliferative states
- Leukaemia
- Neonatal polycythaemia
- Neonatal thrombocytopenia

Dermatological
- Dry skin
- Folliculitis
- Vitiligo
- Alopecia

Neuropsychiatric
- Infantile spasms and other myoclonic epilepsies
- Autism
- Depressive illness
- Dementia (adults only)

SUBSEQUENT MEDICAL MANAGEMENT

Regular paediatric review to monitor health and development.

Screen for common associated problems, e.g. cardiac, vision, hearing, growth and thyroid dysfunction. Down's specific growth charts should be used.

Figure 10.1 gives a suggested schedule of medical checks during childhood.

Guidance on surveillance for specific associated conditions is also available (see 'Sources', below).

THERAPY

Many treatments proposed over the years claim to ameliorate the 'symptoms' of Down's syndrome. Recent interest has been around nutritional supplements.

To date, none is of proven benefit.

Treatment of associated medical problems, especially sensory impairment, is essential to optimise development and prevent unnecessary secondary handicap.

Physiotherapy, speech therapy and educational early intervention programmes all have a role in promoting the child's development.

KEY POINTS FOR PARENTS

The common public image of Down's syndrome is often pessimistic, based on those who have not experienced the opportunities for healthcare and education available to children today. Many children with Down's

DOWN'S SYNDROME

DOWN'S SYNDROME – Suggested schedule of health checks

The following are suggested ages for health checks. Checks at any other time if there are parental or other concerns

	Birth to 6 weeks	6–10 months	12 months	18 months to 2½ years	3–3½ years	4–4½ years
Thyroid blood tests	Routine Guthrie test		Thyroid blood tests including antibodies		Thyroid blood tests including antibodies	
	If your area has introduced fingerprick blood tests these should be done every year.					
Growth monitoring	Length and weight should be checked frequently, using Down's syndrome growth charts from age 3 months. Head circumference should be checked at each routine medical check			Length and weight should be checked at least annually using both Down's syndrome and standard charts		
Eye check	Visual behaviour Check for congenital cataract	Visual behaviour, Check for squint	Visual behaviour, Check for squint	Orthoptic examination, refraction and opthalmic examination		Visual acuity refraction and ophthalmic examination
Hearing check	Neonatal screening if locally available	Full audiological review (Hearing, impedance, otoscopy)		Full audiological review (Hearing, impedance, otoscopy) annually)		
Heart check and other advice	Echocardiogram 0–6 weeks **or** chest x-ray **and** ECG at birth 6 weeks			Dental advice		

FROM AGE 5 TO 19 YEARS	
Paediatric review	Annually
Hearing review	2 yearly audiological review (as above)
Vision/Orthoptic check	2 yearly
Thyroid blood tests	At age 5 years. Every 2 years afterwards. At least annually for people with thyroid antibodies.

Detailed recommendations for Medical Surveillance Essentials for children with Down's syndrome are available.
For further information contact your local community paediatrician.

Down's syndrome insert © DSMIG 1998

Fig. 10.1 Schedule of suggested health checks: special insert for Personal Child Health Record.

syndrome are in good health, or experience treatable medical problems, and with the right support can live healthy fulfilling lives.

New parents should be given the Down's syndrome insert for the Personal Child Health Record (PCHR), which contains general and medical information on Down's syndrome, a suggested schedule of health checks and Down's syndrome specialist growth charts. The DfES publication "Information for parents – Down Syndrome" is a useful overview.

HEALTH PROMOTION

People with Down's syndrome should have a programme of health promotion and preventative medical care based on their special medical needs, but not forgetting to include all aspects of health promotion important for the general population. Preventative programmes including screening should continue throughout life.

Obesity is a particular problem, frequently assumed 'part of the syndrome'; however, this is not an inevitable consequence and should be addressed.

ADDITIONAL POINTS

Children with Down's syndrome can experience the same range of medical problems as the general population, and benefit from similar treatments. Parents and carers often feel they are discriminated against in not receiving optimal medical care. Health professionals should ensure that this does not happen.

SUPPORT ORGANISATIONS

Down's Syndrome Association
Langdon Down Centre
2a Langdon Park
Teddington
Middlesex TW11 9PS
Tel: 0845 230 0372
www.downs-syndrome.org.uk

SOURCES

Basic medical surveillance essentials for people with Down's syndrome. Down's syndrome Medical Interest Group (DSMIG) 2000. Available from DSMIG, Children's Centre, City Hospital, Nottingham, Tel: 0115 9627658, or at www.dsmig.org.uk

Information for parents – Down syndrome, DfES 2005, available at www.earlysupport.org.uk

PCHR insert for babies born with Down's syndrome (DSMIG) 2000. Can be ordered via DSMIG website or from Harlow Printing Ltd, Maxwell Street, South Shields, Tyne and Wear NE33 4PU, or at www.harlowprinting.co.uk

11

CEREBRAL PALSY

DEFINITION

Cerebral palsy (CP) is an umbrella term for a group of disorders. There is a permanent but not unchanging disorder of movement and/or posture and motor function, due to a non-progressive interference/lesion/abnormality of the developing immature brain. (based on SCPE 2000)

EPIDEMIOLOGY AND AETIOLOGY

Incidence

Approximately 2 per 1000 live births in industrialised countries. Incidence has decreased in term and moderately preterm babies, but there is an increased incidence in the survivors of extreme preterm birth <1000 g birth weight.

Aetiology

There are multiple aetiologies.
The origin may be multifactorial (Box 11.1).
CP is often associated with a series of suboptimal conditions between conception and the perinatal period.
There may be no definite aetiological factor.

Classification of CP

Spastic (bilateral/hemiplegic) 85%; dyskinetic 10%; ataxic 5%.
There may be a mixed picture but it is usually possible to classify by dominant type.

PRESENTATION

Congenital hemiplegia

Should usually be identified in the first year of life.
The baby starts reaching out at 4–5 months of age, always using the same arm.
Hand preference under 1 year of age suggests hemiplegia.
There may be fisting of the hand on the affected side.

BOX 11.1

Predisposing factors
- Preterm birth
- Foetal malnutrition and intrauterine growth retardation
- Birth trauma and asphyxia

Predictive factors
- Maternal diabetes mellitus
- Pre-eclampsia
- Twin pregnancy
- Threatened abortion

Prenatal factors
- Genetic and chromosome disorders
- Damaging agents such as intrauterine infections or drugs
- Problems with blood supply to foetus

Perinatal factors
- Hypoxia
- Sepsis
- Haemorrhage/infarction

Postnatal factors
- Sepsis
- Trauma
- Prolonged seizures

The baby is unlikely to develop a pincer grip (8–10 months) on that side.

Involvement of the leg may not be detected until the baby starts to walk; the baby will then usually be on tiptoe on that side, with internal rotation of the leg.

The face is rarely affected.

Later presentation
Very mild congenital hemiplegia or acquired hemiplegia.

May present in an older child with mild motor problems, mild learning difficulties or epilepsy.

There will be asymmetry, mild neurological signs and hypoplasia of one side of the body.

Bilateral spastic cerebral palsy
Many babies have transient neurological problems in the first weeks of life; however, if problems persist and motor development is delayed, the child needs further assessment.

Abnormal signs might include:

- increased or decreased muscle tone
- abnormal posture
- excessively sleepy
- poor sucking
- irritability, convulsions
- persistence of primitive reflexes beyond 3 months of age
- delayed and disordered motor development, e.g. lack of head control by 3 months, not sitting unsupported by 10 months
- floppy in the trunk and stiff in the limbs.

ASSESSMENT

History

Pregnancy, mother's health and previous obstetric history; birth history, including gestation and birth weight; neonatal problems.
Any illnesses/operations/hospital attendances.
Medication, immunisations.
Developmental history.
Family history.
Detailed feeding and growth history.
Current developmental levels.

Associated conditions

- Epilepsy (30%)
- Squint (30%)
- Visual problems (20%)
- Hearing problems:
  - sensorineural (20%)
  - glue ear
- Speech problems
- Learning disorders (60%)
- Spatial perception difficulties
- Constipation
- Incontinence
- Recurrent respiratory infection
- Behaviour problems
- Sleep difficulties

Examination

Developmental assessment – consider quality of movement as well as whether task is achieved.
General physical examination:

- Length/height, weight and head circumference, and plot on charts.
- Dysmorphic features
- Skin lesions

- Spine
- Chest shape

Neurological examination:

- Visual responses and eye movements (squint).
- Response to sound.
- Posture and symmetry
- Gait
- Motor coordination
- Unwanted movement
- Muscle tone and power
- Tendon reflexes
- Range of joint movement.

Diagnostic tests
Diagnosis of cerebral palsy is clinical.
Consider the following investigations:

- Neuroimaging – MRI brain scan and spinal cord
- Investigation for congenital infection – TORCH
- Metabolic studies
- Genetic studies.

DIFFERENTIAL DIAGNOSIS
- For hemiplegia:
    - branchial (Erb's) palsy
    - intrauterine moulding can lead to temporary asymmetry of posture
    - torticollis
    - sternomastoid tumour
    - congenital monoplegia is very rare and more likely to affect a leg.
- For bilateral spastic cerebral palsy:
    - metabolic/neurodegenerative disorders, e.g. leucodystrophies
    - if legs more affected than arms: familial spastic paraplegia, spinal cord lesions.
- For dyskinetic cerebral palsy:
    - dopa-responsive dystonia.
- For ataxic cerebral palsy:
    - incoordination as part of generalised learning difficulties
    - progressive ataxias.
- – CNS malformations

> **ALERTS**
> Hand preference under 1 year of age suggests hemiplegia.
> Bottom shufflers can have cerebral palsy.
> Ataxic CP – consider progressive ataxias.
> Dystonic CP – consider dopa-responsive dystonia.

WHO TO TALK TO

Health visitor.
Community/neurodisability paediatrician.
Child development team coordinator.
Paediatric physiotherapist.
Paediatric neurologist.

WHEN TO REFER

All children with suspected CP need multidisciplinary assessment and
ongoing support.
Refer to locality community paediatrician or disability paediatrician as
soon as possible.
Tell parents of concern re development but do not use the term 'cerebral
palsy' unless absolutely certain.

THERAPY

Motor therapy

Physiotherapy and occupational therapy – to promote normal motor
development, to inhibit abnormal motor development and to prevent
joint contractures.
Advice on how to handle and position the child, inhibiting primitive
reflexes.
Aids, equipment, buggy or wheelchair, seating, home adaptations.
There are different therapy models (e.g. Bobath, Peto) but most teams use
an eclectic approach to the individual child.

Other treatments for spasticity

Baclofen, dantrolene, diazepam.
Intramuscular botulinum toxin.
Intrathecal baclofen.
Dorsal root rhizotomy.
Managed jointly with physiotherapist and orthopaedic surgeon, as splints,
serial plastering, tissue or tendon releases may be necessary.

Feeding and growth problems

These are common and require a multidisciplinary approach – paediatrician,
dietitian, speech and language therapist.
Gastro-oesophageal reflux is a common problem.
Children with severe feeding difficulties may need gastrostomy with or
without fundoplication.

Speech and language therapy

For communication problems.
May need communication aid.

Behaviour therapy

Counselling

FOLLOW-UP

Continuous follow-up by paediatrician is essential.
Review diagnosis.
Medical management of associated conditions.
Monitor hips and spine – hip x-rays at 30 months (dysplasia).
Liaison with education (medical advice for statementing process).
Liaison with social services and voluntary agencies re family support, including respite care.

KEY POINTS FOR PARENTS (from Scope)

Cerebral palsy means that part of the child's brain is either not working properly or has not developed normally. The part affected is usually one of the parts that control the muscles and body movements.
Children with cerebral palsy are entitled to a range of benefits and support services.
Parents of children with cerebral palsy need to be able to take a break sometimes.

HEALTH PROMOTION

Dental health is important.
Annual influenza vaccine if recurrent respiratory infections.

SUPPORT ORGANISATIONS

Scope
6 Market Road
London N7 9PW
Tel: 020 7619 7100
www.scope.org.uk
Local support groups.

SOURCES

Mutch LW, Alberman E, Hagberg B, Kodama K, Perat MV (1992) Cerebral palsy epidemiology: where are we now and where are we going? Developmental Medicine and Child Neurology 34: 547–555
SCPE Collaborative Group (2000) Surveillance of cerebral palsy in Europe: a collaboration of cerebral palsy surveys and registers. Developmental Medicine and Child Neurology 42: 816–824

See also

Chapter 93, Special educational needs; Chapter 94, Checklist for advice to Local Education Authorities.

12

PROBLEMS WITH HEARING

DEFINITION

Threshold levels of hearing between 0 and 20 dBHL across the speech frequency range (500–4000 Hz) on both sides are classified as normal on pure tone audiometry (Fig. 12.1).

Hearing loss is either sensorineural or conductive, or a mix of the two, and varies in degree. Mild loss is between 20 and 40 dBHL, moderate loss between 40 and 60 dBHL, severe loss between 60 and 90 dBHL, profound loss greater than 90 dBHL.

Sensorineural hearing loss is due to defects in the cochlea or retrocochlear pathway – presents with various configurations on audiometry but

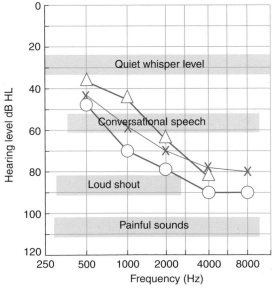

Fig. 12.1 Audiogram with typical everyday sounds superimposed.
○ right ear   X left ear   △ bone conduction

tends to have higher threshold levels at high frequency. Can be mild, moderate, severe or profound.

Conductive hearing loss is due to defects in the conduction mechanism across the external and middle ear. Can be permanent (e.g. defects in the ossicular chain) or temporary (e.g. with middle ear effusion in glue ear). Tends to be mild or moderate with approximately the same degree of loss across the speech frequency range

EPIDEMIOLOGY AND AETIOLOGY

The commonest cause of hearing loss in children is glue ear – a temporary conductive hearing loss associated with middle ear effusion. It is extremely common under the age of 5 years. Peak incidences occur around 2 and 4 years, with around 1 in 8 children having an episode of significant hearing loss by age 5 years. Down's syndrome and cleft palate children are especially prone.

Prevalence of permanent hearing loss is low – approximately 1–2 per 1000 live births.

Permanent conductive losses may be genetic (e.g. Apert's, Treacher Collins), chromosomal (e.g. Down's) or acquired (e.g. trauma – head injury, perforated ear-drum).

Sensorineural hearing loss may be congenital – including genetic, which can be syndromal (e.g. Waardenburg's, Pendred's) or non-syndromal, infection in utero (e.g. CMV) or prematurity – or acquired, including bacterial meningitis, head injury and ototoxic therapy.

PRESENTATION

Includes:
- failure at neonatal screen
- parental concern
- professional concern, e.g. craniofacial abnormalities, ear pits, extreme prematurity
- babble does not develop or ceases
- delay in speech and language acquisition
- behavioural problems
- learning difficulties.

ASSESSMENT

History
Family history – relatives hearing aid wearers?
Birth history.
Response to loud and domestic sounds.
Babble or speech present (quality?).

Examination

General physical examination, including face, neck and external ears.

Hearing testing to assess degree of loss

May be possible in the community at certain ages using behavioural tests if personnel specially trained. Includes distraction testing from 7 months, cooperative testing at 2–3 years, speech discrimination test and performance test from 3 years, and pure tone audiometry from 4 years.

(*Note*: testing before 2–3 years requires two-handed behavioural tests so refer directly to local Audiology Department if personnel not available in the community. Beware temptation to use tympanometry! This is not a diagnostic tool for hearing loss as it merely measures middle ear function and not hearing level!)

Diagnostic tests

All children should be referred to specialist audiology units if their age precludes community testing or community clinics are not available locally. Refer if tests performed in the community indicate hearing loss.
Audiology Department tests might include:

- visual reinforcement audiometry (rewarding turn to sound with visual stimulus)
- pure tone audiometry ('headphones')
- auditory brain stem response (measuring 'messages' in the auditory nerve)
- otoacoustic emissions (measuring the activity of the cochlea)
- steady-state audiometry (measuring brainwaves in 'hearing' part of the brain).

> **ALERTS**
>
> ⚠ All children presenting with speech and language problems must have their hearing tested before referral to speech and language therapy.
>
> All children with permanent hearing loss will require referral for visual assessment.
>
> Hearing loss is often thought by parents to be present when in fact autistic spectrum disorder, severe developmental delay or specific speech and language disorders exist.

WHO TO TALK TO

Health visitor.
School nurse.
Audiologist.
Community paediatrician.
Speech and language therapist.

WHEN TO REFER
Refer to Audiology Department as soon as hearing loss is suspected.

THERAPY
Hearing aids.
Grommet insertion.
Sign language.

FOLLOW-UP (Hearing aid wearers)
In Audiology Department for amplification needs.
Community paediatric input for educational placement and to monitor
  development.

KEY POINTS FOR PARENTS
- Glue ear children:
  - enhance listening skills
  - recognition of temporary and recurrent nature
  - alert class teacher.
- Hearing aid wearers:
  - consideration of alternative means of communication, i.e. sign
    language
  - correct educational placement for child is dependent on preferred
    methods of communication
  - child should have regular input from Teachers for the Hearing
    Impaired.

HEALTH PROMOTION
Access to other deaf children and adults.
Early introduction to hearing children in nursery/playgroup.

ADDITIONAL POINTS
Deaf parents will mostly view their deaf children as normal and so may
  not welcome hearing aid advice or cochlear implant and 'talk' with
  their children in the 'family' sign language.

SUPPORT ORGANISATIONS
Advice for parents and Helpline in National Deaf Children's Society
  (www.ndcs.org.uk).

See also
Chapter 13, Problems with talking.

PROBLEMS WITH TALKING

EPIDEMIOLOGY AND AETIOLOGY

Problems with talking can be classified by cause:

- Structural or sensorimotor defects, e.g. brain dysfunction or damage, global developmental delay, cerebral palsy, hearing loss and cleft palate.
- Possible genetic factors in specific speech and language disorders and in social communication disorders.
- Emotional and behavioural disorders, e.g. elective mutism.
- Environmental deprivation.

PRESENTATION

Presentation can include lack of babble or delayed babble, delay of first clear words, poor phonology, poor progression of clear speech, poor understanding of speech, loss of speech skills, stammering.

ASSESSMENT

This must include history, examination, a formal test of hearing and assessment of developmental progress.

History

Birth and development.
Previous hearing tests/screen.
Parent's opinion of hearing.
Family history of hearing problems, speech and language problems, learning difficulties.

Examination

Physical examination of tongue and palate, syndromal features, neurological examination.

Age-appropriate hearing test

May require referral to specialist audiology clinic (see Chapter 12).

Developmental assessment
Using materials such as Griffith's Mental Scales.

WHEN TO REFER
Refer to Audiology Department if hearing loss suspected on testing or testing results are felt not to be reliable.
Refer to speech and language therapist (*Note*: hearing must be shown to be satisfactory) if:

- suspicion of disordered expressive language (phonology) and/or delay in receptive (comprehension) language
- suspicion of global developmental delay – consider for baseline assessment
- delay in speech and language greater than development in other areas
- speech and language skills behind those of peers in school-age children
- behavioural difficulties with poor speech and language
- continuing problems with stammering (dysfluency).

> **ALERTS**
> ⚠ Hearing across the speech frequency range must be assessed before further action.
> Complete loss of speech and language skills is sometimes seen in autistic spectrum disorders as well as lack of speech and delayed speech and language.

WHO TO TALK TO
Health visitor
Speech and language therapist
Developmental paediatrician
Neurologist
Educational psychologist
Audiologist

THERAPY
Formal speech and language therapy.
Speech and language programme in nursery/school.
Educational placement in special units.
Hearing-impaired children may need manual form of communication (e.g. British Sign Language) in addition to hearing aids.

FOLLOW-UP

Community paediatrician.
Speech and language therapist.
Audiology.
Educational psychology.

KEY POINTS FOR PARENTS

Specific speech and language problems may look like hearing and listening difficulty.
Literacy problems are often experienced by those children with a previous history of speech and language problems.
Balance and coordination problems may also be seen in children with verbal dyspraxia (motor difficulties with tongue and palate).
Statement of special educational need may be required in those with communication difficulties.
Specific speech and language problems often run in families.

HEALTH PROMOTION

Children need constant conversational practice to develop good speech and language skills – don't rely on the TV for listening practice!
Hearing-impaired children may benefit from bi-lingualism (BSL and written English).

ADDITIONAL POINTS

Dysfluency (stammering) is often seen transiently while young children are developing speech skills.
Semantic–pragmatic language disorder may be associated with Asperger's syndrome.

SUPPORT ORGANISATIONS

Afasic – www.afasic.org.uk
I CAN – www.ican.org.uk
Talking Point – www.talkingpoint.org.uk

See also
Chapter 12, Problems with hearing.

PROBLEMS WITH BEHAVIOUR

EATING PROBLEMS – YOUNG CHILDREN

The commonest eating problem in young children is *faddy eating*, which is covered in this section.

Young children may also overeat (see Chapter 31).

Eating problems may also occur in children with acute or chronic illness, and in children with developmental problems.

DEFINITION

Faddy eating is when a restricted variety of foods is consumed.

EPIDEMIOLOGY AND AETIOLOGY

Many toddlers go through phases of food reluctance/refusal, which is often part of their overall behaviour pattern and attention-seeking strategy, commonly associated with the 'terrible two's' period. Transient food refusal may be associated with minor illnesses or emotional upset.

PRESENTATION

By the time the family presents with a child with faddy eating, mealtimes may have deteriorated to 'being a nightmare battle', family relationships strained and considerable emotional distress engendered. Faltering growth only occurs in extreme cases, although weight gain may be suboptimal.

ASSESSMENT

History

A detailed dietary assessment, including attention to past and present feeding behaviour and other social and environmental issues, is vital in identifying the underlying root of the problem, and highlighting any potential nutrient deficiencies. Faddy eating is often associated with *iron deficiency* (see Chapter 29).

Examination

General review for signs of underlying illness.

Weight and height should be measured and plotted on the centile chart.

WHO TO TALK TO

Health visitors and nursery nurses are key personnel who can support families in making changes to children's behaviour.

Community programmes such as Sure Start and Healthy Living Centres provide family support and address parenting skills.

Community dietitians can be involved in dietary and behavioural assessment of more extreme cases.

WHEN TO REFER

Occasionally, input from a clinical psychologist may be required.

THERAPY

Attempts to allay parental anxiety are paramount. If appropriate, normal growth and development should be emphasised and a multivitamin and mineral supplement recommended to cover any potential nutritional deficiencies. Key points include:

- making sure mealtimes are relaxed
- avoiding force feeding or giving undue attention
- eating together
- offering drinks with regular meals and snacks, and no food or drink in between (about 2 hour gaps)
- not giving alternatives if a meal is refused
- ignoring food refusal and removing the child from the table if disruptive
- giving lots of non-food related attention at the end of a meal if eaten well.

FOLLOW-UP

If there are no concerns regarding growth or nutrient deficiencies, discharge following assessment to health visitors, unless extreme eating behaviour, whereby a clinical psychologist may be involved (see 'When to refer').

KEY POINTS FOR PARENTS

Leaflets for the management of faddy eating are available nationally: *Help, my child won't eat*, and *Help, my child still won't eat*, from the Paediatric Group of the British Dietetic Association; and locally, e.g. *Gaining more control at mealtimes*, Nottingham City PCT.

There are a number of books available re parenting skills, including *Toddler Taming: A Parent's Guide to the First Four Years*, by Christopher Green.

SOURCES

Wardley BL, Puntis JWL, Taitz LS (eds) (1997) The preschool child. In: Handbook of Child Nutrition, 2nd edn. Oxford: Oxford University Press, pp 54–72

See also

Chapter 29, Nutritional issues – preschool years and older children; Chapter 30, Poor weight gain – weight and growth faltering in young children; Chapter 31, Excessive weight gain.

3

EATING PROBLEMS – OLDER CHILDREN

DEFINITIONS

Anorexia nervosa

Anorexia nervosa is:

- refusal to maintain body weight over a minimum normal weight for age and height (i.e. weight loss leading to body weight 15% below that expected, or failure to make expected weight gain during a period of growth leading to body weight 15% less than expected)
- intense fear of gaining weight or becoming fat even though underweight
- disturbance in the way in which one's body weight, size or shape is experienced, undue influence of body shape and weight on self-evaluation, or denial of the seriousness of low body weight
- in girls, absence of at least three consecutive menstrual cycles when otherwise expected to occur (primary or secondary amenorrhoea).

Bulimia nervosa

Bulimia nervosa usually presents over the age of 18 years, but may present in younger adolescents.

It is characterised by recurrent episodes of binge eating, with recurrent inappropriate compensatory behaviour in order to prevent weight gain, such as self-induced vomiting; use of laxatives, diuretics or other medication; fasting or excessive exercise.

Children and adolescents may have problems of eating control, not reaching diagnostic criteria. Overeating may result in obesity (see Chapter 31).

EPIDEMIOLOGY AND AETIOLOGY

1–2% of young women have a diagnosis of anorexia nervosa or bulimia nervosa.

Anorexia nervosa usually starts in adolescence, but an increasing number as young as 8 years are being diagnosed. In this age group 25% are boys.

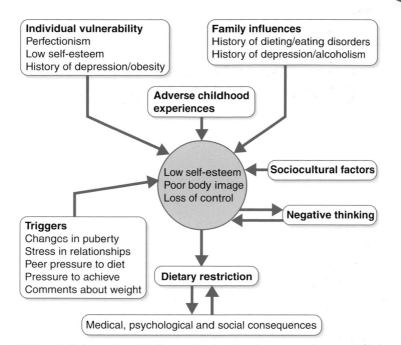

Fig. 15.1 Aetiology: key risk factors in the development of anorexia nervosa.

Over 10% of all young people have problems with eating control. 30–70% of adolescents have engaged in dieting, and a focus on thinness and dieting has become increasingly common in younger children.

The aetiology of anorexia nervosa is outlined in Figure 15.1.

PRESENTATION

Parents, friends or school notice weight loss, excessive exercising, wearing baggy clothes, increasing isolation and loss of friends, moodiness, perfectionism, any obsessions (particularly about food) and ritualistic behaviour, feeling cold, poor circulation, growth of downy hair all over the body.

Young people may also present with amenorrhoea, irregular periods, delayed menarche, or digestive problems such as abdominal bloating and pain, indigestion, nausea, diarrhoea or constipation. They may feel generally unwell, with lethargy and sleeping problems.

In bulimia nervosa there may be secretive behaviour, disappearing to the toilet after meals, vomiting causing tooth erosion and sore throat, dehydration, poor skin.

ASSESSMENT

History

Establish diagnosis based on presentation.

Ask specific questions – e.g. 'Do you think you have an eating problem?' or 'Do you worry excessively about your weight?'.

Document medical, psychological and social/educational consequences of anorexia nervosa.

Offer young people individual appointments separate from family members to obtain a full history.

Assess risk of serious morbidity and mortality (see 'Alerts').

Assess other psychological comorbidity, particularly self-harm.

Examination

Weight, height and calculation of BMI – compare with age and sex norms.

Assess for dehydration, and exclude other causes of weight loss.

Diagnostic tests

Nil specific, but based on BMI and established on assessment (often repeated over time).

ALERTS

⚠ Severe emaciation.
Severe deterioration.
Serious risk of self-harm.
Poor response to treatment.

WHO TO TALK TO

Community paediatrician.

Child and Adolescent Mental Health Services (CAMHS), which may include a specialist dietitian.

WHEN TO REFER

Children and adolescents with established eating disorders are likely to need specialist treatment by CAMHS.

THERAPY

A range of treatments should be available, including cognitive behaviour therapy adapted to suit the young person's age, circumstances and level of development.

Family interventions that address the eating disorder may be helpful, with attention to other psychological factors such as low self-esteem.

Aim for weight gain (variable but likely to be approximately 0.5 kg/week) and healthy eating patterns.

Provide regular monitoring of weight, and assess fluid and electrolyte balance if vomiting is frequent or laxatives are used.
Use oral, rather than intravenous supplementation.
Inpatient treatment may be required.

KEY POINTS FOR PARENTS

Early intervention is important.
Family and friends need support for themselves, both to help the young person and to cope with the impact on their lives.

HEALTH PROMOTION

Within schools – programmes aimed at increasing knowledge about eating disorders and its consequences, changing attitudes towards shape and weight, changing eating behaviour, improving self-esteem, reducing negative thinking.
Aim to counteract media messages, and to develop young people's own ideas about body image.

SOURCES

Eating disorders – a guide to primary care. Online. Available: www.eguidelines.co.uk
National Institute for Clinical Excellence (2004) Eating disorders: core interventions in the treatment and management of anorexia nervosa, bulimia nervosa and related eating disorders. Online. Available: www.nice.org.uk/page.aspx?o=cg009

See also

Chapter 29, Nutritional issues – preschool years and older children; Chapter 31, Excessive weight gain.

EXCESSIVE CRYING

DEFINITION

A clear definition of what is abnormal is difficult and often presentation indicates family/child distress. The quality of the cry and onset are important factors.

PRESENTATION

This will often be a stressful consultation for the parents and may present with a myriad of problems including feeding and sleeping.

ASSESSMENT

History

Important factors to elucidate are:

- character of the cry
- is the current pattern unusual for the child
- is the crying associated with feeding
- maternal feelings/anxieties about the child or within the family.

It is also important to obtain a good medical history of the perinatal period.

Ask about sleeping and feeding patterns which may indicate dysregulation.

Examination

If the character of the cry is abnormal or of recent onset then serious injury or illness may be present and careful examination and investigation should be performed.

Developmental assessment should be undertaken, including assessment for hearing and vision problems.

Diagnostic tests

Careful examination should preclude the need for investigation in those where the cry is 'normal' and follows an established pattern; however, where the cry is abnormal then investigations could include cerebral imaging, radiology, urine microscopy and culture, and other investigations of pain.

DIFFERENTIAL DIAGNOSIS

- Organic disease:
  - cerebral injury or infection
  - fractures
  - gastro-oesophageal reflux
  - urinary tract problems
  - other rare causes, e.g. neuroblastoma.
- Non-organic disease:
  - within child (temperament)
  - teething
  - family/maternal distress (pathology).

> **ALERTS**
>
> ⚠ In most cases the quality of the cry will give a good indication of pathology. Those children in whom the cry sounds abnormal should be investigated promptly and referred to a local paediatrician urgently.

MANAGEMENT

In those children in whom a non-organic cause of the crying has been identified, the management is complex and may need the assistance of other agencies (e.g. health visitors, adult mental health colleagues).

Sympathetic listening and allaying parental anxieties can often be therapeutic. A clear picture of the daily pattern may help to identify areas for intervention (e.g. feeding routine). This needs to be done with the clear recognition that crying is the baby's way of communication.

Working with the parents, particularly around developmental progress, can be a way of developing appropriate responses to the crying behaviour. There may be a need to address parental expectations of the child.

Simple strategies, including sitting the child up (e.g. in a sling) so that they can see what is happening, appropriate stimulation, establishing a routine for the child and family, and also changing the routine, e.g. walking outdoors, are often helpful for parents. Develop strategies to help the family anticipate the baby's needs (e.g. establishment of routine).

It is important to recognise that some children are difficult to parent and ongoing support should be provided to families that may be under considerable stress, especially those that are isolated. In some, day care or nursery placement may provide some respite but does not alter the problem, and management should be undertaken at the same time.

Some nurseries provide parental support through groups for parents as well. In extreme circumstances, respite or admission may be required if the child is thought to be at risk!

FOLLOW-UP

Ongoing support is essential but may not need to be medical once organic disease is ruled out.

KEY POINTS FOR PARENTS

Crying is a form of communication and understanding behavioural and language development is important for management and comfort of the child.

HEALTH PROMOTION

This is a good opportunity with ongoing follow-up to discuss with families the factors of early behavioural management to promote healthy emotional development.

ADDITIONAL POINTS

Support may be required to address the mental health needs of the parent, especially for isolated lone parent families.

TEMPER TANTRUMS

3

DEFINITION

Manifestation of anger, usually involving attempts to get the child to conform to accepted standards of social behaviour and relationships.

EPIDEMIOLOGY AND AETIOLOGY

Peak around 2–3 years of age but common from 2 to 5 years. More common in boys; 10% of 5-year-old boys have tantrums once a week. There is some evidence that about 70% of children with significant behaviour problems at 3 still have them a year later but this diminishes with age. In many, the anger may persist but may manifest in different ways.

PRESENTATION

Tantrums often occur more frequently when a child is hungry or tired.

ASSESSMENT

A detailed assessment of circumstances around the behaviour is valuable. A good family history of the type of behaviour and patterns of behaviour is important, as is evaluation of parenting styles and skills.

History and examination

This should involve close observation of the parent–child interaction, as well as a history of associated features and history/diary of behaviours, interventions attempted and what limited or predicted their success.

Diagnostic tests

Often not required unless associated features suggest alternative diagnoses (e.g. hearing problems).

Child characteristics	Family and social factors
Speech and language problems	Young or elderly mothers
Wetting and soiling	Single parents or step-parents
Feeding or sleeping problems	Poor social conditions
Hyperactive or difficult	Four or more children
Miserable and tearful	Maternal smoking
Frequent aches and pains	Poverty and unemployment
Frequent minor illness	Inner city areas

Associated factors

> **ALERTS**
>
> ⚠ Be aware of potential for emotional, physical and neglect forms of child abuse.

WHO TO TALK TO

The local health visitor may be able to advise about local parenting programmes or services provided by Children's Mental Health Service Teams.

WHEN TO REFER

Significant family psychopathology.

THERAPY

Three main strategies are outlined in Table 17.1.

Table 17.1

The approach	The methods
Prevention	Avoid high risk situations (tired or hungry)
	Plan in advance
	Diversion
	Offering limited choice
Training children to express anger in more acceptable ways	Teach by example
	Rewarding self-control
	Training anger management
Ignoring the behaviour	Remove the audience
	Time out
	Leave until calm

Support to families in distress may take the form of referral to community support agencies for assistance. Emotional support for an isolated parent may be important.

Parenting programmes may be helpful and ongoing support from local workers should be maintained – this may be a health visitor or school nurse.

It is important to get consistency between the parents in their management styles and it may be important to get them together to discuss this.

FOLLOW-UP

Reassurance and a sympathetic ear are often all that is required but where associated factors exist it will be important to see that these factors are managed appropriately.

HEALTH PROMOTION

This is a key time for discussion about normal childhood behavioural development and the development of independence.

KEY POINTS FOR PARENTS

There are many useful resources available, for example:

- Green, G. (1985) Toddler taming: a parent's guide to the first four years. New York: Ballantine Books (ISBN 0449901556)
- Pentecost, D. (2000) Parenting the ADD Child. Can't do? Won't do? London: Jessica Kingsley (ISBN 1 853028118)
- Sanders, M. (1996) Every parent – a positive approach to children's behaviour. Reading, MA: Addison Wesley (ISBN 0201539306)

See also
Chapter 18, Breath holding.

18

BREATH HOLDING

3

PRESENTATION
This is commonly associated with temper tantrums or crying when very upset. The child cannot take a new breath in, the breath is 'held' in expiration, involuntarily and silently. If prolonged, this expiratory apnoea can cause a syncope/transient loss of consciousness.

ASSESSMENT
Consider other causes of apnoea.

Reflex anoxic seizures (sometimes called 'white breath holding') are usually due to reflex asystolic syncope but can be impossible to distinguish without concurrent ECG. Neither is life-threatening. Management depends on education and reassurance.

Pure expiratory apnoea syncope can cause reflex anoxic seizures without asystole. There is no known treatment but, if really troublesome, iron deficiency and/or anaemia (if present) should be treated and reflex asystolic syncope excluded.

SUPPORT ORGANISATIONS
The British Association for Early Childhood Education
www.early-education.org.uk
Syncope Trust And Reflex anoxic Seizures (STARS)
www.stars.org.uk

See also
Chapter 17, Temper tantrums; Chapter 50, Seizures and funny turns.

19

SCHOOL REFUSAL

DEFINITION

School refusal is a condition characterised by reluctance and often outright refusal to go to school in a child who:

1. seeks the comfort and security of home, preferring to remain close to parental figures, especially during school hours
2. displays evidence of emotional upset when faced with the prospect of having to attend school, although this may take the form of unexplained physical symptoms
3. manifests no severe antisocial tendencies, apart from possible aggressiveness when attempts are made to force school attendance
4. does not attempt to conceal the problem from parents (Berg 1997).

EPIDEMIOLOGY AND AETIOLOGY

Boys = girls.
All social classes.
Parenting may be overprotective or anxious.
Children usually do well in school.
Most likely to present at 5 (separation anxiety), 11 (transfer to secondary school) and 15 years (stress and/or depression).
Occurs in about 1% of children.

PRESENTATION

Parent, GP, school, Education Welfare Officer (EWO) may bring non-attendance at school or physical symptoms in child to our attention.

ASSESSMENT

Examine children with physical symptoms to establish those who are genuinely ill, or not being adequately treated (e.g. asthma).

History

Take a standard history and ask about precipitating events and worries about school, individual lessons or teachers, changing for games, using the toilets, games, changes of class teacher, size of school, loss of special friend, bullying, journey to and from school.

Ask about previous school refusal and family's reactions, losses and bereavements, worries about leaving parents (health or child's fears for parent's safety).

Ask about child at school, and any others involved.

Examination

Establish no physical illness and reassure the parent and child.

DIFFERENTIAL DIAGNOSIS

Truanting.
Being withheld from school by parent(s).
Missing school with parent's knowledge or consent

> **ALERTS**
>
> ⚠ School refusal can persist for months or even years if not satisfactorily managed. Exclude an underlying depression that might need treatment.

WHO TO TALK TO

School, school nurse, school support services.
General practitioner.
EWO.
Child and Adolescent Mental Health Service (CAMHS).

THERAPY

Firmly establish absence of illness and reassure. Provide sympathetic support and insist child returns to school. If absence from school is already protracted, move on to the next step.

Discuss with CAMHS team and move to multidisciplinary assessment and detailed planning meeting regarding return to school.

Some children respond better to a full return to school straight away; others benefit from a slower, graduated approach.

FOLLOW-UP

Provide support to parents as long as it is needed and liaise closely with the school.

KEY POINTS FOR PARENTS

Parents may need detailed explanation concerning the child's physical symptoms, and reassurance.

Key to success is early return to school; change of school is usually unhelpful

Parents need to work together and agree a consistent approach.

Good communication with school.

Outlook is good in the long term, when managed well.

ADDITIONAL POINTS

Many children attending infant school experience anxieties (up to 80%). Many children have somatic symptoms in response to an adverse event associated with school. In most circumstances the problem is temporary and responds to firm support of parent and/or teacher. If school refusal is recent, keep in perspective.

SUPPORT ORGANISATIONS

YoungMinds Parent Information Service
Tel: 0800 018 2138
www.youngminds.org.uk/pis

SOURCES

Berg I (1997) School refusal. Archives of Disease in Childhood 76: 90–91

See also

Chapter 20, Anxiety; Chapter 21, Depression and self-harm; Chapter 26, Bullying.

20

ANXIETY

All children experience anxiety – very young children may experience fears and phobias, sometimes precipitated by changes such going to nursery. These are normal and usually settle in a short time. High anxiety levels that continue can be distressing and affect a child's functioning.

EPIDEMIOLOGY AND AETIOLOGY

1 in 10 children experiences anxiety problems that impair their ability to live a normal life. Examples are separation anxiety, school phobia and post-traumatic stress disorder; panic attacks, agoraphobia and obsessive–compulsive disorder are seen in older children. 50% have an additional mental health problem (e.g. depression).
Aetiology is mixed:

- genetic predisposition
- family problems, including child abuse, divorce or separation
- illness of child/carers
- bereavement
- discipline that is harsh, inconsistent or overprotective
- other stressful life events such as bullying or problems at school.

PRESENTATION

Physical symptoms such as headaches, nausea, abdominal pain; restlessness and irritability; difficulty concentrating and sleeping; expressed fears; tires quickly; clinging or regressed behaviour; deterioration in school performance or school refusal; challenging behaviour.
Untreated may progress to low self-esteem, depression, impaired relations with peers, missed school, deliberate self-harm.
May also continue to adulthood.

ASSESSMENT

History and examination
These need to exclude organic illness if there are physical symptoms.

Include psychosocial history, family stresses, information from school, and developmental history when appropriate.

Take account of child's age and developmental level – but identify when symptoms are severe, prolonged, handicapping and developmentally inappropriate.

Some family situations can be quite complex which compounds anxieties.

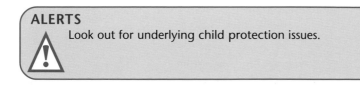

ALERTS

Look out for underlying child protection issues.

WHO TO TALK TO

School – to explore factors that may be contributing.

GP – for up-to-date health information.

Social services – if child protection concern or services needed.

Child and Adolescent Mental Health Service (CAMHS) – for consultation or referral.

WHEN TO REFER

Depression, deliberate self-harm or child protection concerns. Refer to clinical psychology or CAMHS when simple measures to address underlying factors do not help.

THERAPY

This is time intensive.

Need to manage underlying factors and link behaviour and thinking.

Child needs support to gain control of their thoughts in triggered situations – need to be creative in doing this.

Relaxation techniques can be individually tailored for some children.

FOLLOW-UP

Depends on complexity of presentation. If attempting therapeutic intervention, may need to see frequently, and referral made if unsuccessful or more complex factors emerge.

KEY POINTS FOR PARENTS

Anxiety is catching, so parents may need help with how they respond to the child.

If families are going through a lot of stress, encourage them to seek extra support from friends, family members or others.

HEALTH PROMOTION

Parents and teachers can give children information and positive messages
about planned changes in their lives.

There may be books or games that can help children to understand
upsetting things such as serious illness, separation or bereavement.

SUPPORT ORGANISATIONS

Mental Health Foundation
  Tel: 020 7803 1100; fax: 020 7803 1111
  Email: mhf@mhf.org.uk
  www.mentalhealth.org.uk
  Produces a booklet 'The Anxious Child'
Parentline
  Helpline: 01702 559900
  www.parentlineplus.org.uk
  Offers help and advice to parents on bringing up children and
  teenagers
YoungMinds Parent Information Service
  Tel: 0800 018 2138
  Email: enquiries@youngminds.org.uk
  www.youngminds.org.uk/pis

See also

Chapter 15, Eating problems – older children; Chapter 19, School refusal;
  Chapter 21, Depression and self-harm; Chapter 22, Hyperactivity;
  Chapter 23, Tiredness and fatigue – chronic fatigue syndrome; Chapter 24,
  Sleep problems; Chapter 25, Autistic spectrum disorders; Chapter 26,
  Bullying; Chapter 57, Recurrent abdominal pain – medical approach;
  Chapter 58, Abdominal pain – surgical aspects; Chapter 60, Soiling and
  constipation; Chapter 86, Children looked after.

21

DEPRESSION AND SELF-HARM

DEFINITION

- *Deliberate self-harm (DSH)* – 'A deliberate non-fatal act, whether physical, drug overdose or poisoning, done in the knowledge that it was potentially harmful and in the case of overdose, that the amount taken was excessive' (Morgan 1979). (There is often uncertainty about motivation.)
- *Childhood depression* – A mood disorder that resembles depression in adults, but presents differently in children.

EPIDEMIOLOGY AND AETIOLOGY

- *DSH* – female:male 7:1. Figures difficult to assess, may be as high as 1 in 10 teenagers. Many who cut/burn themselves hide the injuries.
- *Depression* – 1 in 33 children and 1 in 8 adolescents at any one time. Boys = girls, but during adolescence twice as many girls as boys. Occurs with other psychological problems. Significant depression probably exists in about 5% of children and adolescents.
- *Suicide* – 13 suicides per 100,000 15–19 year olds per year; males more at risk; sixth leading cause of death for 5–14 year olds and third leading cause of death for 15–24 year olds.

Common factors in aetiology

Family dysfunction, family history of psychiatric illness, depression or other psychiatric illness in the young person, relationship problems, alcohol abuse/substance misuse, history of care and/or physical and sexual abuse, custody (Youth Offending Institutions/prisons), bereavement or other experience of loss, high levels of family stress, examination pressure, bullying, socioeconomic factors.

Children who develop depression are more likely to have a family history of the disorder in childhood.

Children with longstanding illness or who have learning disorders are at a higher risk for depression:

- DSH risks are higher – if personal knowledge of DSH/suicide victim, post-traumatic stress disorders. A common trigger is an argument with a parent or close friend.
- Suicide risks are higher – in males, older age, high suicidal intent, psychosis, depression, hopelessness, an unclear reason for act of deliberate self-harm, use of drugs or alcohol when upset, has a relative or friend who tried to kill themselves. 40% who attempt suicide do so again.

PRESENTATION

Injury, knowledge of DSH or depression may be from young person directly or a friend, family member, youth worker, teacher, school nurse, social worker, etc.

Children with depression may appear persistently sad, no longer enjoy activities, or may appear agitated or irritable.

Depressed children may present physical symptoms, e.g. headaches and tummy aches, miss school or perform less well in school. They may appear bored or low in energy, have problems concentrating and/or a changed eating or sleeping pattern.

They may present at A&E Departments from a drug overdose, with injuries from cutting, burning, self-strangulation, jumping in front of vehicles or from high places.

Also may come to attention indirectly from substance abuse, eating disorders, promiscuous behaviour, as children who are looked after or children who break the law.

ASSESSMENT AND MANAGEMENT

DSH

Needs urgent medical assessment if has taken an overdose, even if they appear all right. Harmful effects can be delayed. Small amounts of some medications can be fatal.

Young people who need hospital treatment for self-harm should be admitted and have a full specialist mental health assessment, looking at psychosocial and risk factors.

Child and Adolescent Mental Health Services (CAMHS), A&E Departments and paediatric services need clear, mutually agreed protocols.

Strategies are needed to address identified issues and prevent recurrences.

Good liaison between services and child and family is imperative.

Induction training is needed for new staff and continuous training for established staff.

Depression

Recognition and diagnosis of depression is more difficult in children because of the way symptoms are expressed, and it varies with developmental age.

Response to methylphenidate is not a diagnostic test.

Assessment of degree of problem in each of three areas using observation and rating scales, e.g. Connors' Teacher and Parent Rating Scales, Strengths and Weaknesses Questionnaire.

Need information about behaviour in different settings. Information from school or nursery is essential.

Cognitive profile is helpful.

FBC is a useful baseline.

Consider fragile X in children with other learning difficulties.

DIFFERENTIAL DIAGNOSIS

General learning disability.

'Ill disciplined and overtired.'

Emotional abuse and neglect.

WHO TO TALK TO

Community paediatrician.

School nurse or health visitor.

Class teacher.

School Special Educational Needs Coordinator.

Local Child and Adolescent Mental Health Services.

Local parent support group.

WHEN TO REFER

Consider diagnosis likely and child might benefit from medication.

Medication should only be initiated by a paediatrician with expertise in ADHD or a child and adolescent psychiatrist.

THERAPY

Coordinated support from health, education and social services.

Advice and support to parents and teachers.

Parent support groups.

Behaviour programmes/therapy.

Specific educational support.

Medication

There is evidence from placebo-controlled RCTs that methylphenidate is effective at reducing hyperactivity, inattention and impulsiveness in the short term while children are taking the medication.

The US Multimodal Treatment Study for Children with ADHD (the MTA trial) found that medication was superior to behavioural treatment.

NICE guidance – Methylphenidate is recommended as part of a comprehensive treatment programme for children with a diagnosis of severe ADHD or HKD, and in some cases may be appropriate for children with severe problems due to inattention or hyperactivity/impulsiveness. Generally start at 5 mg daily and gradually increase to 10 or 15 mg two or three times a day, monitoring effects, including BP weekly. Once on an effective dose children should be monitored 3 monthly for efficacy, adverse effects, growth and BP.

A slow release preparation (e.g. Concerta) allows a once daily regimen. *Start at 18 mg daily and increase weekly up to 54 mg daily.* Equasym XL is an alternative preparation.

Treatment with medication should only be started by a child and adolescent psychiatrist or a paediatrician with expertise in ADHD.

GPs can participate in the ongoing prescribing and monitoring of the medication under shared care agreements.

Methylphenidate may cause or worsen tics. Clonidine may be a useful alternative in children with tic disorder/Tourette syndrome. Need baseline ECG.

Atomoxetine – a newly available noradrenaline reuptake inhibitor – has potentially fewer adverse effects than methylphenidate. It is a sustained release preparation that allows single daily dose and may help sleep. Need to monitor growth and BP. Long-term efficacy and in particular whether treatment can improve educational outcomes are not yet known.

KEY POINTS FOR PARENTS

Medication is not a cure, but may reduce the symptoms and allow the behaviour programmes to take effect.

Things tend to improve as the child matures.

Maintaining the child's self-esteem is vital.

Parent support groups can be very helpful.

ADDITIONAL POINTS

Methylphenidate is a controlled drug therefore prescriptions need to be written accordingly.

SUPPORT ORGANISATIONS

ADDISS (The National Attention Deficit Disorder Information and Support Service)
10 Station Road
Mill Hill
London NW7 2JU
Tel: 020 8906 9068
www.addiss.co.uk

SOURCES

American Psychiatric Association (1994) Diagnostic and statistical manual of mental disorders, 4th edn. Washington DC: APA

Connors CK (1973) Rating scales for use with drug studies with children. Psychopharmacology Bulletin 9: 24–84

Green C, Chee K (1997) Understanding ADHD – a parent's guide to attention deficit hyperactivity disorder in children. London: Vermillion

Hill P, Taylor E (2001) An auditable protocol for treating attention deficit/ hyperactivity disorder. Archives of Disease in Childhood 84: 404–409

MTA Cooperative Group (1999) A 14-month randomised clinical trial of treatment strategies for attention-deficit/hyperactivity disorder. Archives of General Psychiatry 56: 1073–1086, 1088–1097

National Institute for Clinical Excellence (2000) Technological appraisal guidance No. 13. Guidance on the use of methylphenidate (Ritalin, Equasym) for attention deficit/hyperactivity disorder (ADHD) in Childhood. Online. Available: www.nice.org.uk

Taylor E, Sergeant J, Doepfner M et al (1998) Clinical guidelines for hyperkinetic disorder. European Society for Child and Adolescent Psychiatry 7: 184–200

World Health Organization (1992) International classification of diseases (ICD-10): classification of mental and behavioural disorders, 10th edn. Geneva: WHO

3

23

TIREDNESS AND FATIGUE – CHRONIC FATIGUE SYNDROME

Tiredness can be caused by a wide range of conditions. These may occur alone or coexist with chronic fatigue syndrome (CFS). Careful history, examination, investigation and review are needed to ensure that other causes are not overlooked.

DEFINITION

Severe fatigue affecting physical and mental functioning causing significant disability. Symptoms are not explained by medical or psychiatric illness, and are present for at least 6 months for more than 50% of the time. 3 months' duration is often accepted as a level for earlier intervention in children and young people.

EPIDEMIOLOGY AND AETIOLOGY

CFS involves a spectrum of disease from mild to severely affected children. It affects all social classes and ethic groups.

The prevalence of CFS depends upon how cases are defined:

- RCPCH/RCGP Community Survey suggested a prevalence of 0.066%, of whom two-thirds were girls.
- The Chief Medical Officer's Report for the UK cites a prevalence up to 0.2–0.4%; others give estimates of up to 3%.
- Approximately 51% of all long-term sickness absence in a studied school population (Dowsett & Colby 1997) was due to CFS.

Up to a quarter of adolescents may report experiencing the symptom of fatigue.

Although there is no clear aetiology, research has demonstrated immune, endocrine, muscle, skeletal and neurological abnormalities.

PRESENTATION

The commonest age of onset is between 13 and 15 years of age but cases can occur as young as 5 years.

The severe fatigue is both physical and mental (involving poor concentration and unclear thinking) and is associated with:

- non-specific musculoskeletal pains
- sleep disturbance
- depression
- other non-specific pains including headaches and abdominal, chest and joint pain.

The main impacts are:

- restrictions in mobility – patients can be in bed for most of the day, and in severe cases may be wheelchair dependent
- absence from school
- educational underachievement
- stress upon the family
- disruption of social relationships.

Symptoms may develop in the course of a protracted recovery from a mild viral illness.

Patients' activity commonly follows a cycle of 'boom and bust', with fatigue and sedentary behaviour alternating with increases in activity that cause exhaustion.

ASSESSMENT

Diagnosis is clinical, based upon the presentation described above, and the exclusion of:

- a disease likely to cause fatigue
- psychiatric disorders, including substance abuse, bipolar depression, psychoses, eating disorder, organic brain disease.

Depression and anxiety disorder are not exclusion criteria.

History

Medical and psychosocial circumstances at the onset of fatigue.
Symptoms of depression or anxiety?
Presence of another psychiatric disorder, including substance abuse?
Previous episodes of medically unexplained symptoms?
Also consider the very rare possibility of carbon monoxide poisoning (in areas of social deprivation) and Lyme disease (a tick-borne disease and endemic to parts of the world).

Examination

A thorough physical examination is important to look for signs of disease, and to provide reassurance to both the young person and parents. This includes height, weight, head circumference, neurological examination, lymphadenopathy, liver, spleen and blood pressure (lying and standing).

Mental status examination – to identify abnormalities in mood, intellectual function, memory and personality.

Diagnostic tests

There are no diagnostic tests. The following tests may help to both reassure and exclude other problems:

- a minimum level of tests including a full blood count, erythrocyte sedimentation rate, c-reactive protein, liver function tests, urea and electrolytes, thyroid function, creatine kinase, blood glucose and urine analysis.

Further tests can be conducted depending on the clinical presentation. These include serological tests for Epstein–Barr virus and tests of immunological function.

DIFFERENTIAL DIAGNOSIS

Endocrine – hypothyroidism, diabetes, Addison's disease.
Anaemia.
Autoimmune disease.
Chronic infection.
Drug induced, e.g. substance misuse.
Gastrointestinal, e.g. coeliac.
Musculoskeletal disease, e.g. myasthenia.
Early onset juvenile chronic arthritis or connective tissue disorder.
Neurological problem (exceedingly rare) but consider early onset of multiple sclerosis.
Cardiac disorder.
Occult malignancy.
Psychological causes – depression (it can also be a comorbidity), school refusal.
Sleep disorder – obstructive sleep apnoea, narcolepsy.
Young carers frequently present with fatigue as a result of caring for a disabled parent.

> ### ⚠ ALERTS
> There are often difficult clinical decisions to be made about children with unexplained symptoms, as in CFS, when suspicions of child abuse may arise. Unexplained symptoms and child abuse are not synonymous and expert advice should be obtained.

WHO TO TALK TO

Teachers.
School nurse and paediatrician.
Child and adolescent mental health services (CAMHS).
Social worker.

WHEN TO REFER

Teenagers presenting with a short history of fatigue and minimal associated symptoms can be appropriately managed within primary care. If symptoms persist beyond 3 months, or school absence becomes a problem, they should be referred to a local community paediatrician. Referral may also be driven by parents demanding a diagnosis.

THERAPY

Therapy involves:

- *A graduated increase in activity (pacing)* – Managing teenagers involves supporting and channelling their efforts to recover using a system of 'stepwise targets'. Small targets are set, which involve a gradual increase in activity, usually over several months. This is akin to building stamina in athletes by progressively increasing their physical demands. Daytime schedules of rest and activity need to be carefully structured and supervised.
- *Cognitive–behaviour therapy.*
- *Education* – The focus is to minimise disruption to education. Milder cases may require brief periods of home tuition aimed at gradual reintegration into mainstream education; severely affected children may need home tuition and/or distance learning on a longer term basis. The focus of reintegration is to minimise the isolation of children from their peers in addition to the educational benefits.
- *Support of the family* – There is invariably a change in family dynamics and this in turn has an impact on the child. The main carer's problems often mirror that of the child, and can include social isolation, work difficulties, loss of leisure, coping with the misconception of others, perceived blame, loss of confidence, depression and anxiety. These problems need to be addressed by the supervising clinician, and may require informal clinic and home support or family therapy.

An integrated multidisciplinary approach is required, provided locally and coordinated by a paediatrician in partnership with the teenager and family/carer. This may involve:

- Social Work to support the family and professionals.
- Education – schoolteachers or home tuition in addition to the educational welfare officer.
- CAMHS, school nurse, physiotherapy, dietetics.

FOLLOW-UP

Children require frequent clinical contact (often weekly at first) and followed until complete recovery is achieved.

Progress often follows an undulating course with four out of five children achieving a good outcome. The duration of symptoms is from months to years.

Research has not demonstrated prognostic factors at onset that predict the severity of illness. Treatment was associated with increased school attendance. A shorter duration of the fatigue (less than 6 months) appeared to have a better outcome (Patel et al 2003).

KEY POINTS FOR PARENTS

Outlook for children with CFS is much better than for adults.

Progress is made in small, controlled steps.

Parents and children need continuing explanation and support over this period.

HEALTH PROMOTION

Healthy lifestyles – sleep, diet, graduated exercise routines – are a key part of recovery.

SOURCES

Baird GM (1869) Neurasthenia or nervous exhaustion. Boston Medical and Surgical Journal 80: 213–221

Department of Health (2002) A report of the CFS/ME Working Group. Report to the Chief Medical Officer of an independent working group. London: Department of Health

Dowsett EG, Colby J (1997) Long-sickness absence due to CFS/ME in UK schools: an epidemiological study with medical educational implications. Journal of Chronic Fatigue Syndrome 3: 29–42

Fukuda K, Strauss SE, Hickie I, Sharpe MC, Dobbins JG, Komaroff A. International Chronic Fatigue Syndrome Study Group (1994) The chronic fatigue syndrome – a comprehensive approach to its definition and study. Annals of Internal Medicine 121(12): 953–959

Hutchinson A (Chair) (2002) A report of the CFS/ME Working Group: report to the Chief Medical Officer of an independent working group. Online. Available: www.youngactiononline.com/docs/dohrep.htm

Patel MX, Smith DG, Chalder T, Wessely S (2003) Chronic fatigue syndrome in children: a cross sectional survey. Archives of Disease in Childhood 88(10): 894–898

Royal College of Paediatrics and Child Health (2004) Evidence based guideline for the management of CFS/ME. London: RCPCH

Skapinakis P, Louis G, Mavreas V (2003) One year outcome of unexplained fatigue syndromes and primary care: results from an international study. Psychological Medicine 33: 857–866

Walford GA, McNelson W, McCluskey DR (1993) Fatigue, depression and social adjustment in chronic fatigue syndrome. Archives of Disease in Childhood 68: 384–388

See also

Chapter 87, Young carers.

24

SLEEP PROBLEMS

3

DEFINITION

Where a child is not getting enough sleep for normal daytime functioning this may be related to not enough sleep, disturbed sleep or abnormal sleep. It is important to define whether it is a problem for the child or is the timing of sleep impacting on family functioning.

EPIDEMIOLOGY

Approximately 20–30% of children will have a sleep problem at some stage:

- Settling problems – 22% at 9 months, 20% at 2 years, 16% at 3 years.
- Night waking – 42% at 9 months, 25% at 2 years, 14% at 3 years.
- Snoring – 10–12% with habitual snoring.
- Obstructive sleep apnoea syndrome (OSAS) – 1.5–2% of population.

ASSESSMENT

History

It is imperative that a good history is taken, including a very detailed history of night waking and events surrounding the waking episode.

Night-time routines or lack of should be examined in detail; daytime behaviour and routines should be examined thoroughly.

A clear description of noise and movement during the night is important.

Social and environmental factors are also important, particularly maternal depression, illnesses that might keep a child awake (e.g. asthma, eczema, seizures, pain, etc.), marital discord and substance abuse.

Medication may affect sleeping, particularly stimulants and antiepileptics.

Examination

This should be aimed at excluding medical causes for sleeping difficulties, and should include:

- dysmorphology, especially with regard to mid-face structures
- ENT and upper airway examination
- thorough respiratory and neurological examination
- cardiovascular examination, including markers of pulmonary hypertension and hypertension as complications of severe OSAS
- general examination to exclude other causes (e.g. arthritis, hypotonia and obesity)
- recording of height and weight, particularly where OSAS is suspected.

Diagnostic tests

- *Sleep diary*: A useful tool both diagnostically and for monitoring treatment.
- *Oximetry* (oxygenated haemoglobin): Marginally useful as a screening tool; however, is not diagnostic of OSAS or central apnoeas.
- *Actigraphy* (monitoring of movement): Very useful for circadian rhythm disorders or for quantifying amount of sleep and sleep disturbance.
- *Polysomnography* (measurement of multiple physiological functions during sleep): Remains the gold standard of investigation and for distinguishing the presence of obstructive versus central apnoeas where this is indicated. This is important in a number of disorders where there is a high incidence of both, including Down's syndrome and other neurological disorders.
- *Multiple sleep latency testing*: Measures daytime sleepiness; used in the diagnosis of narcolepsy. (*Multiple wakefulness test – generally only used to assess adults for driving.*)
- *HLA typing*: Narcolepsy.

DIFFERENTIAL DIAGNOSIS

- *Behavioural*: Night waking/night settling problems/nocturnal drinking or eating disorders.
- *Obstructive*: Obstructive sleep apnoea – neurological (tone), structural (craniofacial abnormalities), tonsils and adenoids, overweight, familial, etc.
- *Central*:
  - nocturnal epilepsy
  - circadian rhythm disorders (e.g. advanced sleep phase in adolescents)
  - abnormalities of central control of breathing (e.g. central hypoventilation syndrome)
  - neurological disorders (e.g. Duchenne muscular dystrophy).

ALERTS

Children with:
- disorders of tone
- neurological abnormalities
- craniofacial abnormalities
- infants with family history of SIDS.

WHEN TO REFER

The child should be referred if a respiratory or upper airway disorder is suspected, if there is a suspicion of nocturnal epilepsy, if a neurological or craniofacial disorder is present.

Sleep-disordered breathing can present with multiple waking and should be evaluated appropriately.

Children should be referred to a local sleep unit that deals with children or, if not available, the local relevant respiratory or neurological colleagues.

The staging of children's sleep is different from that of adults as is the pathophysiology of OSAS in children.

THERAPY

This is dependent on the diagnosis.

- *Night settling*: Behavioural techniques are the most successful.
- *Night waking*: Drug treatment is not justified as first line treatment but may be used for a short period of time to break a cycle of parental sleep deprivation. It is often more effective for difficulties initiating sleep rather than maintaining sleep. Promethazine and alimemazine have been commonly used in the past, but there is a danger of idiosyncratic reactions such as hyperactivity the next day and a risk of them slipping into inappropriate long-term use.
- *Circadian rhythm disorders*: Advancing the sleep phase is the treatment of choice. Melatonin and light therapy have been used in this circumstance with good supporting evidence. Pure behavioural methods are well known to work but require a high level of commitment.

The following should be instigated by appropriate specialists

- *OSAS*: Various treatments exist. These include weight loss (for the overweight), continuous positive airways pressure (CPAP), dental appliances, mandibular advancement. Check if a central or muscular component to sleep-disordered breathing requires nocturnal ventilation (e.g. Duchenne muscular dystrophy, Arnold–Chiari malformation, etc.).
- *Sleep-disordered breathing*: Dysregulated breathing during sleep may require various therapies such as oxygen or ventilatory support.
- *Nocturnal epilepsies*: Evidence for drug treatment being effective is variable.

FOLLOW-UP

Families will often need intense support to modify a child's night-time behaviour, particularly where the parents' sleep has been disturbed for some time. Phone contact weekly and sometimes daily may be required to support parents through change.

HEALTH PROMOTION

Early postnatal education of families about childhood sleep and regulation may anticipate and prevent establishment of later long-term difficulties.

SOURCES

Ferber R (1985) Solve your child's sleeping problems. New York: Simon & Schuster

Ferber R, Kryger MH (eds) (1995) Principles and practice of sleep medicine in the child. Philadelphia: WB Saunders

National Sleep Foundation – www.sleepfoundation.org

Pearce J, Bidder J (1997) The new baby and toddler sleep program. London: Vermillion

Stores G (2001) A clinical guide to sleep disorders in children and adolescents. Cambridge: Cambridge University Press

Stores G, Wiggs L (eds) (2001) Sleep disorders in children and adolescents with disorders of development. Clinics in Developmental Medicine No 155. London: Mac Keith Press

25

AUTISTIC SPECTRUM DISORDERS

DEFINITION

Autistic spectrum disorder is the term used to describe a group of pervasive developmental disorders that are characterised by a 'triad of impairments', namely:

- impairment of social interaction
- impairment of communication
- impairment of thought and imagination, together with a rigid, repetitive pattern of behaviour.

These difficulties are best thought of as being on a spectrum, as there is enormous variability in the presentation, both between different children, and in the same child at different stages of development. Childhood Autism, Asperger's Syndrome and atypical autism are all considered part of the spectrum.

EPIDEMIOLOGY AND AETIOLOGY

Prevalence depends on definition and diagnostic criteria.

	Per 10,000
Traditionally quoted	4–5
Average prevalence from studies	
Before 2000	10
Recent studies	
Baird et al (2000) (children up to 7 years)	57.9
Chakrabarti & Fombonne (2001) (4–7 year olds)	62.6

Apparent increase clearly in part due to increased awareness, and widening of the concept of autistic spectrum disorders.
Commoner in males than in females. Occurs in all societies and across social classes.

AETIOLOGY

There is no single identified cause and, in most cases, it will be multi-factorial.

Factors that seem to play a part include the following:

- Environmental
- Pre- and perinatal problems more common
- Possible drugs in pregnancy (thalidomide, anticonvulsants)
- Congenital infection (e.g. rubella, cytomegalovirus)
- Encephalitis/meningitis
- Genetic
  - 60% concordance in monozygotic twins
  - 2–6% recurrence in siblings
  - Candidate genes on chromosomes 2, 7, 16, 17
  - Commoner in children with single gene disorders/chromosomal abnormalities.

Overall, a medical 'explanation' will be found in around 10% of cases.

PRESENTATION

Concerns about possible autistic spectrum disorder may arise at any age, but commonly in the second year of life with concerns about language delay or behaviour. In older children, difficulties may only become apparent as the demands for social interaction or communication become more sophisticated.

May present to health professionals because of parental concern, be picked up during development surveillance, or because of educational concerns.

ASSESSMENT

Assessment should be multidisciplinary, and may include paediatricians, psychologists, psychiatrists, speech and language therapists and education professionals.

Should include:

- medical and developmental history
- description of current functioning – get details from parents, other carers and professionals (e.g. teachers)
- medical examination
- developmental assessment (if possible – often difficult in this group of children!)
- observation in more than one setting, including with peers
- information from all involved professionals.

Recommendations including content and time scales can be found in NAPC 2003.

History
Medical
- Pregnancy – infections, bleeding, drugs
- Perinatal – birth trauma, asphyxia, neonatal seizures
- Infancy – significant illness, seizures, vision or hearing problems
- Current health – growth, diet, seizures, vision, hearing.

Developmental history
- Autism specific
- Standardised questionnaires such as the ADI or DISCO may be used by those specifically trained in their use.

Examination
Physical examination should be undertaken to look for possible associated medical or sensory problems, and may give clues to underlying diagnosis. This should include:

- height, weight and head circumference
- dysmorphic features as in fragile X or Williams' syndrome
- skin markings (include examination under Woods light) for signs of tuberous sclerosis or neurofibromatosis
- abdominal examination for organomegaly (metabolic disorders)
- genitalia – large testes may suggest fragile X
- eyes – check for squints, visual acuity, pigmentary retinopathy (congenital rubella)
- phakomas (TS), Lisch nodules (neurofibromatosis)
- ears – glue ear, hearing loss.

Neurological examination should include:

- 'soft signs' – associated movements, gait and clumsiness
- speech – intonation and pitch.

Diagnostic tests
These are outlined in Table 25.1.

DIFFERENTIAL DIAGNOSIS
Learning disability, Rett's syndrome, receptive language disorder, Landau–Kleffner syndrome, ADHD, developmental coordination disorders, sensory impairment may all be considered.

Must also take into account comorbidity, i.e. there is overlap between conditions and more than one diagnostic label may apply.

WHO TO TALK TO
Every stage of assessment and management should be multidisciplinary, and requires close consultation between the parents, health professionals and education staff.

Discuss family support with social services.

Table 25.1

Test	Description	Which children?
Vision and hearing	Formal assessment appropriate to age and ability	All children
Blood	Chromosomes	Dysmorphic features, severe disability
	Molecular genetics for fragile X	As above, significant language delay, family history
	Molecular genetics MECP2 gene (Rett's syndrome)	Regression, severe learning disability
	FBC, ferritin	Faddy diets, pica
	Lead	Pica
	TFT TORCH screen Calcium Amino acids	Significant learning disability, clinical pointers
	CPK	Boys with language delay, general developmental delay and delayed walking
Urine	Metabolic screen including amino acids, purine, pyrimidine, mucopolysaccharides	Severe learning disability, dysmorphism, history of encephalopathy
EEG		History of seizures, loss of previously acquired language, developmental regression or fluctuating symptoms
MRI scan		Neurological signs, evidence of specific diagnosis (e.g. tuberous sclerosis) or focal EEG abnormalities

WHEN TO REFER

Autistic spectrum disorders are common, so there should be a local multidisciplinary child development team capable of assessment in every area.

Referral to tertiary services should be reserved for complex cases, diagnostic uncertainty, second opinion or professional disagreement.

THERAPY

There is no specific treatment. Although various diets and drug treatments have been suggested, sometimes claiming to 'cure' core symptoms, there is no good evidence of efficacy of any specific treatment. Medication may be appropriate for specific symptoms or associated problems (e.g. hyperactivity).

Educational approaches including early intervention programmes are of proven benefit, though no specific programme is recommended.

FOLLOW-UP

Regular contact around the time of diagnosis and until the child's needs are being met.

Routine follow-up after this is often difficult and inappropriate because of the child's difficulties, and keeping in touch via multidisciplinary review meetings may be better.

Open access to advice is appreciated by parents, particularly as the nature of the child's problems may make accessing routine healthcare difficult.

HEALTH PROMOTION

Accessing healthcare is often difficult. May need special support to complete routine immunisation, access dental care, etc.

Health education (including sexual health) is a challenge and often best met by close liaison with experienced specialist education professionals.

SUPPORT ORGANISATIONS

Contact with voluntary sector and local parents support groups is often invaluable.

National Autistic Society
393 City Road
London EC1V 1NG
Tel: 0207 8332299
www.nas.org.uk

SOURCES

Baird G, Charman T, Baron-Cohen S, Cox A, Swettenham J, Wheelwright S, Drew A (2000) A screening instrument for autism at 18 months of age: a 6-year follow-up study. Journal of the American Academy of Child and Adolescent Psychiatry 39(6): 694–702

Chakrabarti S, Fombonne E (2001) Pervasive developmental disorders in preschool children JAMA 285(24): 3093–3099

Department for Education and Skills (2002) Autistic spectrum disorders: good practice guidance. Nottingham: DfES

National Autism Plan for Children (2003) Online. Available: www.cafamily.org.uk/NAPExec.pdf

26

BULLYING

DEFINITION

Bullying is an action by one or more persons against others that they know or ought to know will cause the victim hurt or distress. It can be verbal, emotional, physical, racist, sexual or homophobic.

EPIDEMIOLOGY AND AETIOLOGY

In 2003 ChildLine reported >20,000 children called about bullying, the most common problem. In this 2003 study, 51% of year 5 and 28% of year 8 children were bullied in the previous term.

Aetiology complex – factors in the bully, victim, families or both; peer group relationships, school policy, social acceptance, etc. Often no apparent reason for being bullied. Child may be both victim and bully.

PRESENTATION

Includes:

- physical symptoms such as unexplained headaches, abdominal pain, nausea and/or vomiting, particularly in the morning
- school refusal
- changes in mood, attitude, anxious and tearful or aggressive, stammering
- change in school performance
- belongings damaged, missing
- asking for money or stealing.

ASSESSMENT

Include in differential diagnosis for anxiety states, school refusal, depression and physical symptoms.

Other causes eliminated by full history and examination, and talking to child, parents and school.

> **ALERTS**
>
> ⚠ Risk of suicide.
> Many young people do not tell.
> May hide clues about how clothes torn/bruises/where money/
> belongings have gone.

WHO TO TALK TO

Child
Family
School
GP
School nurse
Governors
Education Welfare Officer

WHEN TO REFER

Consider mental health support for school refusal, continued depression, additional family stresses, self-harm or risk of suicide.

THERAPY

End bullying.
Counselling and support for child in/out of school.
Ask about anti-bullying policy in school.
Support parents and provide information, e.g. Kidscape, online anti-bullying information.

KEY POINTS FOR PARENTS

Bullying is not a natural part of growing up, and the children need their complaints taken seriously. Includes text messages and e-mail.

HEALTH PROMOTION

All schools need effective anti-bullying strategies and policies for promoting emotional health of all children.
Policies need to be revisited and children's views listened to. Lunchtime supervisors need training.
ChildLine for young people who cannot tell – 0800 1111.

ADDITIONAL POINTS

Anti-bullying policies will still not stop bullying.
Children carry the effects of bullying into their adult lives.

SOURCES

Department for Education and Skills (2004) Bullying – don't suffer in silence. Online. Available: www.dfes.gov.uk/bullying

Kidscape Anti-bullying Policy for Schools – www.kidscape.org.uk

See also

Chapter 19, School refusal; Chapter 20, Anxiety; Chapter 21, Depression and self-harm.

27

CHILDREN WHO BREAK THE LAW

3

LEGAL ISSUES

The age of criminal responsibility is 10 years. Three main pieces of legislation are relevant to children who break the law: Crime & Disorder Act 1998 – Orders & Schemes; Crime & Disorder Act 1998 – Youth Justice Provisions; and Youth Justice & Criminal Evidence Act 1999.

EPIDEMIOLOGY AND AETIOLOGY

Average age is 13.5 for boys and 14 for girls. Similar proportion of boys and girls until 14, then boys > girls until ratio is 3:1 at 17.

50% of children who break the law commit one or two minor offences; persistent offenders (10%) commit 50% of crimes. They are twice as likely to live in an inner city rather than a rural locality and deprivation is a factor (1998/99 Youth Lifestyles Survey).

Aetiology for persistent offenders is complex. Main risk factors include:

- drug use (in the last year)
- disaffected from school
- hangs around in public places
- delinquent friends
- poor parental supervision
- persistent truant (at least once a month).

Also relevant are low family income, poor housing, parental conflict, history of bullying. Most risk factors coincide and are interrelated.

Traumatic experiences are common (49%). This can have a significant impact on young people and may link to offending behaviour. Many experience symptoms of post-traumatic stress disorder (PTSD).

Some evidence that untreated ADHD may be a risk factor.

ASSESSMENT

Full medical history and examination are needed.
Immunisations, hospital appointments, etc. may have been missed.
Need to include physical and mental health and health promotion.

25–33% of young people in prison are likely to have a chronic physical complaint.

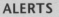

> **ALERTS**
> Mental health:
> - 9 in 10 young offenders aged between 16 and 20 years showed evidence of a mental health problem
> - 38% of young men on remand contemplated suicide
> - 40% of prisoners under 21 have been in care at some stage in their lives.

WHO TO TALK TO

Depends on stage:

- Child and Adolescent Mental Health Service (CAMHS) – for further assessment or consultation.
- Education – may be able to offer more support or adapt curriculum to suit needs.
- School nurse – for immunisation and health promotion.
- GP – for more complete picture.
- Youth Offending Team (YOT) – for many kinds of support to reduce risk of re-offending.
- Child's solicitor – with consent, to give information to present in court.
- Community paediatrician – for further assessment of health problems and links with school.
- Substance misuse team – if relevant.

THERAPY

For those at high risk of re-offending, this will depend on what needs have been identified in assessment, available resources, and trying to involve the young person and listening to their views.

There are effective treatments for trauma and PTSD symptoms.

YoungMinds stress the need for practical support and informal methods in community settings.

YOTs need to be responsible for monitoring young people with mental health problems. CAMHS may need to be available in the YOTs rather than outside them. Successful intervention requires reliability and continuity, as this repairs the child's negative attachment experiences. YOTs are in a better position to provide this and listen to the young person's experiences and view of what happens to them.

www.youngminds.org.uk

KEY POINTS FOR PARENTS

Know where your children are and who they are with. Spend time with them.

Parents may have limited personal resources and need support/help for themselves.

HEALTH PROMOTION

Include whatever is identified from the history.

If not at school, may have missed input on sexual health, drugs, dental health, etc.

Prevention

Strategies need to address specific risk factors mentioned and, where possible, to enhance known protective factors.

Action needed to promote healthy parental attachments to children, give support on parenting, and address social and community issues.

ADDITIONAL POINTS

Young people are more likely to be victims of crime.

Many think our courts, trials and sentencing procedures are not appropriate for children and treat them as adults too soon.

Children who break the law are not treated according to the same principles and philosophy that underpin wider children's law and policy.

The Children's Act applies to young people in prison (judgment late 2002). A greater proportion of young people are in prison in England and Wales compared to other European countries.

SOURCES

Campbell S, Harrington V (2000) Findings from the 1998/99 Youth Lifestyles Survey. Home Office Research Study 209. London: Home Office

See also

Chapter 21, Depression and self-harm; Chapter 22, Hyperactivity; Chapter 26, Bullying; Chapter 86, Children looked after; Chapter 89, Problems in deprived areas; Chapter 93, Special educational needs.

GROWTH AND NUTRITION

28

NUTRITIONAL ISSUES – 0–1 YEARS

DEFINITION

Key nutritional issues in this age group are:

1. *Preterm infants* (born <36 weeks' gestation) discharged into the community.
2. Nutritional management of infantile colic (for definition, see 'Presentation', below)
3. *Cow's milk protein hypersensitivity* (CMPH), which can be IgE or non-IgE mediated (see Chapter 37).

EPIDEMIOLOGY AND AETIOLOGY

1. See below.
2. *Infantile colic* affects 10–30% of babies aged 3–13 weeks, whether breast or formula fed. The aetiology is unclear, but is thought to be associated with painful gut contractions, lactose intolerance and/or gas.
3. In 2002, *CMPH* was reported to occur in 2–3% of infants, and 0.5% in breast-fed infants. For infants with a dual heredity of allergy, there is a 60–80% chance of inheriting atopic disease, and 30–50% chance with single heredity. If neither parent has allergies, a child's risk of atopy is 10–15%.

PRESENTATION

1. *Preterm infants* are often discharged into the community with body weights half that of the term infant, and a weight and height corrected for gestational age <2nd centile. They may have a history of poor feeding and/or poor weight gain or development.
2. *Infantile colic* is defined, based on its presentation, as inconsolable crying and limb flexure, lasting >3 hours a day, ≥3 days a week in otherwise healthy, thriving infants aged 1–3 months.
3. Symptoms of *CMPH* usually occur before 1 month of age, often within 1 week of starting a cow's milk containing formula. Symptoms include atopic dermatitis, GI symptoms (diarrhoea, bloody stools,

vomiting, abdominal distension, constipation), recurrent wheeze in infancy, and asthma and allergic rhinoconjunctivitis in later childhood. It has been estimated that 16–42% of infants with gastro-oesophageal reflux (GOR) have CMPH. Faltering growth is occasionally observed as a consequence of CMPH.

ASSESSMENT
History
1. For *preterm infants* obtain a detailed feeding history, including positioning for feeding, feeding environment and feeding times. Ascertain degree of possiting/vomiting and bowel habits. Ensure accurate plotting of growth charts using corrected age and check developmental stage.
2. *Infantile colic*: Determine whether there is an organic reason for the infant's symptoms. It may be associated with impaired parent–child bonding, and can occasionally contribute to faltering growth.
3. *CMPH*: A detailed feeding and clinical symptom history is required to establish a link between CMPH and symptoms, with particular focus on dermatological and GI symptoms and growth. Consider the role of other potential allergens, e.g. house dust mite, animals, washing powders, etc.

Examination
2. *Infantile colic*: Exclude any organic cause for the symptoms, e.g. intestinal obstruction, hernia, constipation, GOR, infection, etc.
3. *CMPH*: Exclude other causes of faltering growth, dermatological and GI disorders.

Diagnostic tests
2. *Infantile colic* may respond to a 24-hour trial with lactase preincubation of milk (or foremilk in breast-fed infants), e.g. Colief, or trial a lactose-free infant formula, e.g. SMA LF or Enfamil Lactofree. (Lactase drops are preferable to low lactose milks, as they maintain breast feeding, leave low levels of lactose in the feed to induce lactase activity and are cheaper; however, they are less easy to use.) If symptoms abate, colic is probably due to transient lactase deficiency.
   This is not yet established in routine practice, but may be helpful. Non-lactase responders could be given a trial on a hypoallergenic formula, e.g. Nutramigen, before determining that food intolerance is not the cause of colic (Prodigy Guidance 2004).
3. *CMPH* can only be diagnosed by skin tests and RAST tests if IgE mediated, with greater false-negative results seen in infants and very small children. The best form of diagnosis is to remove the suspected allergen, i.e. cow's milk infant formula or cow's milk products in breast-feeding mothers, and to monitor symptoms over a period of up to 3–4 weeks. If symptoms resolve, assume CMPH.

WHO TO TALK TO AND WHEN TO REFER

1. *Preterm infants* may still be under the care of a hospital paediatrician and in some cases a hospital paediatric dietitian. If there is no hospital involvement, and there are concerns about growth or adequacy of nutritional intake, refer to a community paediatric dietitian or local paediatrician (see Chapter 30).
2. *Infantile colic* is usually managed in the community by GPs, health visitors or a community dietitian, particularly if transient lactase deficiency is being considered. Refer to a specialist paediatrician or gastroenterologist for further evaluation of aetiology if symptoms are severe, and not settling.
3. Simple *CMPH* can be managed in the community by GPs, health visitors and community dietitians. Referral to allergy clinics or hospital paediatricians/dietitians is recommended if the infant continues to suffer from unresolving GI symptoms, severe dermatitis and/or faltering growth. Rechallenging of CMPH may be necessary in hospital if there is a risk of anaphylaxis.

THERAPY

1. Although demand breast feeding is preferred for *preterm infants,* nutrient-enriched post-discharge formulas are available on prescription until 6 months' corrected age (e.g. Nutriprem 2 or Premcare) to promote catch-up. These can be continued to 12–18 months of age or changed to standard or follow-on infant formula. Multivitamin supplements containing vitamin D (e.g. Department of Health Welfare vitamin drops) should be given to breast-fed infants or those taking less than 500 ml of a standard infant formula, until 1–5 years of age, as recommended for all term children. Iron supplementation is required for breast-fed premature infants and those with a limited dietary intake (1 ml of Sytron provides 5.5 mg elemental iron).
   A premature baby should be weaned between 4 and 7 months' uncorrected age.
2. In *infantile colic,* lactase responders (see 'Diagnostic tests', above) should continue lactase treatment until 3 months and then reduce the dose over 1 week to ensure that treatment has not masked permanent lactose intolerance. Non-lactase responders whose colic settles on a hypoallergenic formula should remain on this until weaning. Management should include supporting the parents with encouragement and practical advice. Dimeticone is one of the most commonly used treatments for colic, but there is little evidence to support its use.
3. Once *CMPH* is assumed, a hypoallergenic formula, e.g. Nutramigen, should be used for all children under 6 months of age. Soya formulae are no longer recommended for this age group, due to the presence of phytoestrogens and cross-reactivity risk of soya with cow's milk

protein. Nutramigen should be introduced gradually over 1 week to promote compliance, due to its unpleasant taste and smell, and continued until 1 year of age. Weaning foods should be cow's milk protein free, and detailed dietary information will be required to ensure that the diet remains nutritionally adequate.

FOLLOW-UP

1. *Preterm infants* should be reviewed regularly by either a hospital or community paediatrician until normal growth and development are assured. A paediatric dietitian, once involved, will regularly review the progress of a preterm infant until satisfied that their nutritional intake is sufficient to sustain growth and nutritional status.
2. For *infantile colic*, once treatment is established, review by a health professional is necessary to ensure the family has returned to a normal infant formula and an appropriate feeding regime before discharge.
3. For *CMPH*, a trial of cow's milk free formula should be assessed within 1 month by the health professional involved and, if established on Nutramigen with all symptoms resolved, discuss rechallenging of cow's milk products at 1 year of age. If symptoms persist, regular medical review will be necessary. Other than with the risk of anaphylaxis, rechallenging can be done at home, using a stepwise process as agreed by the dietitian or other health professional. Families should be advised to rechallenge on a 6-monthly basis until 3 years of age, then yearly until 5 years. Expected remission rates are 45–50% at 1 year, 60–75% at 2 years and 85–90% by 3 years of age.

KEY POINTS FOR PARENTS

1. BLISS, the premature baby charity, provides a parent support helpline and a range of useful resources, including the leaflet 'Weaning your premature baby', usually provided by neonatal staff.
2. For *infantile colic*, ensure that feeding times are as relaxed as possible and avoid force feeding. Try to have a few hours' break by leaving the infant with a relative.
3. *CMPH*: Avoidance of all traces of cow's milk protein is not straightforward, and parents should be provided with a suitable cow's milk free diet sheet, usually produced by dietitians.

SOURCES

Host A, Koletzko B, Dreborg S et al (1999) Dietary products used in infants for treatment and prevention of food allergy. Archives of Disease in Childhood 81: 80–84

King C (2001) Preterm infants. In: Shaw V, Lawson M (eds) Clinical paediatric dietetics. Oxford: Blackwell Science

Prodigy Guidance (2004) Colic – infantile. Online. Available: www.prodigy.nhs.uk/guidance.asp?gt=Colic%20—%20infantile

See also
Chapter 30, Poor weight gain – weight and growth faltering in young children; Chapter 37, Allergy.

NUTRITIONAL ISSUES – PRESCHOOL YEARS AND OLDER CHILDREN

PRESCHOOL YEARS

DEFINITION

Key nutritional issues in these age groups are:

1. *iron deficiency* – inadequate iron stores as a result of suboptimal dietary iron intake
2. *rickets* – failure to mineralise new bone tissue (osteoid) due to lack of vitamin D (from diet and sunlight) and calcium (see also 'faddy eating', Chapter 14).

EPIDEMIOLOGY AND AETIOLOGY

1. *Iron deficiency* is the most commonly reported nutritional disorder in the UK. The National Diet and Nutrition Survey (1995) revealed that 84% of 1–4 year olds had dietary iron intakes < reference nutrient intake (RNI, an amount sufficient for 97.5% of the population) and 16–24% had intakes < lower reference nutrient intake (LRNI) (meeting only 2.5% of the population's requirements). 1 in 12 of all children and 1 in 8 of 1–2 year olds were anaemic. This tends to be higher in inner city populations.
2. The prevalence of *rickets* was estimated to be 1.6% in non-Caucasian children in Manchester during 2002, equivalent to 60 children. Reported increases in rickets are associated with promotion of exclusive breast feeding for long periods without vitamin D supplementation, reduced vitamin D production in the skin due to use of sun creams, clothing, reduction in outdoor activities, and increase of immigrant groups in temperate regions.

PRESENTATION

1. *Iron deficiency*, as well as causing anaemia, may lead to pica, tiredness, apathy, impaired exercise capacity, possible increased risk of infection and reduced educational achievement.

2. *Rickets*: Frontal bossing in early infancy, delayed closure of fontanelle, enlarged wrists (specificity 81%), rickety rosary (specificity 64%), skeletal deformities (particularly 'bow legs' once walking), delayed eruption of teeth (deciduous incisors not present by 9 months of age and first molars by 14 months). Vitamin D deficiency can also affect intrauterine and infant growth, cause proximal myopathy and symptomatic hypocalcaemia with convulsions (particularly in infants <6 months).

ASSESSMENT
History and examination
1. Faddy eating is often associated with iron deficiency. This can initially be assessed from a diet history focussing on haem and non-haem sources of iron accompanied by vitamin C-rich foods or drinks (Box 29.1). Tea and coffee inhibit iron absorption. Check for pica, exercise capacity, degree of tiredness, progress at nursery and general reported health.
2. *Rickets*: Look for signs of rickets in osseous tissues as described in 'Presentation', above. Weight and height should be measured and compared to norms on centile charts. Determine regular level of exposure to sunlight, past and present intake of vitamin D-fortified

4

BOX 29.1 Sources of iron and vitamin C

Good sources of iron
- Haem iron:
  - red meat, e.g. beef, lamb, pork, corned beef, minced meat dishes such as spaghetti Bolognese, cottage pie, meatballs
  - offal, e.g. liver, kidney
  - eggs (yolks)
  - fish, especially sardines, pilchards, tuna, salmon, mackerel
- Non-haem iron:
  - fortified breakfast cereals (check that iron has been added)
  - bread, pitta bread, chapatti and other products made from flour
  - pulses, e.g. lentils, peas and beans (including baked beans)
  - nuts and seeds, e.g. peanut butter, hummus

Good sources of vitamin C
- Citrus fruits, e.g. oranges, fresh orange juice, grapefruit
- Blackcurrants and blackcurrant squash
- Mangoes and other fruits
- Vegetables, especially if still crunchy
- Potatoes
- Tomatoes

foods (infant formula, weaning foods, breakfast cereals, margarines), oily fish, vitamin D-containing supplement and adequacy of calcium intake (portions of dairy products: ⅓ pint milk is equivalant to 1 pot yoghurt or matchbox piece of cheese).

Diagnostic tests

1. *Iron deficiency* can be diagnosed from haematology tests: low MCV, MCH and serum ferritin concentrations suggest iron deficiency. The WHO classification for anaemia is a haemoglobin concentration <11 g/dl for children aged 6 months to 6 years. Many health centres have access to haemacue monitoring, providing an instant Hb result from a blood spot.
2. Clinical diagnosis of *rickets* is unreliable and should be confirmed with a wrist x-ray. Cupping, splaying and fraying of the metaphysis in the ulna and radius are classic findings. Blood tests will highlight raised parathyroid hormone and alkaline phosphatase concentrations and low calcidiol (25-hydroxycholecalciferol) concentrations.

DIFFERENTIAL DIAGNOSIS

1. For *iron-deficiency* anaemia, exclude any serious underlying cause of anaemia (e.g. gastric bleeding).
2. In *rickets*, exclude physiological bowing, vitamin D-resistant rickets and renal rickets.

WHO TO TALK TO AND WHEN TO REFER

1. Simple *iron deficiency* is often associated with faddy eating (see Chapter 14). It should not require further referral.
2. Rickets requires evaluation by a paediatrician.

THERAPY

1. Subclinical *iron deficiency* can usually be treated by increasing intake of iron-rich foods (see 'Assessment', above). If unable to make a substantial change, recommend a micronutrient supplement containing a prophylactic dose of iron (i.e. 5–12 mg elemental iron). For iron-deficiency anaemia, prescribe a 3-month course of an iron-based syrup, usually 2.5 ml three times a day for children 1–5 years of age, providing 40 mg elemental iron daily. Repeat blood test and, if still uncorrected, continue with another 3-month course. Establish compliance with medication and reported side effects. Ensure an adequate dietary iron intake and address faddy eating if appropriate.
2. *Rickets*: 150 µg (6000 IU) ergocalciferol daily for 2–4 months until lesions are corrected and stores replenished, followed by a prophylactic dose of 5–10 µg/day (present in many vitamin supplements, including vitamin drops). Continue until pubertal

growth has been completed. Ensure an adequate calcium intake, providing 400–600 mg calcium daily (equivalent to ⅔ to 1 pint milk or equivalent – see 'Assessment', above).

FOLLOW-UP

1. Review children with *iron deficiency* after 3 months of treatment and discharge once corrected.
2. Discharge children with *rickets* once lesions have healed and normal growth ensured.

KEY POINTS FOR PARENTS

1. *Iron deficiency*: Most community dietetic departments have dietary information regarding iron-rich foods, which should be available for use by a range of health professionals for families.
2. *Rickets*: There should be similar information available for families regarding calcium- and vitamin D-rich foods.

SOURCES

Wardley BL, Puntis JWL, Taitz LS (eds) (1997) The preschool child. In: Handbook of child nutrition, 2nd edn. Oxford: Oxford University Press, pp 54–72
Wharton B, Bishop N (2003) Rickets. Lancet 362: 1389–1400

OLDER CHILDREN

DEFINITION

This section covers:

1. *lacto-ovo-vegetarianism* (no meat or fish, but milk and eggs are consumed) and *vegan* (no animal products whatsoever)
2. nutritional intervention in *hyperactivity*, a lasting pattern of inattentive and chaotic overactivity. This includes attention deficit hyperactivity disorder (ADHD), characterised by three core symptoms: inattention, hyperactivity and impulsivity (see Chapter 22).
3. nutritional intervention in *autism*. The *autistic spectrum* describes a wide clinical range of disorders associated with a life-long triad of impairments in social interaction, communication and behaviour (see Chapter 25).

EPIDEMIOLOGY AND AETIOLOGY

1. From the National Diet and Nutrition Survey, 4–18 year olds (2000), 10% of 15–18 year old girls and 1% of boys claimed to be *vegetarian* or *vegan*. People follow a vegetarian diet for a number of reasons, including ethical and ecological concerns, beliefs in health-promoting

properties and peer pressure. Young females are particularly influenced by body image-related issues.

2. Approximately 1% of school-age children meet the diagnostic criteria for *hyperkinetic disorder* (see Chapter 22). Dietary factors are not thought to be causal, although there is a belief that food triggers can exacerbate symptoms.

3. No clear aetiology has been established in *autism*, but some researchers believe diet may be an important factor.

PRESENTATION

1. Poorly managed *vegetarian* and *vegan* diets may result in children presenting with iron deficiency anaemia and possible rickets in non-Caucasian adolescents undergoing puberty (see Preschool section, above). The growth of vegan children may be impaired due to a poor dietary energy and protein intake, whereas the lack of dietary vitamins B_6 or B_{12} rarely presents with the symptoms of peripheral neuropathy and microcytic hypochromic anaemia in B_6 and megaloblastic anaemia and/or neuropathy (subacute combined degeneration) in B_{12}.

2. *Hyperactivity*: Parents may request advice on excluding certain foods from the diet.

3. *Autistic* children may present with dietary problems as part of their overall difficulties, e.g. difficulty with transition to textures, increased oral sensitivity, difficulty in accepting new foods, restricted intakes due to colour, texture, packaging, food temperature, decreased selection of food over time and difficulty with changes in mealtime environment.

ASSESSMENT

History and examination

1. The National Diet and Nutrition Survey (2000) reported that 45% of 11–14 year old and 50% of 15–18 year old females had iron intakes below the LRNI (meeting only 2.5% of the population's requirements). Zinc intakes were also low, being commonly associated with the same foods. Calcium intakes were also suboptimal, with approximately 20% of 11–18 year olds having intakes < LRNI. *Vegetarians/vegans* are at greater risk of deficiencies of all the above nutrients, especially vegans in relation to calcium and vitamins B_6 and B_{12}. A detailed diet history focusing on the dairy and meat alternative food groups is essential to highlight areas of potential deficiency (see Preschool section, above, for iron and calcium). Weight and height should be plotted on centile charts. Serum levels for vitamin D (25-hydroxycholecalciferol), B_6 (plasma pyridoxal phosphate and erythrocyte transaminase activation coefficient) and B_{12} (radiometric assay), ferritin and haemoglobin should be measured where concerns are raised.

2. *Hyperactivity*: As part of the multidisciplinary assessment of hyperactivity, explore any apparent triggers for certain behaviours.
3. *Autism*: As part of overall assessment, measure weight and height and plot on centile charts. Obtain a diet and feeding history to review whether there is a range of foods from all food groups present to ensure nutritional adequacy.

WHO TO TALK TO AND WHEN TO REFER

1. If concerned about the nutritional adequacy of a *vegetarian/vegan* diet, a dietitian can conduct a computer-based nutrient analysis from a detailed food diary or assess the adequacy from dietary recall.
2. Management of *hyperactivity* requires a multiprofessional approach. A dietitian can ensure the child has an adequate nutritional intake and explore potential food triggers.
3. Nutritional issues in *autism* may require referral to a dietitian, especially in children eating fewer than 20 different foods and those <5 years of age, to ensure that restricted dietary intakes are nutritionally adequate, and for providing information on elimination of certain foods/nutrients from the diet if requested.

THERAPY

1. Any identified nutritional deficiencies in *vegetarian/vegan* children should be corrected by either improving the balance of foods in the diet or, if not possible, recommend a suitable micronutrient supplement (see Preschool section, above, for iron and vitamin D). An iron supplement containing 60 mg elemental iron once or twice daily will be required for older children with iron deficiency anaemia. Older children should consume 700 mg calcium per day, equivalent to 1 pint of cow's milk. For good sources of vitamin B_6 and vitamin B_{12}, see Box 29.2.

   As there are few non-animal sources of vitamin B_{12}, vegans should take a supplement containing approximately 1 µg vitamin B_{12}.
2. A multiprofessional approach is usually required for management of *hyperactivity*, If parents feel there is an exacerbation of hyperactive behaviour following consumption of certain foods, it is reasonable to try to exclude them one at a time. The Feingold diet involves avoidance of artificial colours (azo dyes) and certain preservatives, particularly benzoates, sulphites and nitrites.

   Parents commonly report worsening behaviour following sugary drinks and certain sweets, which could be attributed to the above ingredients, although this has not yet been confirmed in clinical studies. Nevertheless, adoption of such a diet can only improve overall dietary intake, as it restricts use of many squashes and fizzy drinks, sweets and highly processed foods.

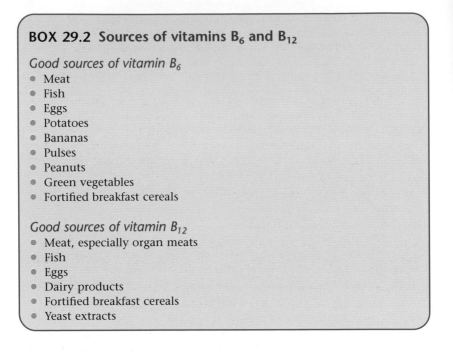

BOX 29.2 Sources of vitamins B$_6$ and B$_{12}$

Good sources of vitamin B$_6$
- Meat
- Fish
- Eggs
- Potatoes
- Bananas
- Pulses
- Peanuts
- Green vegetables
- Fortified breakfast cereals

Good sources of vitamin B$_{12}$
- Meat, especially organ meats
- Fish
- Eggs
- Dairy products
- Fortified breakfast cereals
- Yeast extracts

Recent work has focused on the benefits of micronutrient and omega 3 fish oil supplementation as a means of improving behaviour and attention span. Anecdotal reports have shown a benefit in some cases, but there are few published studies available as yet. Use a complete micronutrient supplement such as Junior Forceval capsules, which are prescribable, or adult chewable Centrum. Omega 3 fish oils are recommended in a dose providing approximately 500 mg eicosapentanoic acid (EPA) for the first month, reducing to 150–200 mg thereafter, e.g. Eye Q, Boots Omega 3 or Haliborange high DHA.

3. *Autism*: A number of children with restrictive behaviours will have restricted diets, and some will eat only a very small number of foods. A computer analysed dietary assessment by a dietitian can be helpful in defining any nutritional deficiencies. Ensure the eating environment is appropriate for the individual, such as fixed mealtimes in the same place/situation, use/avoidance of distractions, absence or company of other family/friends. Attempts should be made to broaden the variety of already accepted foods, e.g. different types of bread.

Many parents are aware of 'The Sunderland Protocol' by Shattock and Whiteley (2000), which recommends removal of casein for 3–4 weeks, followed by a gluten-free diet for 3–6 months. Gluten- and/or casein-free products are not available under ACBS for this condition as there is no good research evidence to support this. Some doctors will take the pragmatic view that if parents wish to exclude casein and gluten they should be supported in doing this safely.

FOLLOW-UP

1. Once correction has been made of any nutrient deficiencies observed in *vegetarian/vegan* children, follow-up is not necessary.
2. Children with *hyperactivity* will have follow-up into adolescence.
3. The majority of children with *autism* will remain under the care of a paediatrician and multidisciplinary team throughout their childhood. Their dietary intake may need to be reviewed at intervals to ensure that the diet continues to be nutritionally adequate.

SUPPORT ORGANISATIONS

1. *Vegetarian/vegan*: The Vegetarian Society (www.vegsoc.org) is a reliable source of information. Dietetic departments should be able to provide some basic dietary information for families.
2. *Hyperactivity*: – the British Hyperactive Children's Support Group (www.hacsg.org.uk) is a registered charity. www.addiss.co.uk has useful general information on ADHD.

   The hyperactive child: a parent's guide by Dr Eric Taylor is a useful reference book. Dietary information on avoidance of artificial colours and preservatives may be available from some dietetic departments.
3. *Autism*: The National Autistic Society (www.nas.org.uk) is a useful site for families and professionals alike. Dietary information regarding gluten- and/or casein-free diets can be obtained from dietetic departments.

SOURCES

Department of Health (1995) National diet and nutrition survey. London: DH
Department of Health (2000) National diet and nutrition survey. London: DH
Shattock P, Whiteley P (2000) The Sunderland Protocol: a logical sequencing of biomedical interventions for the treatment of autism and related disorders. Online. Available: http://osiris.sunderland.ac.uk/autism/durham2.htm
Taylor E (1985) The hyperactive child: a parent's guide (positive health guide). London: Martin Dunitz

See also

Chapter 14, Eating problems – young children; Chapter 22, Hyperactivity; Chapter 25, Autistic spectrum disorders.

POOR WEIGHT GAIN – WEIGHT AND GROWTH FALTERING IN YOUNG CHILDREN

DEFINITIONS

- *Weight faltering* – weight falling through centile spaces, low weight for height or no catch-up from a low birth weight (LBW).
- *Growth faltering* – crossing down through length/height centile(s) as well as weight. A low height centile or a height less than expected from parental heights.

Assessment by the primary health care team should be made if:

- a weight or height below the 0.4th centile is noted for the first time
- there is a sustained fall through two centile spaces, for weight and/or height
- weight or height is below the 2nd centile, or below the target centile range.

Infants commonly show some weight faltering in the first 2 years, but it may also affect older children.

EPIDEMIOLOGY AND AETIOLOGY

Faltering growth occurs in 2–5% of children, and is readily resolvable in the majority.

It occurs in all socioeconomic groups and cultures. Children with disabilities are also affected.

Babies of LBW should show catch-up growth in the first 3–6 months of life, and need a high nutrient intake to do so.

Aetiology

The early years are a time of nutritional vulnerability due to young children's rapid growth and high nutrient requirements.

Faltering weight and/or growth is usually caused by inadequate energy intake, in association with a number of factors:

- Inadequacy of the content or frequency of meals.
- Interactional difficulties between parents or carers and children.

- Poor inherent feeding drive.
- Oral motor dysfunction.
- Developmental difficulties.
- Illness (although it is rare for serious illness to present with weight and/or growth faltering alone).
- Abuse and/or neglect.

PRESENTATION

Growth surveillance (Health for all Children).
Opportunistic measurement.
Parental concern.

ASSESSMENT (see Fig. 30.1)

Initial assessment by the family health visitor, ideally at a home visit at meal/feed time to allow observation.

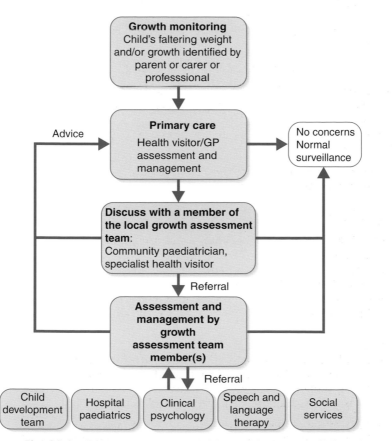

Fig. 30.1 Response to young children's faltering weight/growth.

Information should be collected on:

- feeding and symptom history since birth
- growth history since birth
- details of mealtime routines, including observation of food preparation and mealtime interactions.

Interaction between parents and child, with description of any behavioural problems (see Chapter 14), recording of family's concerns/anxieties.

A food diary should be obtained outlining both food/drinks offered and taken, and times offered.

The health visitor will identify areas where there is potential for change, and offer advice and ongoing support (e.g. strategies to address faddy eating, excess drinking, poor parent–child interaction, lack of knowledge or skills on good nutrition or stressful social situations). Progress should be monitored by periodic weighing (1–3 monthly) and assessment of family functioning. Height/length should be measured 6 monthly.

The paediatrician should assess for a medical cause for poor growth, provide expertise in interpretation of the growth pattern, assess development, and provide diet and behavioural advice with the health visitor and dietitian.

The community paediatric dietitian should establish food attitudes, value systems and beliefs, explore drinking habits, prolonged use of the bottle, advise on appropriate structured mealtimes, snacks and drinks, increase nutrient density of meals, identify any micronutrient deficiencies, and consider use of supplements only if there is no improvement in growth.

Examination

Height, weight, head circumference.

Assessment for syndromatic features, or disproportion.

Developmental assessment.

General review for systemic or endocrine disease.

Diagnostic tests

FBC and ferritin.

Others if suggested by history or examination – U&E, Cr, Ca, P, LFT, TFT, coeliac screen.

ALERTS

Child may need hospital-based investigation if unwell, or of exceptional low weight.

Extreme height faltering suggesting an endocrine cause.

Very low birth weight (VLBW) babies with poor growth may require assessment for growth hormone treatment.

WHO TO TALK TO

Paediatrician with interest in growth problems.

WHEN TO REFER

Referral for further assessment, ideally to a community-based growth team (paediatrician/dietitian/specialist health visitor) should be made if there is continuing cause for concern.

For children with more complex needs, referrals may be made to other professionals, including:

- speech and language therapist for assessment and management of feeding problems
- clinical psychologist for further assessment of psychological factors and family processes
- the child development team if the child has a neurodevelopmental condition
- social services (child protection concerns/assessment of need)
- hospital paediatrician (see 'Alerts', above).

FOLLOW-UP

Growth measurements – weighing 1–3 monthly, height 6 monthly.

5% thrive lines may be a useful adjunct for interpreting weight gain in infants, and identify the slowest growing 5% of infants (Wright et al 1998).

KEY POINTS FOR PARENTS

Growth faltering is highly stressful for parents and the child.

Normal patterns require reassurance, growth faltering timely and effective interventions.

HEALTH PROMOTION

Height and weight review at childhood health episodes.

Documentation in the parent-held record.

Need for high energy intake in the first 3–6 months for catch-up growth in LBW babies.

ADDITIONAL POINTS

Importance of accurate measurement and good equipment, including reliable scales that are checked and calibrated regularly.

Measurements should be plotted accurately on UK 1990 nine-centile standard cross-sectional growth charts.

SOURCES

Didcock E, Waddell L 2004 The Nottingham Integrated Care Pathway for the management of weight and growth faltering in young children.

Health for All Children – http://shop.healthforallchildren.co.uk/pro.epl
Paediatric Information and Education Resource. Recommendations for best practice for weight and growth faltering in young children. Online. Available: http://pier.shef.ac.uk/home.htm
The Children's Society – www.the-childrens-society.org.uk
Wright C, Avery A, Epstein M, Burks E, Croft D (1998) New chart to evaluate weight faltering. Archives of Disease in Childhood 78: 40–43

See also

Chapter 14, Eating problems – young children; Chapter 32, Short stature and abnormal growth.

EXCESSIVE WEIGHT GAIN

DEFINITION

Body mass index [BMI: weight (kg)/height (m^2)] should be calculated and compared with BMI for age centile charts to identify childhood overweight and obesity (see 'Sources', below). Obese children have a BMI >98th centile, and overweight children have a BMI >91st centile of the UK 1990 reference charts for age and sex.

EPIDEMIOLOGY AND AETIOLOGY

Analyses of the Health Survey for England (2002) suggested that 6% of schoolchildren were obese, and a further 18% were overweight. On this basis some 1.8 million children in the UK are overweight with a further 700,000 obese. Between 1996 and 2001 the proportion of overweight children aged 6–15 years increased by 7%.

Aetiology

Obesity is an imbalance between energy consumption and energy expenditure. For the majority, obesity is simply due to a greater intake of high energy foods and a reduction in physical activity (simple obesity).

The rise in obesity in children is likely to be related to increases in snack consumption, soft drinks, energy-dense ready meals, fewer home-cooked family meals, larger portion sizes, less physical activity and increases in sedentary behaviours, e.g. television viewing and use of computers.

There is also a wider societal and political context to these changes, with loss of school playing fields and a lack of safe environments for walking, cycling and play near home.

The food industry targets children with advertisements for high energy foods.

Obesity/overweight is more common in lower socioeconomic groups.

Uncommonly, there is a medical cause for obesity, e.g. Down's syndrome, Prader–Willi syndrome or endocrine disorders. Some children are at special risk, e.g. physical disability.

PRESENTATION

Growth surveillance (*Health for All Children*; see 'Sources', below).
Opportunistic measurement.
Parental concern.
Weight crosses centiles upwards, and exceeds height centile by at least two centiles. Child appears clinically overweight, although may otherwise be well.
Children may present with medical or psychological consequences of obesity, e.g. developing/exacerbation of asthma, sleep apnoea, cardiovascular risks such as raised blood pressure and hyperlipidaemia, diabetes, benign intracranial hypertension, orthopaedic disorders or psychological problems.

ASSESSMENT

History

Full dietary history, levels of physical activity, lifestyle, family/social issues (including parental eating patterns/obesity).
Early history of poor feeding/growth, developmental delay/low tone with current insatiable appetite suggestive of Prader–Willi syndrome.
Poor growth in height suggestive of endocrine disease.
Drug history.
Ask about possible psychological consequences of obesity.

Examination

Weight, height, BMI (waist circumference not useful in diagnosis).
General review for signs of endocrine disease (hypothyroidism/panhypopituitarism/GH deficiency) if *short and obese*
Pubertal stage.
Development.
Fundi/visual fields.
Blood pressure.
Medical consequences of obesity.

DIFFERENTIAL DIAGNOSIS

Simple obesity.
Endocrine (GH deficiency, pituitary dysfunction, hypothyroidism, Cushing's disease)
Genetic, e.g. Prader–Willi syndrome.
Drugs – OCP, steroids, sodium valproate, risperidone.

WHO TO TALK TO

For 'simple obesity', liaise with health visitor, school nurse or community dietitian.
Refer into local community programmes, e.g. the Nottingham 'Go 4 It' physical activity sessions in leisure centres, the 'MEND' (mind, exercise,

nutrition and diet) programme targeted at families with obese children in London, or 'Drop in Weight Clinics' run by the APPLES team in Leeds.

WHEN TO REFER

Children should be referred to a community or hospital paediatrician if:

- BMI >99th centile (higher risk of morbidity)
- <2 years, >99th centile for BMI
- exhibiting obesity-related morbidity
- there is a suspected underlying medical cause (rare).

THERAPY

Only consider if BMI >98th centile *and* child and family are receptive. In most obese children with no comorbidity, weight maintenance is an acceptable goal. For obese children >7 years under secondary care services, a modest weight loss (≤0.5 kg/month) is acceptable. Adopt a whole family approach, and address a combination of:

- reduction in energy intake via a healthier diet
- increase in habitual physical activity (e.g. brisk walking/active play) to a minimum of 30 minutes/day (60 minutes/day in healthy children)
- reduction in sedentary behaviour (watching television and playing computer games) to <2 hours per day or <14 hours per week.

FOLLOW-UP

If there is no underlying medical cause, patients should be referred back to primary care.

Regular support in the community is essential to facilitate families in making lifestyle changes, but ongoing review of simple obesity solely by paediatricians is often unsuccessful.

Include use of BMI and waist circumference centiles for age and sex to monitor progress and provide feedback.

KEY POINTS FOR PARENTS

Family-centred approach. Link up with other families to share activities/ outings etc.

Avoid having energy dense snacks in the house and adopt regular meals to avoid constant snacking.

Avoid undue focus on food.

HEALTH PROMOTION

More effective to target young children and the WHO recommend taking a life course approach, i.e. starting with prenatal nutrition.

At primary care level, provide information on healthy eating and physical activity to all members of the family and support effective parenting skills.

Whole school approaches should support adoption of healthy diets and physical activity, e.g. National Healthy Schools Programme and the Scottish Hungry for Success strategy, based on the successful Fuel Zone programme in Glasgow.

SOURCES

Cole TJ, Freeman JV, Preece MA (1995) Body mass index reference curves for the UK, 1990. Archives of Disease in Childhood 73: 25–29

Gibson P, Edmunds L, Haslam D et al (2002) An approach to weight management in children and adolescents (2–18 years) in primary care. Royal College of Paediatrics and Child Health, National Obesity Forum. Online. Available: www.rcpch.ac.uk and www.nationalobesityforum.org.uk

Hall DMB, Elliman D (eds) (2003) Growth monitoring and nutrition. In: Health for all children, 4th edn. Oxford: Oxford University Press, pp. 169–196

Scottish Intercollegiate Guidelines Network (2003) Management of obesity in children and young people – a national clinical guideline, no. 69. Online. Available: www.sign.ac.uk/pdf/sign69.pdf

Sproston K, Primatesta P (eds) (2003) Health Survey for England 2002. Volume 1: The health of children and young people. London: The Stationery Office

SHORT STATURE AND SUBNORMAL GROWTH

DEFINITION

1. Height less than 0.4th centile (using UK 1990 nine-centile growth charts).
2. Height less than target centile range (TCR) predicted from mid-parental heights adjusted for sex. For males add 7 cm to the mean of the parental heights and in females subtract 7 cm from the mean of the parental heights. TCR = adjusted mean ± 10 cm.
3. Subnormal growth rate – less than 4 cm/year or loss of more than one centile band (0.67 SD) for prepubertal child.
4. A combination of (1) and (2) gives acceptable sensitivity and specificity. The routine use of (3) demands greater resource and adds potential delay before specialist referral.
5. Disproportionate growth identifies skeletal dysplasia.

EPIDEMIOLOGY AND AETIOLOGY

This covers a wide range of conditions.

Common
- Familial short stature
- Familial growth delay
- Small for gestational age (SGA) infants who have persistent small stature (approximately 8% fail to catch up)

Less common
- *Syndromatic*: Typically short with abnormal features, e.g. Turner's syndrome (TS), 1 in 2500 females; Noonan's syndrome (NS), 1 in 1000–1250 births.
- *Systemic*: Typically short and thin, e.g. coeliac disease, chronic inflammatory bowel disease.
- *Endocrine*: Typically short and fat, e.g. growth hormone (GH) deficiency, 1 in 3500 births; panhypopituitarism; hypothyroidism.
- *Skeletal*: Typically short with limb–trunk disproportion, e.g. achondroplasia, hypochondroplasia.

PRESENTATION

Growth surveillance

The frequency of growth measurement remains a controversial topic: on the one hand, a single measurement at school entry best satisfies criteria for health screening; on the other, early childhood diagnosis based on measurements between 18 months and 5 years of age allows earlier and more effective intervention in GH deficiency and TS.

Opportunistic measurement at coincidental visits or health episodes as guided by parental concern.

ASSESSMENT

History

Pregnancy and birth history – intrauterine growth failure.

Growth chart review – early or late childhood growth deviation but 2% of normal children cross one centile band or more.

Parental heights (check that short parent does not have a growth disorder).

Familial pubertal pattern as a marker of genetic growth delay.

Environmental factors – diet or inappropriate eating behaviour, emotional status, neglect.

Key symptoms – headaches or visual defects suggestive of pituitary area tumours.

Examination

Accurate height measurement (Fig. 32.1).

Assessment for syndromatic features, or disproportion.

Weight and BMI.

Pubertal staging and testicular size (orchidometer) (see Ch. 35).

General review for signs of systemic or endocrine disease (Fig. 32.2).

Fundoscopy and visual field assessment.

Review growth chart and/or plan repeat measurements at 6-month intervals (growth monitoring).

Diagnostic tests

None required if familial short stature is confirmed.

FBC, E&U, Cr, Ca, Pi, LFT, TFT, coeliac screen.

Karyotype for girls with otherwise unexplained short stature (suspect TS).

Left hand bone age.

Dynamic GH tests reserved for use by specialist endocrine service.

DIFFERENTIAL DIAGNOSIS

Innocent growth patterns amenable to explanation, e.g. familial short ± delay.

Chronic disorders, e.g. GH deficiency and TS.

Short obese children are more likely to have an endocrine basis.

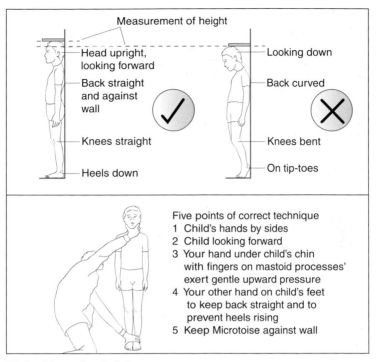

Fig. 32.1   Measuring height

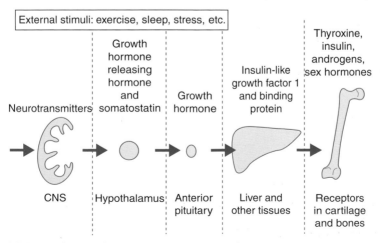

Fig. 32.2   Endocrine factors influencing growth.

> **ALERTS**
>
> ⚠ Signs of visual impairment or raised intracranial pressure needing
>   urgent cranial imaging.
>   Short girls with recurrent ENT problems may have TS.

WHO TO TALK TO

Community/general paediatrician if initial investigations have not been
done.
Paediatrician with an interest in growth problems.

WHEN TO REFER

Infants – see growth faltering guidelines (see Ch. 30).
Preschool children with short stature and/or growth failure.
Older children with growth deviation not explained by familial growth
delay.
Associated features, e.g. lethargy, headaches, weight loss.

THERAPY

Explanation and counselling about projected growth pattern, and the
social pressures of being short.
Growth hormone indications (NICE guidance).
GH deficiency, Turner's syndrome, Prader–Willi syndrome (PWS), SGA
infants with failure of catch-up growth by age 4 years.
GH results in greater height gain if started in early childhood.
GH may benefit the body composition of a PWS child if started before
severe obesity is established (severe obesity and sleep-induced airway
obstruction are relative contraindications).
Low dose androgen therapy (oxandrolone or testosterone) for early
adolescent boys with growth and pubertal delay that results in
emotional or behavioural difficulties.

FOLLOW-UP

Growth measurements at 6- to 12-month intervals (at the same time of
day to avoid diurnal variation). Refer any child, from age 18 months,
whose growth curve continues to fall after three 6-monthly
measurements.
Children receiving GH or other endocrine management require an agreed
shared care plan.

KEY POINTS FOR PARENTS AND CHILDREN

Interpretation of growth charts, prediction of adolescent growth and adult
height.

Reinforcement of 'normality' of familial short stature.
Medical intervention to promote modest height gain does not improve the emotional well-being of a child.

HEALTH PROMOTION

Height and weight review at childhood health episodes.
Documentation in parent-held record.
Parents reminded to make the record available at all health episodes.

ADDITIONAL POINTS

Training in measurement technique, the interpretation of growth charts (including the relevance of parental heights), normal growth and its variants is vital (Hall 2003).

GPs, practice nurses and public health doctors should identify the early signs of childhood obesity and offer interventions at an early stage (Chief Medical Officer for England 2003).

Practices should ensure that they have properly maintained and calibrated equipment and a supply of nine-centile, cross-sectional growth charts (available from Child Growth Foundation, 2 Mayfield Avenue, Chiswick, London W4 1PW). Practices should also aware of the EU directive on weighing scales for medical purposes (90/384/EEC).

SOURCES

Hall DMB, Elliman D (eds) (2003) Health for all children, 4th edn. Oxford: Oxford University Press. Online. Available: www.healthforallchildren.co.uk

eGuidelines (*comprehensive collection of UK clinical guidelines and related information for healthcare professionals and patients*) www.eguidelines.co.uk.

NICE (2002) Guidance on the use of human growth hormone (somatropin) in children with growth failure. Guideline No 42, May 2002. London: NICE.

Royal College of Paediatrics and Child Health & National Obesity Forum (2002) An approach to weight management in children and adolescents (2–18 years) in primary care. (Included in the Nutrition section of eGuidelines; www.eguidelines.co.uk.)

See also

Chapter 30, Poor weight gain; Chapter 35, Late puberty.

33

THE TALL CHILD

DEFINITION

1. Height above the 99.6th centile (using UK 1990 nine-centile growth charts).
2. Height greater than target centile range (TCR) predicted from mid-parental heights adjusted for sex. For males add 7 cm to the mean of the parental heights and in females subtract 7 cm from the mean of the parental heights. TCR = adjusted mean ± 10 cm.
3. Excessive growth rate, gain of more than one centile band (0.67 SD) for prepubertal child.
4. Disproportionate growth, e.g. long limbs

EPIDEMIOLOGY AND AETIOLOGY

Common
- Familial tall stature
- Familial growth advance (early puberty)
- Constitutional growth advance, e.g. associated with obesity

Less common
- *Syndromatic*: Soto (dolichocephalic, learning disability), Klinefelter (hypogonadism, long legs relative to trunk), Marfan (long limbs, joint laxity, chest deformity, eye problems).
- *Systemic*: Homocystinuria, (learning disability, marfanoid appearance).
- *Endocrine*: Congenital adrenal hyperplasia (non-salt losers), premature puberty, thyrotoxicosis, very rarely growth hormone excess.

PRESENTATION

Growth surveillance.
Parental concern.
Associated problems – joint laxity, visual or cardiac signs.

ASSESSMENT

History
Birth weight and length.
Family heights.
Familial pubertal pattern as a marker of genetic growth advance.
Review growth record and onset of height acceleration.

Examination
Accurate height, and assessment for syndromatic features including joint laxity, scoliosis.
Weight and BMI.
Pubertal staging and testicular size (orchidometer).
General review for signs of systemic or endocrine disease.
Fundoscopy and visual field assessment (formal ophthalmic review for lens dislocation as in Marfan).
Review growth chart and/or plan repeat measurements at 6-month intervals (growth monitoring).

Diagnostic tests
None required if familial tall stature.
Investigations directed towards confirmation of suspected endocrine disorder or syndrome – LH, FSH, testosterone/oestradiol, androstenedione, TFT.
Left hand for bone age and metacarpal index (measure of arachnodactyly).
USS to assess ovarian size and follicular activity, and uterine growth.
CXR.
Echocardiography (approximately 30% of Marfan patients have aortic root or mitral valve abnormality).
Karyotype for suspected Klinefelter's syndrome (XXY), or XYY.

DIFFERENTIAL DIAGNOSIS
See above.

ALERTS
Accelerated growth with inappropriate bone age advance and risk of adult short stature.
Growth acceleration may be the first sign of premature puberty.

WHO TO TALK TO
Paediatrician with interest in growth problems/paediatric endocrinologist or, if the investigations highlighted above have not been performed in primary care, an initial referral to a community paediatrician would be indicated.

WHEN TO REFER

Children whose height is above 99.6th centile need be referred only if they have prepubertal height acceleration and/or other symptoms or signs, e.g. inappropriate puberty, heart murmur, headaches.

THERAPY

Explanation and counselling about projected growth curve, and the social pressures of being very tall.

Hormone intervention seldom required other than in confirmed endocrine pathology.

Rare justification for oestrogen treatment in pre-adolescent girls with predicted very tall adult stature.

KEY POINTS FOR PARENTS

Tall stature is seldom a marker of health disorders.

The majority of tall children become acceptably tall adults.

Society and clothes retailers are better prepared for tall girls.

ADDITIONAL POINTS

Growth documentation in parent-held record.

34

EARLY PUBERTY

DEFINITION

The development of secondary sexual characteristics before age 8 years for girls, and 9 years for boys. The trend towards more frequent childhood obesity and earlier growth acceleration has blurred this definition, especially in girls from age 6 years. Afro-Caribbean girls also tend to have earlier onset from age 6 years.

- *Premature complete (isosexual) puberty* due to progressive activation of the hypothalamic–pituitary gonadal axis, and with appropriate sexual maturation, needs to be differentiated from so-called incomplete puberty. The majority of the latter are normal variations of puberty.
- *Premature adrenarche,* comprising pubic and axillary hair growth together with increased apocrine secretion and a modest growth spurt, reflects maturation of the adrenal cortex and increased production of adrenal androgens. It is relatively common in children from age 6 years.
- *Premature thelarche,* comprising isolated, cyclical and self-limiting breast development, may occur in girls during infancy or later childhood, and is due to temporary FSH pulsatility with resultant elevation of oestradiol. Typically it is not accompanied by full progression or growth acceleration.
- *Pathological incomplete early puberty* due to abnormal hormone pathways is suggested by variation from the normal order and pace of sexual maturation, and notably by contrasexual development – virilisation of girls or feminisation of boys.

EPIDEMIOLOGY AND AETIOLOGY

The majority of children with early puberty represent the early part of the normal distribution curve (Box 34.1).

Girls are more susceptible to central premature puberty and less likely to have a definable neurological basis.

BOX 34.1 Onset of Puberty

Activation of gonadotrophin pathway (central or complete)
- Constitutional or familial
- Secondary to disorder of brain–pituitary pathway
  - congenital, e.g. hydrocephalus
  - acquired, e.g. postencephalitis, hamartoma, optic nerve glioma, postcranial irradiation

Independent of gonadotrophin pathway (peripheral or incomplete)
- Gonadal
  - tumour
  - activating mutations of gonadotrophin receptor
- Adrenal
  - tumour
  - congenital adrenal hyperplasia
- Ectopic source of gonadotrophin activity
  - germinoma
- Exogenous source of sex steroid

Incomplete forms of puberty
- Isolated adrenarche
- Isolated thelarche

PRESENTATION

Early or inappropriate development of secondary sexual characteristics. Growth acceleration.

ASSESSMENT

History

Birth history and early childhood health and growth.

Congenital or acquired intracranial disorders may trigger early puberty, e.g. girls with spina bifida and hydrocephalus.

Family pattern of puberty.

Drug history.

Associated symptoms, notably headache and visual disturbance.

Examination

Height and weight.

Puberty staging using the Tanner scheme for recording the stage of maturation of the genitals, breast and pubic hair (Figs 34.1, 34.2). It is possible to examine a child and, using the Tanner scheme, describe which stage of puberty they are approaching.

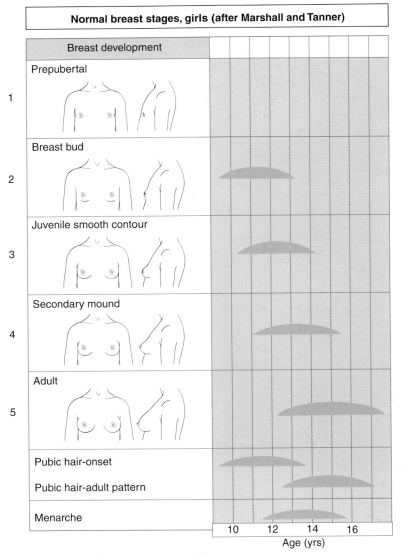

Fig. 34.1 Normal breast stages in girls.

Testicular size (with Prader orchidometer, i.e. a set of 12 ellipsoids that vary in volume, allowing the clinician to estimate the volume of the testicles): bilateral testicular growth suggests central puberty; small testes with penile and pubic hair growth point to adrenal disorder; asymmetrical testes point to a gonadal tumour.

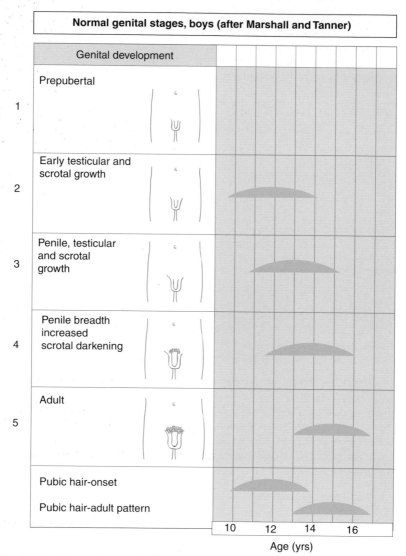

Fig. 34.2   Normal genital stages in boys.

Inappropriate virilisation, e.g. clitoromegaly in girls, or feminisation, e.g. breast development in boys.

Abnormal skin pigmentation suggestive of neurofibromatosis or McCune–Albright syndrome.

Increased blood pressure and/or cushingoid features in adrenal disorders.

Signs of raised intracranial pressure or visual disturbance.

Signs of associated endocrine disorder, e.g. hypothyroidism.

Diagnostic tests

Left hand and wrist x-ray for bone age.
Abdominal/pelvic ultrasound scans for ovarian and uterine maturation.
Baseline hormone profile guided by clinical features – LH, FSH, oestradiol,
testosterone and adrenal androgens.

DIFFERENTIAL DIAGNOSIS

Is puberty likely to be innocent, e.g. familial, and girls more than boys?
Is the sexual maturation appropriate for gender and following a normal (if
early) progression?
Are there any worrying features?

ALERTS

CNS symptoms and signs.
Contrasexual development.

WHO TO TALK TO

If the initial investigations have not been performed, a community
paediatrician may be able to help in the first instance.
Paediatric endocrinologist.
The key issues for children with early puberty are:

- To define the cause, potentially requiring cranial MRI or detailed
  abdominal imaging.
- If the cause is central, is there a brain lesion requiring intervention?
- If the cause is peripheral, adrenal or gonadal disorders must be excluded.
- Is the pace of puberty such that it is detrimental to the child's
  well-being and/or adult height potential? There may be a role for
  suppression of puberty.

WHEN TO REFER

Puberty not in keeping with normal early pattern or with suspect
character.
Puberty that is unacceptable to child and family.

THERAPY

In central puberty, there may be a role for gonadorelin agonist agents.

FOLLOW-UP

The diagnosis of innocent forms of early puberty can usually be
consolidated by observation for 6 months. Pathological forms or those
requiring intervention will require regular specialist review.

KEY POINTS FOR PARENTS

That onset of puberty in girls does not dictate that menarche is imminent.
Discuss likely growth and pubertal pattern together with potential adult
  height.

ADDITIONAL POINTS

Growth documentation in parent-held record.
Booklet: Premature sexual maturation. Serono/Child Growth Foundation.
  Online. Available: www.bsped.org.uk/patients/serono/index.htm

See also

Chapter 32, Short stature and subnormal growth; Chapter 33, The tall child

35

LATE PUBERTY

DEFINITION

Girls who have not started breast development (breast bud and areolar enlargement) by age 13 years, and boys without testicular growth (volume 4 ml or more, length above 2.5 cm) by 14 years. Incomplete puberty, e.g. failure of menarche, or puberty protracted beyond duration of 4–5 years also requires assessment.

Short stature is often a component of delayed puberty.

EPIDEMIOLOGY AND AETIOLOGY

A majority represent the late part of the normal distribution curve. This is more striking in boys who have later puberty, and growth acceleration as a component of the second half of puberty (Box 35.1).

PRESENTATION

Delayed sexual development with or without short stature.
Associated emotional and behavioural problems.

ASSESSMENT

History

Birth history – hypospadias and undescended testes favour pathological hypogonadism.

Growth pattern – late childhood growth delay is a common association with constitutionally delayed puberty.

Family pattern of growth and puberty.

General health, e.g. repeated ENT problems in girls with TS, or headaches and visual deficit linked to pituitary area tumours.

Assessment of smell as a clue to Kallmann syndrome.

Eating and exercise behaviour.

> **BOX 35.1 Familial or constitutional delay of growth and puberty (CDGP)**
>
> *Disorders of the hypothalamic–pituitary pathway (hypogonadotrophic hypogonadism)*
> - Primary
>   - congenital, e.g. isolated gonadotrophin deficiency, Kallmann syndrome (associated hyposmia), multiple pituitary hormone deficiency, Prader–Willi syndrome
>   - acquired, e.g. pituitary area tumour (e.g. craniopharyngioma)
> - Secondary
>   - chronic systemic illness, e.g. coeliac disease, chronic inflammatory bowel disease, malnutrition, anorexia, over-training
>
> *Disorders of gonads or genitalia (hypergonadotrophic hypogonadism)*
> - Congenital
>   - sex chromosome disorders, e.g. Turner's syndrome (TS) and Klinefelter's syndrome (KFS)
>   - gonadal disorders, e.g. dysgenesis, vanishing testes syndrome
>   - androgen insensitivity
> - Acquired
>   - infarction after torsion, autoimmunity, irradiation

Examination

Height and weight.

Puberty staging using Tanner scheme for breast, male genital and pubic hair maturation (see Figs 34.1, 34.2).

Testicular size (with Prader orchidometer).

Signs of raised intracranial pressure or visual disturbance.

Signs of associated endocrine disorder, e.g. hypothyroidism.

Dysmorphic including features of TS; long limbs and gynaecomastia of KFS.

Diagnostic tests

Formal investigations have little role in children where there is a high probability of familial delay.

Left hand and wrist x-ray for bone age if short stature is a feature.

Girls who are short by comparison with their family require karyotype to exclude TS.

Boys with persisting hypogonadism also require karyotype to exclude KFS.

Elevated LH/FSH levels point to disorders of gonads or genitalia. Low levels can be difficult to interpret as they do not clearly differentiate between innocent delay and disordered secretion unless there are other features of hypopituitarism. The GnRH test does not necessarily help this distinction.

Plasma testosterone or oestradiol levels add to the picture.

Pituitary dedicated MRI is indicated if pituitary pathology is suspected.

Ultrasound imaging is guide to ovarian status.

DIFFERENTIAL DIAGNOSIS

The challenge is to recognise the minority who do not have innocent delay and who require specialist review.

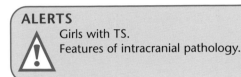

ALERTS

Girls with TS.

Features of intracranial pathology.

WHO TO TALK TO

Paediatrician with an interest in growth, or paediatric endocrinologist.

WHEN TO REFER

Observation of otherwise healthy children is in order but failure of progress over 6–12 months merits referral, especially if the delay is fuelling psychological issues.

THERAPY

Boys with constitutional delay, especially if emotionally troubled, can benefit from limited courses of weak androgen preparations. Oxandrolone 2.5 mg/day for up to 6 months improves height growth without detracting from adult stature. For older boys concerned about height and puberty, testosterone formulations are helpful, e.g. Sustanon 50 mg/month for up to 6 months or overnight transdermal patch.

Teenagers with confirmed hypogonadism require staged sex steroid replacement in order to match normal puberty and ensure bone mass development. Boys with anorchia can be offered prosthetic implants. Fertility issues need review.

FOLLOW-UP

Long-term sex steroid replacement necessitates specialist supervision either with endocrinologist or gynaecologist.

Women with TS benefit from multidisciplinary review directed at endocrine, cardiac, ENT and potential fertility issues.

KEY POINTS FOR PARENTS

The normality of most teenagers with delay and potential for catch-up growth.

Potential assistance available to those with underlying disorders.

ADDITIONAL POINTS

Growth documentation in parent/patient-held record.

Booklets: Growth and growth disorders (Serono/Child Growth Foundation/BSPED) and Constitutional delay of growth and puberty (Serono/Child Growth Foundation/BSPED). Online. Available: www.bsped.org.uk/patients/serono/index.htm.

COMMON CLINICAL PROBLEMS

36

INFECTIOUS DISEASES

DEFINITION

The term 'infectious disease' can be used synonymously with 'communicable disease' to describe a disease that can be communicated from one person to another.

EPIDEMIOLOGY AND AETIOLOGY

With the improvement in drugs and vaccines, many have thought that the threat of diseases in the developed world is now absent. Common childhood illnesses are still very prevalent, difficult to eradicate and remain a challenge for the medical profession.

PRESENTATION

Diseases can only be controlled if there is accurate information on incubation periods (time between being exposed to a pathogen and onset of the clinical disease) and periods of infectiousness (time during which the infection may be transmitted to others). Based on this information advice on periods for exclusion from school or preschool can be provided (see Table 100.1). In some cases the exclusion from school is unnecessary and can be avoided.

ASSESSMENT

History

Date of onset of symptoms
Description of any rashes
Upper respiratory tract symptoms
Evidence of lymphadenopathy
Diarrhoea
Vomiting
History of cough
Known contact
Travel history
Contact with farm animals
Obvious focus of entry for infection, e.g. wound

Examination

Full examination looking for evidence of above.

May require blood pressure and urine dipstick if considering haemolytic uraemic syndrome (characterised by thrombocytopenia, microangiopathic haemolytic anaemia and renal failure, usually caused by *E. coli* 0157:H7 presenting as an acute illness with bloody diarrhoea).

Diagnostic tests

Dependent on differential diagnosis; may only require clinical diagnosis.

Other investigations include full blood count, blood culture, viral culture, polymerase chain reaction, monospot, liver function tests, throat swab; antibodies; stool for viruses, bacteria, ova and parasites.

> **ALERTS**
> ⚠ Child with diarrhoea and blood in urine (investigate for haemolytic uraemic syndrome).
> Child with non-blanching petechial rash – refer for urgent assessment.
> Ask about pregnant contacts.
> Look for hidden sources of infection such as sanitary towels.

WHO TO TALK TO

Nursery and school nurses for contact information.

Microbiologist for information re investigations and appropriate drugs.

Paediatrician if referral or management information required.

Public health for notification.

WHEN TO REFER

If concerned about systemic symptom(s) or sequelae.

If evidence of serious disease such as meningococcal disease.

THERAPY

Depends on diagnosis.

FOLLOW-UP

Most children with minor common childhood illnesses will not require follow-up. For more serious diseases follow-up for identification or management of sequelae to the illness will be required.

KEY POINTS FOR PARENTS

Parents can be reassured that most infectious diseases are common and self-limiting.

Symptomatic treatment is usually all that is required, e.g. monitoring of fluid intake, keeping the child comfortable and relieving any itching caused by the rash, use of antipyretics for fever control.

Parents should be appropriately advised about exclusion periods from school or preschool. They should also be informed about symptoms that should alert them to contact health professionals for further advice or review, such as signs of dehydration, reduced conscious level, fever that does not settle and changing appearance of any accompanying rash.

HEALTH PROMOTION

Families may need advice on the risk of transmission and methods for prevention of the disease. They may require guidance about hand washing and exclusion periods to help reduce the risk of transmission.

ADDITIONAL POINTS

Schools and nurseries need advice about exclusion periods so that children are not inappropriately kept at home.

SUPPORT ORGANISATIONS

Health Protection Agency – www.hpa.org.uk/infections/topics_az/schools/summary.htm (*full guide*);www.wiredforhealth.gov.uk/PDF/pocketg.pdf (*useful summary*).

See also

Chapter 100, Infectious diseases – reference tables

ALLERGY

DEFINITION

- *Allergy*: IgE-mediated hypersensitivity reaction with activation of mast cells and release of histamine.
- *Food intolerance*: Usually temporary symptoms with certain foods – not IgE mediated, e.g. lactose intolerance following gastroenteritis.
- *Anaphylaxis*: Severe allergic reaction – angioedema, hypotensive shock and rapid onset of breathing difficulty – life threatening.
- *Eczema*: Chronic inflammatory skin disorder of children, young people and adults which remits and relapses.
- *Hay fever*: Seasonal allergic rhinitis.

EPIDEMIOLOGY AND AETIOLOGY

Allergy is increasing, particularly in more highly developed populations worldwide:

- Asthma – 1 in 5 school-age children
- Eczema – 5–10% of children and young people
- Hay fever – 1 in 5 people, most common in teenagers
- Food allergy – 1–2% of general population.

Food allergy is particularly common in childhood, approximately 3% in preschool period:

- Most children with milk allergy grow out of it by 3 years
- Most children with egg allergy grow out of it by 5 years
- Most children with peanut allergy remain allergic (1 in 5 may resolve)
- Prevalence nut allergy = 1% of schoolchildren
- Siblings of children with nut allergy have 7% risk of nut allergy.

Aetiology

Genetic predisposition and then environmental factors, including early exposure to allergens. '

'Hygiene theory' – modern lifestyle in highly developed countries prevents exposure of young children to worm infestation and childhood illnesses which would in the past have occupied this part of the immune system.

Younger children in a large family have less allergy than their older siblings. In theory their more frequent exposure to viruses may protect them. Smaller families lead to relatively more allergy.

Exclusive breast feeding may protect against eczema.

PRESENTATION

- Eczema:
  - under 3 months of age with itchy, red rash on face, distribution becomes flexural.
- Food allergy
  - cow's milk, egg, nuts; occurs on first-known exposure
  - there must have been previous sensitisation, but usually not an identifiable event
  - there may be tingling tongue, urticarial rash, angioedema, wheeze
  - in a severe reaction there may be rapid onset of breathing difficulty due to laryngeal oedema, even signs of 'shock' – pale, clammy, floppy, sleepy
  - usually atopic child/family.

ASSESSMENT

History

Identify provoking agents.

Details of all reactions – number/frequency.

Are symptoms clearly and consistently linked to particular allergen(s)?

Diet – is child already on an exclusion diet?

Is the diet a healthy one? (Need for dietetic advice.)

Severity and speed of onset of symptoms, particularly rapid onset of breathing difficulty or any indication of shock.

Treatment history – intramuscular adrenaline needed in previous reactions?

Personal and family history of atopy is usual.

General health of the child.

Often has asthma – very important to identify and treat effectively as this will lessen the risk of a severe food allergic reaction.

Level of anxiety in the family.

Examination

Eczema – severity and distribution.

Growth – plot on growth charts.

Signs of poorly controlled asthma – chest shape, wheeze, peak flow.

Cardiovascular, including BP – *important if considering prescribing adrenaline.*

Diagnostic tests

Rarely helpful in eczema.

Often in food allergy the history is very clear and no diagnostic tests are needed.

Skin prick tests and RASTs (allergen specific IgE levels in the blood) can be misleading, particularly in young children or those with severe eczema.

Generally a negative result is highly reliable, but there are often false positives.

Oral challenges are the only way to be sure a child has outgrown an allergy, but must be conducted in hospital if there is any risk of a severe reaction.

Tests cannot reliably identify the severity of the allergy

DIFFERENTIAL DIAGNOSIS

Eczema

Psoriasis.

Contact dermatitis – nickel allergy, latex allergy.

Juvenile plantar dermatosis – eczema on the soles of the feet due to friction from footwear.

Fungal infection.

Scabies/lice.

Food allergy

Food intolerance.

C1 esterase deficiency.

Viral or idiopathic urticaria.

Hay fever

Perennial rhinitis – symptoms all year round.

Allergens – house dust mite and pets.

ALERTS

Eczema and herpes – danger of severe infection.

Potent topical steroids used long term will cause skin atrophy and growth suppression.

Oral challenges for nut allergy should always be carried out in hospital.

Prescription of adrenaline without support is unacceptable.

Risk of dying from food allergy is small – 1 in 800,000 children with food allergy per year.

Food allergy is common but it is not possible to predict who is at risk, either from severity of previous reaction or tests.

Underlying asthma is a risk factor; therefore make sure asthma is as well controlled as possible.

Two-thirds of fatal cases had adrenaline before hospital.

Need salbutamol and rapid transfer to hospital as well as adrenaline.

WHO TO TALK TO

Health visitor/school nurse
Community paediatrician/school doctor
Paediatrician with special interest in allergy
Paediatric immunologists are rare/adult immunologist
Paediatric dermatologist
Paediatric dietitian
Anaphylaxis Campaign
Allergy Foundation

WHEN TO REFER

Children with nut allergy need prompt assessment.
Refer to paediatrician those children with:

- frequent severe reactions
- unidentified triggers
- multiple allergies and difficult diet
- high anxiety
- poorly controlled asthma.

May need referral to specialist allergy assessment clinic.
Severe eczema with failure to respond to conventional treatments – refer
    to paediatric dermatologist.

THERAPY

Food allergy

Avoidance of allergen(s) if possible – more straightforward if one or two
    clear triggers.
For full treatment guidelines including indications for adrenaline pen –
    see *Drug and Therapeutics Bulletin*. Mild, moderate and severe reactions,
    and their treatment, are outlined in Table 37.1.

Table 37.1

Reaction	Signs/symptoms	Treatment
Mild	Itchy eyes Tingling tongue Urticaria	Oral antihistamine
Moderate	Angioedema Wheeze	Oral antihistamine Bronchodilator
Severe	Laryngeal oedema Severe bronchospasm Hypotensive shock	IM adrenaline* Bronchodilator Antihistamine Paramedic ambulance

* Adrenaline dose (from BNF):
   6 months–6 years: Junior pen (0.15 mg adrenaline)
   6 years onwards: Adult pen (0.3 mg adrenaline)

Personal emergency management

Each child needs a personal emergency management plan, e.g.

- *Name* may suffer an allergic reaction if he/she eats ....
- In a *mild* reaction, with itchy eyes, tingling tongue, blotchy rash, give chlorphenamine (Piriton) liquid 4 mg, i.e. 2 × 5 ml. Can be repeated 4–6 hourly if necessary.
- In a *severe* reaction, with rapid onset of breathing difficulty, faintness or collapse, give adrenaline EpiPen 0.3 mg intramuscularly and call paramedic ambulance. Also give chlorphenamine as above and salbutamol inhaler – 1 puff every 1 minute up to 10 puffs, preferably via volumatic. Tell ambulance staff what he/she has been given.

Training of child and family

Training of school staff by school nurse/school doctor, using child's own emergency plan as above incorporated into the school protocol provided by the Anaphylaxis Campaign.

Eczema

It is essential that parents understand the relapsing nature of the condition and the need to keep in the skin's natural oils by avoiding irritants such as soap and tight clothing and by avoiding foods that have been identified as relevant allergens.

Use emollients and moisturisers daily instead of soap.

Ointments for dry eczema, creams for moist areas.

Steroids: 1% hydrocortisone 3–4 times per day for inflamed skin. Can be used long term, even on the face. Prescribe enough quantity to avoid treatment gaps.

Stronger steroids may be needed short term, e.g. 1–2 weeks? Use the least potent that is effective (see childrens *BNF*). Avoid the face and avoid in children under 2 years. Once daily may be enough.

Bacterial infection with *Staph. aureus* often exacerbates eczema. Treat with topical or oral antibiotics depending on severity.

Herpes simplex infection can lead to eczema herpeticum with punched out erosions and vesicles. If suspected, treat promptly with oral and topical aciclovir.

Avoidance of scratching:

- Light cotton clothing, including gloves at night.
- Avoid overheating.
- Keep fingernails short.
- Antihistamines at night

Other treatments for eczema

Wet wraps and occlusive bandages – may need nursing assistance.

Topical immunosuppressants for acute treatment of flare-ups:

- Tacrolimus ointment, twice daily – 0.03% for 2 years and over, 0.1% for 12 years and over – for moderate to severe eczema unresponsive to conventional therapy.
- Pimecrolimus 1% cream twice daily for 2 years and over for mild to moderate eczema.

Systemic steroids, azathioprine, ciclosporin, prescribed only under specialist supervision.
Phototherapy.
Chinese herbal medicine – effective but may cause liver damage.

Hay fever
Decongestants
Non-sedating antihistamine
Sodium cromoglicate
Steroid nasal sprays
Steroid tablets – 14 days
Hyposensitisation

FOLLOW-UP
Ongoing support for child, family and school is very important
Eczema – review frequently if needing potent steroids
Food allergy – ideally annual review with community paediatrician or GP:

- Monitor frequency of reactions.
- Change level or dose of medication if necessary.
- Prompt repeat training for schools etc.
- School protocol needs review annually.
- Rewrite on transfer to secondary school.
- School training updates should be offered annually.
- Parents and children need repeat adrenaline pen training with repeat prescription, by practice nurse or pharmacist.

Asthma/hay fever – 6 monthly in GP asthma clinic.

KEY POINTS FOR PARENTS
- Eczema
  - dry skin condition
  - keep natural oils in
  - fluctuates
  - 80% of children will grow out of it
  - avoid biological washing powders.
- Food allergy
  - common
  - rarely life threatening but difficult to predict who is at risk.

HEALTH PROMOTION

Atopic women should avoid peanuts in pregnancy.
No peanuts to children under 3 years.
Helpful labelling of food.
Awareness of restaurant staff.
School training.
Nut-free school meals.

SUPPORT ORGANISATIONS

The Anaphylaxis Campaign
    PO Box 275
    Farnborough
    Hants GU14 6SX
    Tel: 01252 377140
    www.anaphylaxis.org.uk
The British Allergy Foundation
    Deepdene House
    30 Bellegrove Road
    Welling
    Kent DA16 3PY
    Helpline: 0891 516500

SOURCES

British Medical Association/Royal Pharmaceutical Society of Great Britain. British National Formulary. London: BMA/RPSGB. Online. Available: www.bnf.org

Drug and Therapeutics Bulletin. Online. Available: www.dtb.org.uk/idtb

Furue M, Terao H, Rikihisa W et al (2003) Clinical dose and adverse effects of topical steroids in daily management of atopic dermatitis. British Journal of Dermatology 148: 128–133

Macdougall CF, Cant AJ, Colver AF (2002) How dangerous is food allergy in childhood? Archives of Disease in Childhood 86: 236–239

38

HEAD SIZE AND SHAPE

DEFINITION

Abnormal head size is defined as greater or less than 2 SD from the mean for age. Abnormal head shape or size may indicate underlying brain abnormalities, bony abnormalities or positional effects.

PRESENTATION

Concern about shape or size may be the presenting factor but more often it is recognised as part of an examination for another reason.

ASSESSMENT

It is important that all children, particularly under the age of 2 years, have their head growth monitored. Their head size should be plotted using a 'lasso tape' on the growth centile charts available from the Child Growth Foundation.

History

It is important to get a good family history of head abnormalities as well as factors that may give clues to the differential diagnosis.

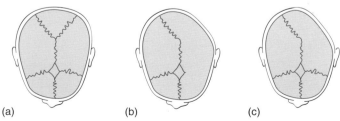

Fig. 38.1 Plagiocephaly: flattened forehead due to: (a) deformation; (b) unilateral coronal stenosis; (c) unilateral lambdoid stenosis.

Examination

This should include a thorough neurological and developmental examination as well as parental head circumferences. It should also look at the shape of the head.

Diagnostic tests

These may include imaging of the skull and/or brain, as well as TORCH screening and genetic or metabolic testing (see 'Differential diagnosis').

DIFFERENTIAL DIAGNOSIS

Abnormal head size

Macrocephaly
- Familial/genetic.
- Hydrocephalus – particularly if circumference is crossing centiles upward.
- Subdural effusions (possible non-accidental injury).
- Megalencephaly (large brain size).
- Skeletal dysplasia/achondroplasia – specific growth charts are available.

Microcephaly
- Prenatal:
  - genetic (AD/AR)
  - chromosomal (especially trisomy 13 and 18 as well as associations with holoprosencephaly, midline defects and other migrational disorders)
  - intrauterine infections (TORCH)
  - foetal alcohol syndrome
  - placental insufficiency, e.g. smoking, maternal systemic disease
  - undiagnosed or untreated maternal PKU.
- Postnatal
  - hypoxic ischaemic encephalopathy
  - CNS infections
  - severe chronic disease causing malnutrition.

Abnormal shape

Craniosynostosis
Look for ridging of sutures and premature closure of fontanelles.

Plagiocephaly
More commonly seen since babies have been lying on their backs to sleep.
Is due to external pressure, i.e. sleeping on same side or intrauterine position.
Most improve with time but does need to be distinguished from craniosynostosis, usually by skull x-ray.

WHEN TO REFER

If concerned about abnormal head shape then initial referral should be made to paediatrician who will decide whether a paediatric neuro-surgeon (craniofacial clinic) or a neurologist (if abnormal head size) is needed.

THERAPY

Depends on diagnosis.

FOLLOW-UP

Consistent and frequent measurements can alert to crossing centiles upwards or downwards which may have a more sinister outcome.

KEY POINTS FOR PARENTS

Cosmetic procedures are available for some of the more severe deformities. Early contact with craniofacial clinics is important where an abnormal shape exists.

SUPPORT ORGANISATIONS

Child Growth Foundation
    2 Mayfield Avenue
    London W4 1PW
    Tel: 020 8995 0257
    Email: cgflondon@aol.com
    www.childgrowthfoundation.org

5

39

SPOTS IN BABIES

Many transient vesiculopapular rashes occur in babies, and are generally harmless. Always check that the baby is systemically well, and ask about family history of blistering skin conditions to avoid missing rare cases of infection or genetic skin conditions

Differential diagnosis of vesiculopapular or pustular eruptions in babies

5

INFECTIVE
- Bacterial pustules – bullous impetigo, systemic bacterial sepsis
- Viral – herpes, varicella, CMV
- Fungal – congenital cutaneous candida

NON-INFECTIVE
- Milia
- Miliaria
- Erythema toxicum neonatorum (ETN)
- Transient pustular melanosis
- Infantile acropustulosis
- Incontinentia pigmenti
- Omenn's severe combined immunodeficiency
- Mastocytosis
- Acne

The commonest will be described in detail.

MILIA

EPIDEMIOLOGY AND AETIOLOGY

Approximately 50% of all newborn infants develop milia. Sebaceous glands are thought to be overstimulated following exposure to maternal androgens in utero. Keratin plugs impair oil secretion and papules form.

PRESENTATION

Pin-point papules, approximately 1–3 mm diameter (white/yellow), mainly on nose, cheek, upper lip and forehead. Also rarely seen on upper trunk, areola and genitalia.

ASSESSMENT

History
Usually present within the first 48 hours of life.
Completely asymptomatic.
Usually disappear within a few weeks.

Examination and diagnostic tests
Diagnosed on clinical examination; no tests necessary.
Larger papules are called pearls.

DIFFERENTIAL DIAGNOSIS

Erythema toxicum neonatorum.
Miliaria.
Transient neonatal pustulosis.

ALERTS

⚠ If exceptionally extensive or persistent and associated with other abnormalities, consider orofacial–digital syndrome or a Marie–Unna type congenital hypotrichosis.

ERYTHEMA TOXICUM NEONATORUM (ETN) (Fig. 39.1)

EPIDEMIOLOGY AND AETIOLOGY

Affects approximately 50% of all infants.
Unknown aetiology but rarely seen in preterm and small-for-date infants.
An eosinophil-rich exudate fills papules.
It is unsightly but neither contagious nor dangerous.

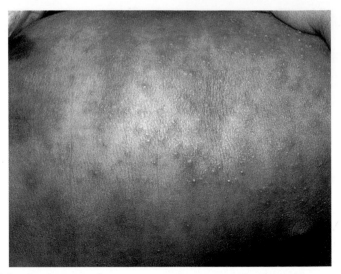

Fig. 39.1 Erythema toxicum neonatorum on an infant's trunk.

PRESENTATION

Rarely present at birth but develops within 48 hours of birth.
Can occur up to 14 days of age with a peak incidence at 2 days of age.
Resolves spontaneously with no complications.

ASSESSMENT

History

Occurs in a *well* infant who develops numerous erythematous patches,
  many of which will have yellow/white papules in their centres.
Patches can be confluent and develop rapidly within hours, while older
  patches fade without residual skin changes.

Examination and diagnostic tests

The rash affects any part of the body but only rarely the palms and soles.
Diagnosed on clinical examination; no tests necessary.

DIFFERENTIAL DIAGNOSIS

Milia.
Miliaria.
Herpes simplex.
Infantile acne.

ALERTS

⚠ An unwell infant requires immediate investigation for sepsis as this will not be erythema toxicum. Consider herpes simplex.

TRANSIENT NEONATAL PUSTULOSIS (Fig. 39.2)

EPIDEMIOLOGY AND AETIOLOGY
0.1–0.35% in white Caucasian infants and 4–5% in African–American infants within the US. There is no familial predisposition or any known aetiology.

PRESENTATION
Clusters of tiny, 1–2 mm pustules occur on the face, trunk and proximal extremities; more rarely on the palms and soles.

ASSESSMENT
History
Pustules are present at birth and can have some scale around them, but are not red or inflamed. The pustules rupture in the first few days of life, leaving flat dark areas that resemble freckles. These areas will fade in 3 weeks to 3 months without treatment. In darker skinned patients, pigmented freckles can last several months.

Examination and diagnostic tests
Diagnosed on clinical examination with no specific tests.
Mainly present on face, trunk and proximal extremities; more rarely on the palms and soles.
Pustules rupture to leave a brownish crust.

DIFFERENTIAL DIAGNOSIS
Milia.
Miliaria.
Herpes.

ALERTS

⚠ Investigate an ill infant.

THERAPY
None.

5

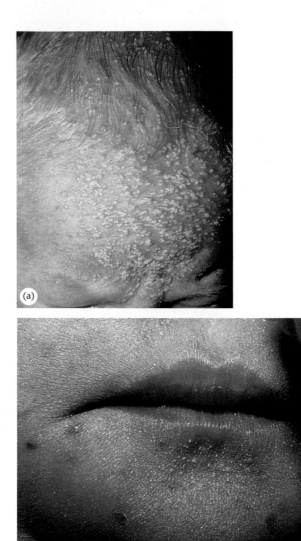

Fig. 39.2   Transient neonatal pustulosis (or pustular melanosis):
(a) numerous pustules on a neonate's scalp and forehead; (b) healing
pustules caused hyperpigmentation on this infant.

Fig. 39.3 Miliaria crystallina – the tiny vesicles soon desquamated in a cooler environment.

MILIARIA

5

EPIDEMIOLOGY AND AETIOLOGY

There are two types of miliaria, affecting around 3% of babies: crystallina and rubra. Both are thought to be caused by eccrine sweat gland obstruction. It is uncertain if the sweat glands are obstructed due to their relative immaturity or due to warmth triggering excessive sweating.

PRESENTATION

- *Crystallina* (Fig. 39.3): Infants have thin-walled superficial vesicles *without* surrounding erythema. These vesicles are delicate and rupture. Present within the first 2 weeks of life.
- *Rubra* (Fig. 39.4): Erythematous papules and papulovesicles on a background of macular erythema. Present any time in the first year of life but common in the neonatal period.

Both disappear in a few days without treatment but are helped by maintaining a cool skin, either through changing the type of clothing worn or lukewarm baths.

ASSESSMENT

History

Both seen in well infants and considered to be secondary to heat and humidity.

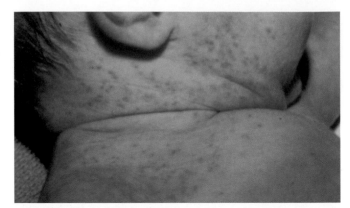

Fig. 39.4 Miliaria rubra – the red papules of prickly heat.

Examination and diagnostic tests

Diagnosed on clinical examination; no tests necessary.
Common in flexures or covered parts of the skin or where there is friction against clothing.
Fever may trigger miliaria but it does not cause fever.

DIFFERENTIAL DIAGNOSIS

Milia.
Erythema toxicum.
Herpes simplex.
Infantile acne.

> **ALERTS**
>
> ⚠ An unwell infant needs immediate investigation as miliaria does not cause systemic symptoms.

EPSTEIN PEARLS

EPIDEMIOLOGY AND AETIOLOGY

Unknown aetiology but seen in 85% of infants.

PRESENTATION

Asymptomatic at birth.

Examination and diagnostic tests

White keratinous painless cysts at the junction of the hard and soft palate that resolve spontaneously without treatment. They do not affect feeding.

DIFFERENTIAL DIAGNOSIS

If infant is unwell, consider herpes simplex.

HERPES SIMPLEX

EPIDEMIOLOGY AND AETIOLOGY

Most babies are infected from the vaginal tract and caesarean section minimises this risk. Unfortunately, mothers may be asymptomatic (up to 70% of cases).

PRESENTATION

Within 1 week of age but may be seen at birth or up to 3 weeks of age.

ASSESSMENT

History

Usually non-specific with fever, irritability, lethargy, poor feeding, vomiting, respiratory distress, convulsions, jaundice and apnoeas.
The blisters affect skin and mucous membranes.

Examination and diagnostic tests

Viral presence in blister fluid confirms diagnosis.

DIFFERENTIAL DIAGNOSIS

In a well infant, consider:

- milia
- erythema toxicum
- transient pustular melanosis.

> **ALERTS**
>
> ⚠ Need aggressive treatment as there is the danger of CNS involvement and consequent serious morbidity and mortality.

WHEN TO REFER

Urgent referral to paediatrics is required whenever herpes simplex is suspected in the newborn.

INFANTILE ACNE

EPIDEMIOLOGY AND AETIOLOGY

Unknown aetiology but there may be a family history of severe parental acne in their adolescence. It is believed that there is hypersensitive end-organ responsiveness to hormones.

PRESENTATION

Pustules, papules, and open and closed comedones.

ASSESSMENT

History

Usually present by 1 month of age and resolve within the first 4 months but persistence noted for months in rare cases.

Examination and diagnostic tests

The acne is usually confined to the face.
Diagnosed on clinical examination; no tests necessary.

DIFFERENTIAL DIAGNOSIS

Miliaria.
Transient neonatal pustulosis.

> **ALERTS**
>
> ⚠ Higher incidence of later adolescent acne.

THERAPY

No treatment is suggested in the neonatal period as spontaneous resolution generally occurs without scarring.
Persistent cases can be treated with topical benzoyl peroxide.

Haemangiomas

EPIDEMIOLOGY AND AETIOLOGY

Up to 10% of infants develop these birthmarks with a preponderance in females (approximately 75% of cases) and preterm infants. There are two types, depending on the depth of the haemangiomas below the skin:

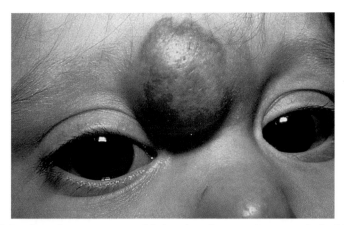

Fig. 39.5 Strawberry naevus – this involuted over a 3-year period without leaving a scar.

- capillary (superficial layers of skin) haemangiomas, e.g. strawberry naevus (Fig. 39.5)
- cavernous haemangiomas which are deeper and have a bluish tinge.

Clumps of abnormal blood vessels gradually distend leading to the haemangiomas.

PRESENTATION

Most are *not* present at birth. They appear over the first 1–3 months and enlarge for up to 1 year, then gradually resolve over the next 2–7 years.

Most resolve completely by adolescence: 70% resolve completely, but 30–50% leave telangiectasia and loose skin.

ASSESSMENT

History
Vary in size from pin-point to a few centimetres across and though most commonly occur in isolation, in some instances can be multiple.

Examination and diagnostic tests
Painless nodule, diagnosed on clinical examination; no tests necessary.

DIFFERENTIAL DIAGNOSIS
Port wine stain.

> ## ALERTS
>
> ⚠ If overlying the eyes, consider referral to ophthalmologist (vision and amblyopia concerns).
>
> If interfering with any vital function, e.g. overlying urethra, anus, mouth and not feeding well or if in airway, consider referral to dermatologist or paediatrician.
>
> Remember that a haemangioma can extend deeper, and compress/invade underlying organs, e.g. if on neck. If over trachea, consider airway obstruction; if overlying spine, check neurology, etc.
>
> Very rarely, Kasabach–Merritt syndrome (haemangioma–thrombocytopenia syndrome) develops from a rapidly growing cavernous haemangioma in the first few months of life. There is rapid consumption of platelets within the haemangioma.

THERAPY

If ulcerated, dermatologists will treat with lasers.

KEY POINTS FOR PARENTS

Most will resolve spontaneously, will not require treatment and will not leave scarring.

PORT WINE STAIN (Fig. 39.6)

EPIDEMIOLOGY AND AETIOLOGY

Unknown aetiology but thought to be secondary to abnormal sympathetic vascularisation of superficial venules. These venules lack vascular tone and become engorged over time, distending the capillary bed distal to the affected venules

PRESENTATION

At birth with well-demarcated red flat birthmark, which may become more prominent when infant cries or gets hot.

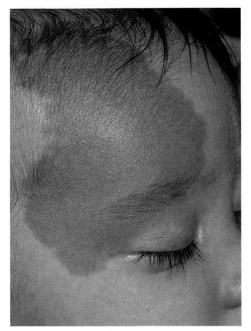

Fig. 39.6 Port wine stain on an infant with Sturge–Weber syndrome.

5

ASSESSMENT

History

Usually present at birth.

The colour changes from red to purple as the child grows to adolescence.

Surface is smooth at birth but in later life may become 'studded' with a cobblestone appearance as venules become prominent.

Associated with hypertrophy of underlying tissues as the child grows older.

Examination and diagnostic tests

Lesions are often confined to the face, but may involve any part of the body.

Diagnosed on clinical examination; no tests necessary.

DIFFERENTIAL DIAGNOSIS

Capillary haemangiomas.

Stork bites/naevus simplex/naevus flammeus neonatorum – these present on the nape of the neck or bridge of the nose but resolve spontaneously within a few years.

ALERTS

⚠

- Approximately 10% of patients with facial lesions develop glaucoma. The risk increases if the lesion involves the skin supplied by both the ophthalmic (VI) and the maxillary divisions of the trigeminal nerve.
- Sturge–Weber syndrome: Association of facial port wine stain with underlying CNS abnormality leading to epilepsy, intellectual impairment and eye abnormalities:
  - suspect if port wine stain in ophthalmic division of the trigeminal nerve (VI distribution)
  - will only be present in <10% of VI port wine stains.
- Lesions over the spine can be associated with vascular malformations (venous or arteriovenous) in the underlying spinal meninges, or with spinal cord abnormalities.
- Klippel–Trenaunay syndrome: Extensive vascular lesions over the limbs may be associated with limb enlargement and should be referred for assessment.

WHEN TO REFER

All port wine stains on the face should be referred to a dermatology centre for consideration of laser treatment (timing according to local policy).

Lesions involving VI distribution of the trigeminal nerve should be referred for ophthalmological assessment.

Large lesions on the limbs and lesions overlying the spine should be referred to paediatrician or dermatologist for consideration of associated problems (see above).

Imaging studies

If Sturge–Weber syndrome suspected:

- CT scan or MRI findings may be absent during the first few years, unless intravenous contrast is administered.
- Skull x-rays traditionally demonstrate 'tram line calcification'.

Patients with port wine stains over the lumbar spine, especially if associated with other skin lesions (see above), should have a spinal MRI scan.

Other tests

Ophthalmologic review to exclude glaucoma in infants with upper trigeminal nerve (1st and 2nd division) or eyelid involvement should be performed semi-annually for the first 3 years of life and annually thereafter.

THERAPY

Cosmetic camouflage.

Pulsed dye laser is the treatment of choice. It emits a yellow light that is preferentially absorbed by oxyhaemoglobin. Treatment is usually carried out by dermatologists under general anaesthetic. Unfortunately there is a poor evidence base for 'when to refer' as certain centres start treatment at 7–14 days and is best discussed with your local dermatologist. Results vary according to a number of factors including darkness of lesion and age of treatment (infants have better results compared to adults).

MONGOLIAN BLUE SPOT

EPIDEMIOLOGY AND AETIOLOGY
Melanocytes fail to migrate to the epidermis and remain in the dermal layer during embryogenesis.

It is completely benign but present in up to 90% of babies in East Asia (China/Indonesia etc.) and 80% of Indian Asian infants.

It is commoner in babies with darker skin.

PRESENTATION
At birth with bluish (as pigment is in the deeper dermal layer) birthmarks, often over the lumbosacral region.

The macules (i.e. not raised) often measure a few centimetres in diameter but can be extensive and involve the buttocks, back and shoulders; they rarely affect the face,

ASSESSMENT
History
Usually resolve spontaneously within 4 years.

Examination and diagnostic tests
Diagnosed on clinical examination; no tests necessary.

DIFFERENTIAL DIAGNOSIS
Bruise – hence useful to document position and approximate size and shape at birth to avoid later confusion with non-accidental injury.

Blue naevi (but these are rarely present at birth and develop in the second decade of life, gradually enlarging into a papule).

WHEN TO REFER
These benign birthmarks resolve spontaneously in the vast majority.

THERAPY

Nil in most cases. Very rarely consider opaque cosmetics.

SUPPORT ORGANISATIONS

The Birthmark Support Group
  PO Box 3932
  Weymouth
  Dorset DT4 9YG
  Tel: 01202 257703
  www.birthmarksupportgroup.org.uk
  Offers information to anyone affected by a birthmark (including port wine stain). The website is regularly updated with the group's activities and provides links to other relevant organisations.
Red Cross Skin Camouflage Service
  British Red Cross Association
  9 Grosvenor Crescent
  London SW1X 7EJ
  Tel: 020 7235 5454
  www.redcross.org.uk
Vascular Birthmarks Foundation –
  www.birthmark.org/babieswithbirthmarks.php – guidelines in the United States
www.emedicine.com/derm/contents.htm – a comprehensive overview

40

RASHES IN OLDER CHILDREN

PRESENTATION

A quick 'look' usually precedes history and examination.

Be clear about the history as patients may use dermatology terminology inappropriately. In Lancashire, wheals are called blisters.

Impact on the quality of life has to be determined within the history. Many rashes are chronic, i.e. eczema, and have an impact on sleep with nocturnal itching and a consequent effect on schooling.

- *Patient perception*: Diet is often implicated and the clinician really needs to distinguish perception, i.e. certain diets affect the rash from a more objective description. Food may hence be inappropriately blamed for flare-ups, and unless the timing between consumption and aggravation of the rash is documented, it may be difficult to formulate a plan.
- *High expectation*: Many parents want complete resolution of rashes and, if not forthcoming, seek alternative therapies and second opinions. Though their concerns are appropriate, patient education is imperative.
- *Poor compliance*: Chronic problems are often associated with poorer compliance and allegations that the previous treatments were 'ineffective'.

ASSESSMENT

History

Does anyone else have a rash now (i.e. infectious) or is there a genetic component?

Examination

- *Site/distribution*: Describe the site of the rash – eczema is classically demonstrated on flexor surfaces whereas psoriasis presents on the knees, elbows and scalp.
- *Characteristics*: Measure their size, shape (round, linear or irregular) and describe their border (well defined as in psoriasis or blurred as in

5

> ### BOX 40.1 Clinical description
>
> *Lesion characteristics*
> - Macule – flat circumscribed area of skin discoloration
> - Papule – circumscribed elevation of skin less than 0.5 cm in diameter
> - Nodule – circumscribed elevation of skin greater than 0.5 cm in diameter
> - Plaque – circumscribed disk-shaped elevated skin
> - Vesicle – small visible collection of fluid less than 0.5 cm in diameter
> - Bulla – small visible collection of fluid greater than 0.5 cm in diameter
> - Ulcer – loss of epidermis (often with loss of underlying dermis as well as subcutis)
> - Wheal – circumscribed, elevated area of cutaneous oedema
>
> *Surface characteristics*
> - Scale – Visible and palpable flakes due to aggregation and/or accumulation of shed epidermal cells
> - Crust – accumulated dried exudates of serum
> - Excoriation – secondary, superficial ulceration due to scratching.
> - Lichenification – a flat top thickening of skin often secondary to scratching

eczema). Also describe their colour (red/purplish etc.). It is also important to describe their surface feature, i.e. crust (dried serum) or scale (hyperkeratosis) (Box 40.1).
- *Describe secondary sites*: i.e. nails in psoriasis, fingers and wrists in scabies, and toe webs in fungal infections.

Rashes can commonly be separated into itchy and non-itchy lesions. This latter category is often harder to define as children may 'pick' at lesions even if they are not itchy (e.g. molluscum contagiosum, acne).

ITCHY RASHES

ATOPIC ECZEMA

EPIDEMIOLOGY AND AETIOLOGY
See Chapter 37, Allergy.

ASSESSMENT
Must have an itchy skin condition in the last 12 months *and* three of the following:

ALERTS

Remember that eczema also affects the ear canal and appropriate treatment averts parents mistakenly ascribing waxy discharge from the ears to being due to an 'ear infection'.

Vulval irritation may be due to atopic eczema

Herpes simplex infections cause eczema herpeticum (Fig. 40.1), and require oral and topical aciclovir. Look for punched-out erosions and vesicles.

Sudden onset itching – don't miss scabies.

Plot growth – systemic steroids are implicated in growth retardation and chronic severe eczema can slow growth.

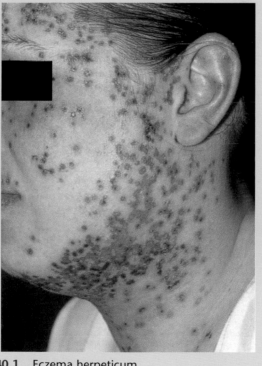

Fig. 40.1 Eczema herpeticum.

5

- History of involvement of the skin creases.
- Personal history of asthma or hay fever (or history of atopic disease in a first-degree relative if the child is under 4 years).
- History of a generally dry skin over the past year.
- Onset under 2 years of age
- Visual flexural dermatitis (includes cheeks and forehead in a child less than 4 years).

History
As above and see Chapter 37, Allergy.

Examination and diagnostic tests
Clinical examination. Tests not required. Look for distribution in flexures.

DIFFERENTIAL DIAGNOSIS
Psoriasis.
Contact dermatitis.
Scabies.
Head lice.
Fungal infection.

WHO TO TALK TO
The National Eczema Society is a good source of information.
Local dermatology nurse who may be attached to a dermatology department or paediatric dermatologist.

THERAPY
Avoidance of scratching, keeping fingernails short, wearing light cotton clothes and avoiding overheating at night all help.
Emollients treat the skin dryness and are the mainstay of maintenance treatment; flare-ups require an active treatment.
First line treatment is with 'short sharp' bursts of topical steroid. Use the weakest preparation that will control the eczema. Start with 1% hydrocortisone ointment and increase to moderate strength, e.g. clobetasone (Eumovate), then potent, e.g. betamethasone (Betnovate), if ineffective. Potent steroids should not normally be used on the face or neck due to the risk of skin thinning and glaucoma. Ointments are better than creams.
If the eczema is not controlled with intermittent treatment, refer to a dermatologist for consideration of second management, e.g. additional investigations, topical immunomodulators, (tacrolimus, pimecrolimus), UV light or systemic therapy.
Secondary infection of the skin is best treated with oral flucloxacillin as opposed to topical preparations.

HYPERSENSITIVITY REACTIONS

DEFINITION
Type 1 hypersensitivity is an immediate wheal-like reaction to skin contact or ingestion of an allergen.
Type 4 is a delayed eczematous reaction to skin contact with the allergen.
They have separate aetiology and clinical presentations.

PRESENTATION
The history is usually clear, i.e. a rapid onset rash on previously normal skin following contact with a particular allergen.

DIFFERENTIAL DIAGNOSIS
Type 4 reaction – eczema.
Type 1 – chronic idiopathic urticaria.

> **ALERTS**
>
> Ask about systemic reactions following contact with allergen – wheeze, feeling of itching in the throat (see Chapter 37, Allergy).
> Type 4 hypersensitivity reactions are commonly associated with nickel and seen around rings, earrings (and other areas where body piercing may occur) in addition to the traditional places from buttons and buckles on clothing and bras. The history and distribution are often sufficient to make the diagnosis but patch tests are the definitive investigations.

WHO TO TALK TO
Type 1 allergy – investigation and management of severe reactions should be carried out by a paediatrician with an interest in allergy.
Type 4 allergy – patch testing by a dermatologist.

THERAPY
Avoidance often resolves the problem.
Type 1 – education involving family and school. Use antihistamine syrup in the acute phase (see also Chapter 37, Allergy).
Type 4 – acute episodes can be treated with a topical steroid. If there is doubt about the causative agent, the patient should be referred to a dermatologist for patch testing.

TINEA PEDIS (ATHLETE'S FOOT)

EPIDEMIOLOGY AND AETIOLOGY

This is the commonest of all fungal infections, with scaling and itchy areas in the toe webs. It is acquired from infected keratin debris on floors or swimming pools/showers.

PRESENTATION

Peeling, maceration and fissures, characteristically starting in the web spaces of the 4th and 5th toes, which may then spread to nails, other toes and soles of the feet.

History, examination and diagnostic tests

Asymmetric involvement of feet helps to distinguish it from eczema. Fungal scrapings are diagnostic but unnecessary in classic cases. Nail involvement will require fungal tests (microscopy, culture), as treatment will be oral and prolonged.

DIFFERENTIAL DIAGNOSIS

Contact dermatitis.
Eczema.
Psoriasis.

WHO TO TALK TO

Dermatologist if persistent and severe.

THERAPY

Treatment is with a topical antifungal. The imidazole group (ketoconazole, miconazole) or topical terbinafine is effective. Topical preparations containing tolnaftate are on sale to the public. Antifungal dusting powders are thought to have little therapeutic value and may cause skin irritation. They may have a role in preventing reinfection.
Nail involvement requires oral griseofulvin for at least 3 months.

SCABIES

EPIDEMIOLOGY AND AETIOLOGY

The scabies mite burrows into the skin and has an asymptomatic phase (4–6 weeks).
Hypersensitivity to the mite and its products (faeces, saliva) eventually lead to itching.
Infection is by close physical contact.

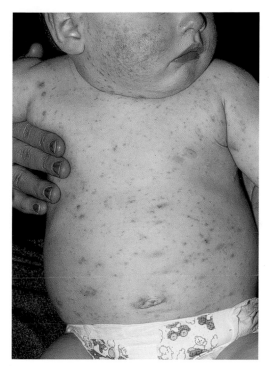

Fig. 40.2 Scabies in an infant.

5

PRESENTATION

Scabies is a very common skin infestation. It should be considered in any child with an abrupt onset of a papular or eczematous rash (Fig. 40.2).

ASSESSMENT

History

It is intensely itchy.

Examination and diagnostic tests

'Burrows' are found on the hands and feet, especially in the web spaces, wrists and instep, and, in infants, in the palms of the hands. The burrow is several millimetres long, tortuous, with a vesicle at one end next to the burrowing mite and surrounding erythema (Fig. 40.3).

There is usually a *secondary* generalised papular rash as an allergic reaction to the mites. Longstanding scabies can cause nodules in the axillae and scrotum.

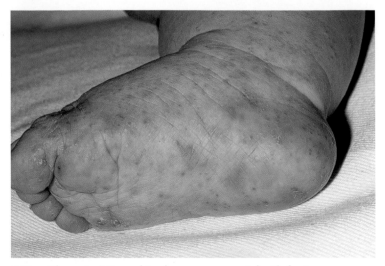

Fig. 40.3 Characteristic scabies burrows on an infant's foot.

DIFFERENTIAL DIAGNOSIS

Eczema

> **ALERTS**
>
> Itching and secondary eczema following the scabies may persist for some weeks after the infestation has been eliminated. Treatment for both the pruritus and eczema may be required.
> Crusted scabies is an uncommon presentation. It is seen in children with Down's syndrome and separately in severely disabled children who may be unable to scratch. The hands and feet are encrusted in thick, fissured, crusty skin with grossly thickened nails. Burrows are often difficult to find. Microscopy of scales demonstrates large numbers of mites and eggs. This condition is highly infectious.
> Scalp itching – see Chapter 41, Itchy head.

WHO TO TALK TO

Local community paediatrician if severe and resistant to treatment.
If at school, parents of other children should be advised to consult their GP if their child has persistent itching.

THERAPY

All family members need treatment *on the same day* with malathion or a permethrin. Malathion must be left on for 24 hours. Aqueous preparations are preferable to the alcoholic lotions as the latter cause irritation of the excoriated skin. Clothing and bedding should be washed.

'NON-ITCHY' LESIONS

Face

ACNE

EPIDEMIOLOGY AND AETIOLOGY

Common in pubescence but also seen transiently in infancy. Acne is a disease of the pilosebaceous unit, and therefore affects the face, back and chest.

ASSESSMENT
History
Onset at puberty with involvement of face (forehead, midface, chin) and, particularly in boys, the thorax (upper chest, deltoid and upper back).

Between 25 and 50% of all girls with acne have exacerbations approximately a week before their periods (unknown aetiology).

Examination and diagnostic tests
There are four basic types of lesion:

- open and closed comedones (Fig. 40.4)
- papules
- pustules
- nodulocystic lesions.

One or more types of lesion may predominate.

DIFFERENTIAL DIAGNOSIS
Usually the acne is obvious but rarely can be confused with:

- flat warts
- folliculitis.

WHO TO TALK TO
Local dermatologist if severe and resistant to treatment.

5

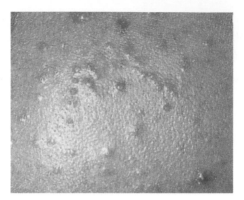

Fig. 40.4 Closed comedones (whiteheads) on the forehead of a 14-year-old.

THERAPY

Treatment depends on three factors:

- the type of lesion (i.e. inflammatory or comedonal)
- the acne severity
- the psychological impact of the disease.

Treatment should be given early if the acne is causing scarring. Patients should be aware that improvement may take 2–3 months.

Topical therapy

Topical benzoyl peroxide is first line therapy for mild to moderate acne of both types. Irritation is a frequent problem.

For comedonal acne, a retinoid should be added at night. Tretinoin or adapalene is equally effective. Skin irritation is a frequent problem, which can be helped by washing off the preparation after 1–2 hours.

For inflammatory acne, topical antibiotics can be effective. Intermittent treatment is recommended to reduce resistance.

Azeleic acid is an alternative in both acne types.

Do not continue treatment for longer than necessary though treatment with topical preparations should be continued for at least 6 months.

Oral therapy

- *Oral antibiotics*: These can be used if the acne is extensive, or if the patient cannot tolerate topical therapy. Tetracyclines are first line treatment in adolescents, but should not be used under the age of 10 due to teeth staining. They are most effective in inflammatory acne.

- *Hormonal treatment*: The contraceptive pill. Dianette can be helpful in female patients who require contraception.
- *Oral isotretinoin*: Treatment with oral isotretinoin is extremely effective for severe and scarring acne. It is a hospital-only drug because of known teratogenicity. Any patient with scarring acne who does not respond quickly to other therapy should be referred to a dermatologist for consideration of isotretinoin.

HERPES SIMPLEX

EPIDEMIOLOGY AND AETIOLOGY

There has to be intimate contact involving mucous membranes or damaged skin between a susceptible person (no previous antibody response) and an individual who is actively shedding the virus. Most acquire infections asymptomatically and approximately 80% of adults are seropositive.
Peri-oral lesions are common in childhood.

PRESENTATION AND HISTORY

Often asymptomatic but can have a prodrome of fever followed by lymphadenopathy of the neck, sore throat and coincident reduced fluid intake. The blisters are painful and can occur anywhere around the mouth. The lesions ulcerate and heal after 2–3 weeks.
In recurrences, the onset is more localised, with burning/paraesthesiae in the mouth and eventual blisters that last a week.

5

ASSESSMENT
Examination and diagnostic tests
Clinical examination, but rarely viral immunofluorescence if in doubt and there are concerns in an immunocompromised child.

DIFFERENTIAL DIAGNOSIS
Chicken pox.
Hand, foot and mouth disease.
Stevens–Johnson syndrome (rare).

> **ALERTS**
> ⚠ Genital lesions are suggestive (but not diagnostic) of sexual abuse.
> Immunocompromised children require immediate antiviral treatment.
> Can develop eczema herpeticum (see above).

WHO TO TALK TO

Local community paediatrician if severe and resistant to treatment.

WHEN TO REFER

Persistent and distressing oral herpes that is unresponsive to oral/topical aciclovir.

Genital herpes should raise suspicion of sexual abuse.

THERAPY

Recurrent eruptions are best treated with topical aciclovir usually as the 'tingling starts'. Triggers include fever, strong sunlight and menstruation.

HAND, FOOT AND MOUTH DISEASE

EPIDEMIOLOGY AND AETIOLOGY

The Coxsackie virus (usually Type A16) causes this transient problem. This is highly infectious and spread by droplet and contact. There is an incubation period of 3–6 days.

PRESENTATION

Blisters on hands, feet and mouth (Fig. 40.5).

ASSESSMENT

Examination and diagnostic tests

Small grey vesicles are seen with a halo of erythema around the hands and feet. The buccal mucosa has erosions resembling aphthous ulcers. They are self-limiting.

DIFFERENTIAL DIAGNOSIS

Chicken pox.
Herpes simplex.
Stevens–Johnson Syndrome (rare).

WHO TO TALK TO

School nurse. There are usually school policies on whether the children can attend school given that they usually feel well but education staff feel wary of the problem.

Local community paediatrician if severe and resistant to treatment.

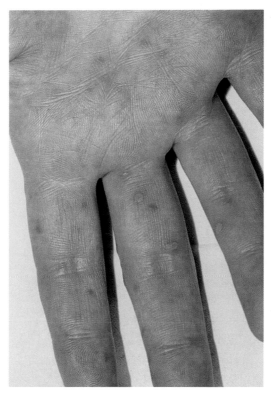

Fig. 40.5 Hand, foot and mouth disease. (From White 2001, Diseases of the skin, with permission of Mosby Ltd.)

THERAPY

None.

Rashes on the trunk

MOLLUSCUM CONTAGIOSUM

A pox virus that causes pearly pink vesicles with an area of central umbilication (Fig. 40.6). This umblication is filled with a keratin plug. It is commonly seen on the head, neck and trunk with more extensive involvement in children with atopic eczema.

Molluscum contagiosum usually resolves spontaneously over 6–24 months, and treatment is not generally recommended. There is no effective treatment. Cryotherapy (liquid nitrogen) is occasionally used, but it is painful and the lesions can recur.

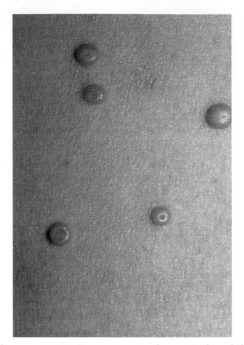

Fig. 40.6   Molluscum contagiosum – note the central umbilication on these mature lesions.

PSORIASIS

Psoriasis is an inherited papulosquamous skin disorder characterised by well-defined pink/red lesions with typical silvery scale. Onset is usually after puberty, but 10% of patients have onset before 10 years. There are various forms but the commonest is the classic plaque psoriasis, with large plaques over the extensor surfaces of the elbows and knees, the trunk, and scalp scaling. Guttate psoriasis often develops suddenly after an infection (especially streptococcal throat infections) and may itch.

THERAPY

Guttate psoriasis is often self-limiting. The sore throat should be treated if streptococci are isolated on throat swab. Emollients and a mild topical steroid, or a tar preparation, can be helpful. Persistent or severe cases should be referred to a dermatologist for consideration of UV light.

Plaque psoriasis in children is often chronic. First line treatment is with a topical vitamin D analogue (e.g. calcipotriol) or a tar-based preparation.

Scalp psoriasis should be treated with a tar-based shampoo. Descaling can be achieved with Cocois ointment left on overnight and washed out in the morning.

Any child with significant psoriasis should be referred to a dermatologist for ongoing management.

ERYTHEMA MULTIFORME

These target lesions are typically round with an area of central paleness. They may be triggered by herpes (and other viruses) in addition to being drug induced. They are self-limiting in a child who is otherwise well.

PITYRIASIS VERSICOLOR

These lesions are seen in the older teenager (Fig. 40.7). It is uncertain why the malassezia fungus multiplies more profusely in some individuals. Fair-skinned children will have light brown macules with a fine surface scale whereas children with pigmented skin have patchy areas of hypo-pigmentation. They are usually asymptomatic but cause cosmetic problems.

DIAGNOSIS

Gently scrape affected areas of skin with a scalpel blade. Collect the skin scrapings and send for mycology.

THERAPY

Selenium sulphide shampoo diluted with water and then left to dry on the skin for at least 30 minutes after a bath. It can be left overnight. It should be applied two to seven times over a 2-week period and the course repeated if necessary.

Complete repigmentation may not occur until after sun exposure.

Topical azole antifungals can also be effective. Occasionally systemic treatment may be required using an azole antifungal and usually requires consultation with a dermatologist.

Recurrence is a frequent problem, which is difficult to manage.

WARTS

EPIDEMIOLOGY AND AETIOLOGY

This human papillomavirus (HPV) infection is usually self-limiting though this may take years to resolve. It has an incubation period of 1–8 months

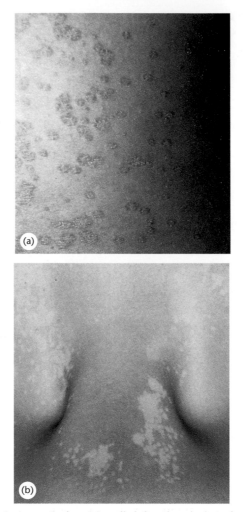

Fig. 40.7 Pityriasis versicolor: (a) well-defined scaly papules on a teenager's back; (b) hypopigmented rash as a result of exposure of papules to sun.

and peak for infection is after 5 years of age. There are many subtypes of the virus but the commonest affects the hands/feet/face while another subgroup affects the genitalia. It is highly infectious and reportedly spread by towels, skin contact and floor surfaces. Transmission by asymptomatic individuals (infected but no visible warts) makes prevention difficult. Susceptible individuals (those without immunity to HPV) are at increased risk if their skin is damaged (e.g. small lacerations).

PRESENTATION

Raised papules with a warty surface which vary in size. The infection is confined to the epidermis.

ASSESSMENT

History

30% resolve spontaneously within 6 months and most within 3 years.

Examination

Clinical examination.

ALERTS

⚠️

Genital warts only

- Genital warts in children can be an indication of sexual abuse. This is not diagnostic of abuse but warrants greater detail in history taking. They can be acquired in infancy following maternal vaginal contact at birth and may take up to 2 years to present (Royal College of Physicians 1997).
- There are high and low risk strains of HPV that predispose to cervical carcinoma and it is impossible to distinguish between the two clinically. Treatment is therefore recommended for genital warts. Vaccines are currently at a developmental stage.

5

WHO TO TALK TO

Non-genital warts – local dermatologist if severe and resistant to treatment.
Genital warts, especially in a child over 2 years – community paediatrician as risk of associated abuse.
Genital warts in a sexually active child – genitourinary medicine clinic.

THERAPY

65% of warts resolve spontaneously within 2 years. If unwilling to wait, persistent (greater than 2 years), spreading, extensive, discomfort or cosmetically unacceptable, consider next step.
Start with least expensive/painful approaches.

Topical therapy – non-genital warts
- Treatment with topical salicylic acid-based preparations has been shown to be as effective as cryotherapy, and should be recommended in patients who want treatment. Can be purchased over the counter. Pare skin (using scalpel) or use emery board prior to application to remove as much dead skin on surface of wart. Best applied on damp skin (after bath) as enhances absorption. Can occlude with band aid/plaster to maximise action. Repeat the following day. Treatment can take weeks and demands perseverance.

- Formaldehyde, glutaraldehyde or silver nitrate are also available over the counter and act similarly.
- Cantharidin is available in the USA and is applied by doctors. It causes epidermal necrosis and blistering, and must be used with caution to avoid damage to surrounding skin.

Topical therapy – anogenital warts

- Soft, keratinised external warts can be treated with podophyllin.
- Cryosurgery–liquid nitrogen is the most effective and is applied using a cotton bud. Freeze the wart and a rim of 1–2 mm of normal skin surrounding the wart. Repeat every 1–4 weeks for 3 months. Caution around sides of fingers/toes as can damage underlying structures. 50–80% cure rate. Plantar warts benefit from being pared prior to treatment (see above).
- Neither cryotherapy nor topical treatment is thought to cause scarring.
- Lasers can be used along with electrocautery but run the risk of scarring and the virus has been identified in the smoke plume, increasing risk of infection to health staff.
- Treatment failure/recurrence is seen more commonly in immunocompromised patients.
- Patient education is important, including risk of treatment failure and recurrence. Spontaneous immunity usually develops and will offer protection but this is difficult to predict at initiation of treatment.

PITYRIASIS ROSEA

There is often a mild prodromal illness followed by a 'herald' patch (Fig. 40.8). This is a large red oval and slightly scaly patch of skin, which resembles ringworm. A few days later, pale pink oval patches appear over the trunk. They start from the spine and almost follow the spinal nerves. These patches have scale on their surface. They resolve spontaneously with no treatment, but can last up to 4 weeks or even longer (up to 8 weeks). They are usually seen in older children in early adolescence.

Parental concern about pigmentation

DEFINITION

Melanoma – a malignant skin tumour arising from melanocytes.

EPIDEMIOLOGY AND AETIOLOGY

It is very rare in childhood and adolescence. Exposure to high levels of sunlight in childhood is a key risk factor for melanoma in adult life.

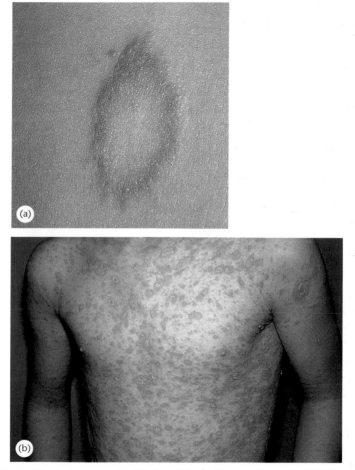

Fig. 40.8 Pityriasis rosea: (a) this herald patch on a 10-year-old mimics tinea corporis; (b) myriad oval lesions on a teenager.

Risk factors:

- Increased number of common moles
- Red or fair hair
- Skin that does not tan easily
- Light coloured skin
- Family history of melanoma
- Atypical moles: >5 mm, irregular border and pigmentation
- Giant melanocytic naevi >20 cm diameter.

PRESENTATION

Commonly present because of concern about growth or change in a mole. Most frequent site in males is the trunk and in females the leg.

Late diagnosed lesions metastasise to lymph nodes, distant skin, lung and other organs.

ASSESSMENT

Examination

Major features

- Change in size
- Irregular pigmentation
- Irregular border

Minor features

- Inflammation
- Itch or altered sensation
- Oozing or crusting
- Lesion larger than other moles

Diagnostic tests

Biopsy of suspicious lesions with a 2 mm surround of normal skin.

DIFFERENTIAL DIAGNOSIS

Other skin diseases.

Excessive pigmentation or hypopigmentation following inflammation, e.g. in eczema.

Pigmented lesions associated with syndromes, e.g. café-au-lait spots in neurofibromatosis, Albright's syndrome, Turner's syndrome.

> **ALERTS**
>
> ⚠ Clinical diagnosis is often difficult and the non-expert paediatrician or general practitioner should have a very low threshold for referral.
>
> The lesions are not always pigmented.
>
> Multiple café-au-lait spots may also be a marker of a more generalised disorder.
>
> Non-dermatological associations should be considered in any child with extensive pigmented lesions.
>
> Areas of hypopigmentation (vitiligo) may be associated with autoimmune disorders.

WHO TO TALK TO

Consultant dermatologist.

WHEN TO REFER

The presence of any major feature requires referral. Many districts have fast track procedures for referral of suspected melanomas.

THERAPY

Most naevi do not require treatment other than when melanoma is suspected.

Some will request excision for cosmetic reasons only.

Treatment is surgical, the extent of the procedure depending upon the staging of the lesion.

FOLLOW-UP

Suspicious lesions that do not require excision or those with risk factors should be kept under review.

KEY POINTS FOR PARENTS

Primary prevention by sun protection and awareness of the need for surveillance for those with risk factors.

HEALTH PROMOTION

Sun protection should be part of the health promotion programme for all children.

Protect children from intense sunlight through:

- clothing
- sunscreens with a sun protection factor (SPF) of at least 15
- sun avoidance, i.e. keep in the shade.

Do not use sun beds.

SOURCES

British National Formulary (2005) London: British Medical Association/Royal Pharmaceutical Society

emedicine (*treatment guide and patient information*).
www.emedicine.com/derm/contents.htm

Royal College of Physicians (1997) Physical signs of sexual abuse in children, 2nd edn. London: RCP

Scottish Intercollegiate Guidelines Network (2003) Cutaneous melanoma: a national clinical guideline. Online. Available: www.sign.ac.uk

See also

Chapter 37, Allergy; Chapter 41, Itchy head.

41

THE ITCHY HEAD

HEAD LICE

EPIDEMIOLOGY AND AETIOLOGY

Lice are seen in all social groups and not isolated to poverty. They follow prolonged head-to-head contact. The lice crawl (as opposed to jump) and hence the required prolonged head contact. The lice sense the heat from another head in close proximity and thus spread.

PRESENTATION

Itching is usually the first sign. This is triggered by a local hypersensitivity reaction to the saliva of the biting lice. Some individuals remain asymptomatic with no itching. These 'non-itchers' fall into two groups: one composed of babies/young children who have an immature immune system and hence do not react to the saliva with no consequent itching; the other composed of those who have had chronic lice infestation, becoming 'immune' to the lice saliva, and therefore do not itch as much. *Both groups remain carriers.*

Nits (egg cases laid by the lice) are present. These white nits are approximately 1 mm in diameter and are glued to the hair. They are usually found around the occipital regions and around the ears. In short hair it may be possible to see the lice crawling.

ASSESSMENT

History
Itching.

Examination and diagnostic tests

Identification of live lice is the gold standard. Treatment should only be commenced if lice are found as opposed to when nits are observed. This criterion is important, as nits are often confused with dandruff.

Identification of lice is best done by 'wet combing' hair, which is damp. Head lice combs are inexpensive and can be purchased from chemists. Hair conditioner helps the fine teeth of the comb slide through the hair.

DIFFERENTIAL DIAGNOSIS

Dandruff.

Seborrhoeic dermatitis – less itching but flaking of scalp.

Dermatitis – includes eczema. Some have local hypersensitivity reactions to hair gels and other products.

> **ALERTS**
>
> ⚠ Public perception, fear and stigma are often out of proportion to the clinical importance. Nonetheless, parents' anxieties should be addressed sympathetically and practically.

WHO TO TALK TO

If persistent following a number of courses of therapy, community paediatrician or school nurse.

THERAPY

- *Insecticides*: Carbaryl, malathion and pyrethroids are all effective. Local policies usually recommend one preferred preparation which is rotated to an alternative if resistance emerges. Alcoholic formulations are effective but inflammable. Aqueous preparations are preferred in patients with severe eczema or asthma and in small children. Treat all affected individuals in the family at the same time. Medical supervision of treatment is recommended in all children under 6 months of age. Medication can be purchased over the counter with advice from pharmacists.

  The treatment is usually massaged into the hair and allowed to dry over a 12-hour period (less time with pyrethroids). The treatment is then repeated 7 days later to kill any nits that survive the initial treatment and hatch.

- *Wet combing*: This technique is similar to the initial identification whereby the plastic detection comb and hair conditioner are used with meticulous combing over a 30-minute period of the whole scalp. This is conducted at 4-day intervals for a minimum of 2 weeks. Initial results from comparative studies suggest that insecticide treatment (malathion) is more effective than wet combing.

- *Dry combing*: There is a proprietary comb, which carries a small electrical current. The lice are 'electrocuted' by this method. There are no published case control studies comparing its effectiveness with insecticide treatment.

FOLLOW-UP

For children with repeated infestation, it is imperative that *all* 'close contacts' who have head-to-head contact be screened. Asymptomatic individuals (see above) go untreated and reinfect the index child; it may therefore not be failure of the initial treatment. Parent education is important.

Assuming these points have been covered, proceed to 'mosaic treatment' using a different insecticide for the retreatment. Drug resistance is thought to be re-emerging in certain areas.

KEY POINTS FOR PARENTS

Treat all affected members of the family at the same time.

Remember to use separate brushes and combs – either replace or treat with insecticide.

TINEA CAPITIS

EPIDEMIOLOGY AND AETIOLOGY

There are different causative organisms internationally but this fungal infection should be identified from a differential diagnosis.

It is common in childhood and thought to be related to changes in fatty acid constituents of sebum around puberty.

Postpubertal sebum contains fungistatic fatty acids.

ASSESSMENT

History

Itching is variable.

Examination

The affected area has fine scales and often partial hair loss. The hair is typically broken just above the scalp, giving rise to a stubby appearance (Fig. 41.1).

Diagnostic tests

Scraping the affected area with the back of a scalpel blade and collecting both hair and scales is imperative. Unfortunately, this is painful, especially in the presence of secondary infection. Some laboratories accept toothbrush samples. Use a disposable toothbrush to gently but firmly brush the affected area. This is less painful and obtains more skin. The toothbrush is then wrapped in clingfilm and sent to the laboratory.

THERAPY

Oral griseofulvin is the only effective treatment. Recent studies have also suggested using it in conjunction with an antifungal shampoo (selenium sulphide).

Treatment is for a minimum of 3 weeks.

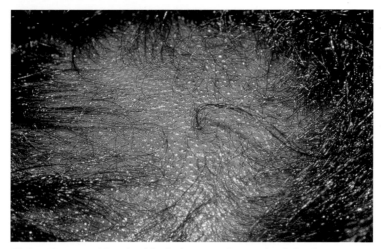

Fig. 41.1 Tinea capitis. The black dots are the result of the fungus invading the hair causing it to break off.

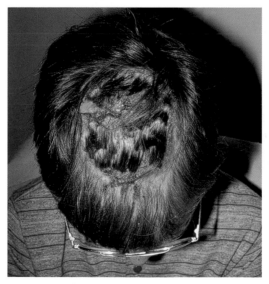

Fig. 41.2 Large kerion on a child's head.

KERION

This is a severe version of tinea capitis and resembles a secondary infection (Fig. 41.2). The scalp is boggy, may have pustules and abscesses, and children are mistakenly given recurrent antibiotic courses. Diagnosis and treatment is as above.

DANDRUFF

This is the commonest cause of an itchy scalp and is more prevalent in dark hair. Treatment with over-the-counter/proprietary brands is effective.

SEBORRHOEIC DERMATITIS

EPIDEMIOLOGY AND AETIOLOGY

This is poorly understood but the malassezia/pityrosporum ovale fungus is thought to be implicated.

PRESENTATION

Itching.

ASSESSMENT

Examination

Diffuse raised scaling on an erythematous background, usually confined to the scalp with poorly demarcated boundaries. It can, however, extend to the face and scaly skin on an erythematous background is typically seen around the nasal labial folds and eyebrows.

THERAPY

Often continues for years with no obvious cure.

Topical steroids, tar-based shampoo and ketoconazole shampoo have all been used, often in rotation.

PSORIASIS

Various forms are present and the scalp version presents with the classic plaque which, when gently scraped, has surface capillary bleeding.

It is difficult to distinguish from seborrhoeic dermatitis on the scalp and may require referral to a dermatologist for advice on diagnosis and treatment.

THERAPY

Tar-based shampoo or topical salicylic acid

PROBLEMS WITH VISION

PRESENTATION

Usually presents from concerns by the parents or health visitor of a young baby not tracking visual stimuli or 'abnormal' eye movements. Parents may have noticed a squint and 1–2% of children under 5 years have a manifest (one that is present most of the time) squint (misalignment of visual axes). Some children are picked up at preschool sight testing or by the orthoptist or optician.

Occasionally schoolchildren complain of poor sight. Many of these are simple refractive errors, which should always be formally assessed with cycloplegic refraction (spectacle test with dilated pupils) in all children below 10 years of age.

ASSESSMENT

History

History should explore the following areas:

- Parents' concerns
- Family history – particularly of any strabismus or refractive errors
- Developmental history – including birth weight and gestation
- Uni- or bilateral
- Neurological symptoms
- Medication.

Examination

Visual acuity.

Eye movements – particularly looking for nystagmus, corneal light reflex, pupil light and red reflex, dilated fundus.

Neurological examination.

Diagnostic tests

- Always enquire from the parents of their experiences with the child, such as fixation on small targets and during feeding.

- *Visual acuity*: In the preschool or older child, test left and right separately, plus with and without pinhole (which eliminates some of the refractive errors). In cases of optic nerve disease, include pupil-light reflex and, if the child is old enough, colour vision (use a red target).
- *Occlusion*: In infants, occlude each eye separately to determine if the infant protests at covering the only seeing eye. The child's interest has to be maintained throughout this test.
- *Spinning baby/rotating head eye movements* identify gross vision in the young infant. Hold the child facing you and rotate yourself quickly over 360 degrees. If the child has vision, it will exhibit normal physiological nystagmus as they try to fixate on objects behind you. The eyes should stop moving as soon as you stop spinning. If vision is grossly impaired, the eyes will only deviate to one side.
- *Direct ophthalmoscope*: Look at the quality of the red reflex and identify any opacities seen within it (usually lenticular). Dilate with 1% tropicamide (0.5% in the under 1 year old), which lasts about 5 hours. In particular, look at the disc margins and pulsation of the blood vessels over the disc.
- *Krimsky corneal light reflex test*: Compare the position of the light reflex image on the two corneas to exclude pseudostrabismus (Fig. 42.1), i.e. normal light reflex positions in pseudostrabismus.

DIFFERENTIAL DIAGNOSIS

No apparent vision at birth
Spinning baby eye movement test may identify gross vision in the small infant. Any concerns with a child or parents complaining of poor sight should be thoroughly investigated by an ophthalmologist.

- *Cataract*: Refer all cases urgently to a paediatric ophthalmologist and to a paediatrician to exclude systemic associations. The child should

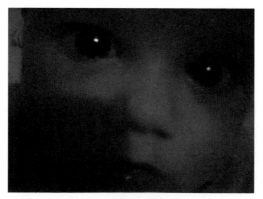

Fig. 42.1   Pseudostrabismus (pseudosquint).

be screened for congenital infections (TORCH test). Significant cataract (i.e. one that is delaying visual development) must be removed as soon as possible and most surgeons would leave the child pseudophakic (with an artificial intraocular lens).

- *Loss of red reflex* or white pupil (leucocoria) can occur with any media opacity obscuring the light path reflected from the chorioretinal blood vessels which give rise to the red colour of the light reflex. Look for nystagmus (present from about 6 weeks of age), with failure of social smiling and other interactions with parents. Causes include persistent hyperplastic vitreous, retinopathy of prematurity, retinoblastoma, Coat's disease, toxocariasis, high myopia and, of course, cataract. Urgent referral should be made to the paediatric ophthalmologist.

- *Delayed visual maturation* also causes failure of social smiling, tracking, etc. but nystagmus is generally absent. The parents may complain that the child rubs their eyes frequently. If not associated with any other neurological abnormalities, the vision usually matures to normal levels.

Nystagmus

Look for rapid eye movements, and whether constant or gaze evoked. A child with nystagmus always requires a full neurological work-up, including imaging, and referral to a paediatric neurologist. Bobbing (vertical) movements are particularly worrying. Always enquire about drug history.

- *Sensory nystagmus* caused by poor vision – usually pendular. Develops at about 6 weeks of age.

- *Motor nystagmus*, caused by abnormalities in ocular–motor centres. Present at birth. Vision usually mildly impaired due to ocular instability. Often associated with cerebellar abnormalities. May be inherited.

- *Spasmus nutans*: Benign head and eye wobble in an otherwise normal baby. May be monocular. Resolves within a few years of life. This diagnosis can only be made retrospectively, and a child with nystagmus always requires a full neurological work-up, including imaging.

Failing vision in childhood

A pinhole or corrected visual acuity test should be carried out to diminish any refractive error.

- *Strabismus (squint) and amblyopia*: Look at the corneal light reflexes and always ascertain parents' concerns. Strabismus is associated with a family history of the condition. Low birth weight children are more at risk of developing squints. Most strabismus can be corrected with spectacles and it is essential that these children are treated promptly as any amblyopia after the age of 8 years is usually permanent. *Any child with suspected squint, regardless of age, should be evaluated by an ophthalmologist. Children with a family history should also have an ophthalmic review.*

- *Amblyopia* (lazy eye) is defined as subnormal vision in the absence of an organic cause and is due to failure of the full development of the visual pathway.
- *Acute* onset of loss of vision generally will present more quickly if both eyes are affected. Causes include optic neuritis, encephalitis and, rarely, optic nerve compression due to tumour, e.g. craniopharyngioma. This tumour compresses the pituitary gland and optic chiasma so might present with hormonal imbalance, visual loss and headache.

  Retinal haemorrhages due to *shaken-baby syndrome* (bilateral, peripheral and dark) is a less common cause, and should always be referred to the ophthalmic paediatric service, if suspected.

  Optic neuritis can be severe but does not warrant steroids unless bilateral or extremely painful, as treatment has not been shown to be directly beneficial. The disc may appear totally normal as most inflammation is retrolaminar, but the child will complain of painful eye movements and may have a central negative scotoma ('something missing' in the vision as opposed to 'something in the way' as seen in retinal disease). Attacks of neuritis should settle spontaneously within 2 weeks, the vision returning to normal in the vast majority of cases.

  Classic migraine can present at any age with acute visual loss (prodrome) and fortification spectra (flashing lights that start from one side and disperse in a circular or horseshoe pattern). The child may be photophobic and nauseous, and later complain of an intense unilateral headache. Ophthalmoplegic migraine (recurrent transient 3rd nerve palsy after headache) typically occurs in children before the age of 10. Attacks usually resolve without any permanent deficit, but can rarely leave permanent visual field defects. The frequency and severity of the attacks usually lessen with time.
- *Gradual* loss of vision may be caused by optic atrophy, a retinal dystrophy or chronic optic disc oedema caused by hydrocephalus.

  Papilloedema (disc swelling due to raised intracranial pressure) tends to affect vision in the later stages and should always be excluded in a child with headache (worst in the morning) and a swollen optic disc. The vessels over the disc loose their pulsations (although 20% of the population do not exhibit this pulsation normally). Visual acuity and colour vision assessment should be made, along with visual fields to confrontation and pupil examination. Remember that children have small crowded discs which can give rise to pseudopapilloedema, but this is a diagnosis of exclusion. Visual loss is also associated with many progressive neurological disorders (see below).
- *Hysterical (non-organic) visual loss* is common in older children, but is a diagnosis of exclusion. In the absence of signs, orthoptic and electrodiagnostic tests can also be helpful.

Colour blindness
Use Ishihara colour plates or red (and green) targets to one eye at a time. Most forms are inherited X-linked but some homozygous females also manifest the disease. If needed, special filters on spectacles may help.

These children may benefit from hospital and specialist clinic evaluation and a routine referral is sometimes appropriate.

There are some occupational restrictions, e.g. certain jobs in the defence services.

Retinal dystrophies

Dilated fundal examination – any abnormality seen should be referred.

Associated with neurological disorders so a full neurological examination is appropriate.

- *Retinitis pigmentosa* (RP, rod–cone dystrophy): Progressive loss of rod function with night blindness; cone function affected later. Fundal changes include vascular attenuation, pigmented 'bone spicules' (Fig. 42.2) following the vascular distribution, and disc pallor. Presentation is usually with night blindness and earlier presentation indicates a worse prognosis, with most patients affected in older childhood or adulthood. Autosomal recessive, autosomal dominant or X-linked inheritance (in order of severity). RP is associated with many systemic disorders and requires full evaluation by a paediatrician and ophthalmologist. When associated with congenital deafness it is known as Usher's syndrome. About a quarter of patients maintain good vision throughout their working lives.
- *Cone dystrophies* are rare and result in severe visual loss and colour blindness. Juvenile Batten's disease must be excluded.

Associated with *drug use* – hydroxychloroquine, vigabatrin.

5

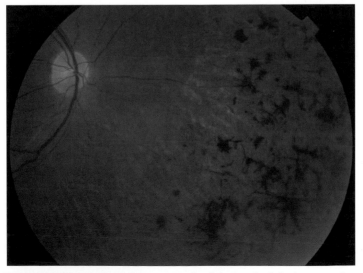

Fig. 42.2 Retinitis pigmentosa – note the 'bony spicule' pigmentation and pale optic disc.

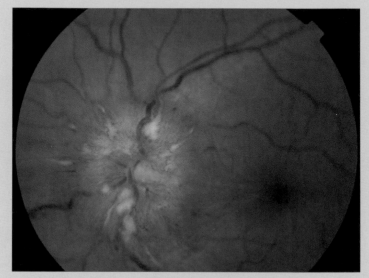

Fig. 42.3 Swollen disc. A child with headache and a swollen disc should always be referred urgently.

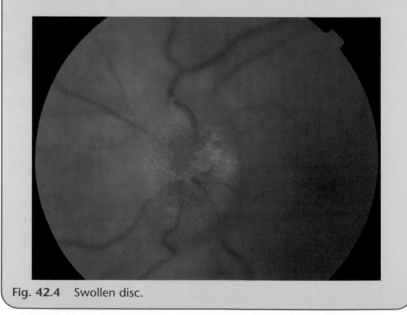

Fig. 42.4 Swollen disc.

WHO TO TALK TO

Paediatrician and/or paediatric ophthalmologist or hospital orthoptist service.

Local social services can provide further help, so registration of the child for visual impairment (blind or partially sighted) should always be completed by the consultant ophthalmologist where appropriate.

Many charities exist locally to provide further help to the visually impaired child and this should be encouraged.

WHEN TO REFER

Any child where clinical concerns arise from the history or examination. It is usually appropriate for most schoolchildren with poor vision, or strabismus, to have an up-to-date (cycloplegic) refraction, either by the local optician or, if appropriate, the hospital Ophthalmology Department.

THERAPY

Involves optimisation of vision by correction of any refractive errors, removal of any significant media opacities and correcting any strabismus.

In strabismus the aim of therapy is to align the eyes correctly and to encourage development of the visual pathways. The child will most likely continue to wear spectacles even after any surgery for squints and it is important to ensure the parents are aware of this.

Visually impaired children and families will need further input from support services and may be eligible for blind registration by a consultant ophthalmologist.

FOLLOW-UP

Ensure all children receive the correct care from a multidisciplinary team approach including educational services.

KEY POINTS FOR PARENTS

Babies can often look like they have a squint due to the wide flat bridge of the nose and wide epicanthic folds. This appearance will diminish as the face develops.

Young children require prompt treatment of any visual impairment as amblyopia is not treatable after the age of 8 years – the earlier it is treated, the better the outcome.

The aim of patching the better-seeing eye for parts of the day (as recommended by the orthoptic service) is to encourage the 'lazy' eye to be used and develop better sight.

The most common cause of a squint is refractive error.

Surgery is not a substitute for spectacles or refractive correction.

Most children would be advised to wear any required prescription spectacles at all times.

5

Cataract surgery in children is very successful but the child will require long-term monitoring to exclude the common complication of glaucoma.

SUPPORT ORGANISATIONS

British Retinitis Pigmentosa Society – www.brps.org.uk
Partially Sighted Society – www.eyeconditions.org.uk/pss.htm
Royal College of Ophthalmologists – www.rcophth.ac.uk
Royal National Institute for the Blind – www.rnib.org.uk

SOURCES

Taylor D, Hoyt C (2004) Paediatric ophthalmology and strabismus, 3rd edn. London: Saunders

See also

Chapter 12, Problems with hearing; Chapter 43, Sticky eyes; Chapter 44, Sore eyes.

43

STICKY EYES

EPIDEMIOLOGY AND AETIOLOGY

Sticky eyes are usually a result of conjunctival irritation either from infection or from tear-film and ocular surface disturbances.

Conjunctivitis is common (2% of all GP consultations), usually bacterial, and self-limiting. Viral conjunctivitis can be extremely infectious and can lead to epidemics. Seasonal allergic conjunctivitis has become more prevalent in recent times.

These common conditions do not affect vision and children who complain of visual loss should be investigated thoroughly by a specialist.

This section relates to a patient complaining of a sticky eye where pain is not a prominent feature and there is little photophobia, if at all. These latter symptoms suggest corneal involvement or uveitis, which are discussed further in Chapter 44.

PRESENTATION

As well as a discharge, the child may also have other symptoms and signs such as discomfort, mild photophobia (dislike of bright light), (intermittent) blurred vision, epiphora (watery eye) and ptosis (due to eyelid swelling). A red eye (representing an inflamed conjunctiva) is common and any localised pathology should be noted.

ASSESSMENT

History
History should explore the following areas:
- Duration, watery/purulent and colour of discharge.
- Recurrence, uni- or bilateral (together or separately?).
- Trauma or foreign body?
- General well-being with temperature, atopy; enquire about other family members.
- In neonates, delivery details are essential.
- Medication is important in cases of suspected Stevens–Johnson syndrome.

Examination

Should include eyelid margins and eyelashes. Look at the distribution of any vascular injection of the conjunctiva, which in most cases of benign conjunctivitis is diffuse and non-specific. Look at the inferior conjunctiva, underneath the lower lid, for deposits or discharge, noting the colour.

Using the direct ophthalmoscope set on high plus lens (+15 or more), a magnified view of the cornea and anterior chamber can be obtained.

Optic nerve examination (visual acuity, pupil light reflex and colour vision) should be performed in cases of suspected orbital cellulitis.

Diagnostic tests

In the older child corrected visual acuity (one with spectacles on) should be possible. Removal of any discharge with cleansing, saline drops or repeated blinking will ensure that the tear film is not disturbing vision. If visual acuity is affected, prompt referral is recommended.

In recurrent cases, with a red medial lower eyelid, look at the punctum to see if there is any discharge by pressing lightly by it to ensure no localised dacrocystitis (a lacrimal sac abscess).

In all cases of a red eye, fluorescein staining of the cornea with cobalt blue light (found on most direct ophthalmoscopes) is helpful in excluding corneal involvement.

Preauricular (non-tender) lymph nodes in viral conjunctivitis.

Swabs for Gram stain, and culture and sensitivities are commonly not helpful in the diagnosis, and are not required in routine cases. However, they are extremely useful in cases with severe discharge, such as in Chlamydia or gonococcal disease.

Differential diagnosis

Bacterial conjunctivitis
Lid disease
Viral conjunctivitis
Allergic conjunctivitis
Nasolacrimal duct obstruction
Preseptal cellulitis
Ophthalmia neonatorum

Bacterial conjunctivitis

This can occur at any age, frequently in conjunction with lid margin disease (blepharitis). A purulent discharge, yellow–green in colour, is common. Treatment with topical chloramphenicol four times a day is sufficient in most cases.

Gonococcal conjunctivitis presents with a very purulent discharge and can rapidly lead to corneal perforation.

Lid disease

Can present with a focal lesion or a generalised 'sticky' discharge.

- *Chalazions* are lipogranulomas caused by blockage of the glands. If a nuisance, they usually require incision and curettage under general anaesthetic, although administration of hot compresses may resolve up to 30% of cases. Infected chalazions usually resolve without any treatment, but if pyrexial or particularly hot and tender, systemic antibiotics (co-amoxiclav or erythromycin) are required.
- *Hordeola (styes)* are infected (tender) sweat glands on the outer eyelid margin. These generally resolve with simple warm compresses without the need for surgery.
- *Blepharitis* is a common chronic irritation from inflamed oil glands on the lid margins, and is associated with a chronic *Staph. aureus* infection. Presentation is with an oily, sticky discharge and the skin around the eyelid margins may be red. The conjunctiva (and cornea) can be irritated from the oily secretions. Treatment is with daily lid cleansing. A 3-month course of systemic tetracycline, with its anticollagenase properties to stabilise lipid production, is beneficial, but should be only used in chronic cases with *children over 12*, and only after specialist opinion has been obtained.

Viral conjunctivitis

Usually caused by adenovirus. Both eyes are affected in 60–70% of cases, although one eye is usually affected before the other, and produces a watery discharge. Symptoms can be asymmetrical with an itchy sensation, and a preauricular lymph node is usually present, along with a watery nasal discharge. It may be preceded by a sore throat or fever.

Pseudomembranes (strips off leaving intact epithelium) in the conjunctiva are occasionally seen and, if the cornea is involved (fluorescein staining may reveal small punctate erosions), the patient usually complains of photophobia. This is a highly infectious disease, so the child should be kept out of school for the course of the disease, and care taken not to infect other family members.

Supportive measures such as artificial tears (preferably preservative-free to decrease toxicity to the already compromised cornea) are helpful. Provide reassurance that the disease is self-limiting and usually resolves within 2–3 weeks.

Chlamydia can cause a bilateral, acute mucopurulent, follicular (on the upper tarsus of the inverted upper eyelid) conjunctivitis or trachoma – a chronic infection leading to scarring of eyelids and keratitis. It is associated with poor hygiene conditions and lack of face washing.

Molluscum contagiosum is an uncommon skin infection caused by a poxvirus presenting with a chronic or recurrent conjunctivitis. Look for a single or multiple, pale, waxy, umbilicated nodule near the lidmargin. Treatment is by excision or destruction using cautery or cryotherapy.

Allergic conjunctivitis

This may be seasonal, or vernal, and can be unilateral. Signs include a chronic white discharge with an uncomfortable, itchy red eye. The eyelids may be swollen. Often associated with atopy, it may require identification of the allergen by allergy testing.

Vernal disease can lead to a severe keratitis (corneal inflammation), which requires immediate specialist attention, but usually burns out by the early teens. Treatment is with allergen removal, artificial tears and antihistamines (systemic and topic). Newer antihistamine eye drops (i.e. Opatanalol and Relestat) have a quicker dual action than traditional mast cell stabilisers (i.e. Opticrom) which take up to 2 weeks to take effect. Steroid eye drops should *never* be administered without an ophthalmic evaluation and, even then, only in the short term.

Atopic or children with rheumatoid arthritis can occasionally produce excessive mucus in their tear film, exacerbating their dry eye condition and leading to repeated mucus fishing. In such cases it is best to advise not to touch or to attempt directly to remove the mucus.

Nasolacrimal duct obstruction

The nasolacrimal ducts are the last portions of the lacrimal system to canalize. They are often non-functional at birth, especially in premature babies. Symptoms include recurrent sticky eyes, especially in the morning, with epiphora (a watery eye), and are often unilateral. The eye is rarely red, and there is rarely any distress. Visual development is unaffected. The role of regular massage over the area is unproven but may be helpful.

Most patients' nasolacrimal ducts become functional before 12 months of age and the symptoms disappear. If the symptoms persist beyond 10 months of age, refer to a paediatric ophthalmologist for consideration of probing of the nasolacrimal ducts under general anaesthesia, which is successful in 95% of cases. Surgery, usually after the age of 12 months, can be performed nasoscopically (to avoid scar formation) and is highly successful.

Supportive measures such as regular cleansing with boiled water will help, with direct treatment of complications such as bacterial conjunctivitis (see above) and, rarely, lacrimal sac abscess. The latter should be referred as an emergency to the paediatric ophthalmic service.

It is important to consider congenital glaucoma in infants with a watery eye. Look for large corneal dimensions and for Haab's striae (horizontal lines representing breaks in the inner corneal Descemet's membrane). Optic disc examination may reveal a cupped disc. A child with suspiciously large 'watery' eyes may have glaucoma and ophthalmology opinion should be sought.

Preseptal cellulitis

As preseptal cellulitis (Fig. 43.1) affects only the eyelids and anterior tissues, there is usually no restriction of eye movement, and pupil reactions should always be normal. In the apyrexial child oral antibiotics such as co-amoxiclav are effective. Swelling and redness of the hot eyelid, conjunctivitis, chemosis (conjunctival swelling) and nasal discharge are common.

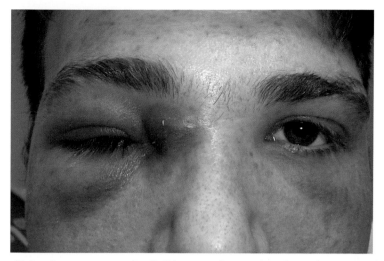

Fig. 43.1 Severe preseptal cellulitis secondary to an ethmoid sinusitis. This patient required drainage surgery and intravenous antibiotics.

If the child is systemically unwell with fever, urgent IV antibiotics are recommended. Admit and obtain opinion from an ophthalmologist.

Extension of the infection through the septum or from the ethmoid and frontal sinuses can lead to orbital, or postseptal, cellulitis. This is much more serious and threatens vision and, in severe cases, life. The rare complication of cavernous sinus thrombosis from spreading infection must be prevented. If the lids are so swollen that the eye cannot be examined, it must be assumed that the postseptal orbit is involved, and the child should be referred as soon as possible. Organisms are usually streptococci or staphylococci, although *Haemophilus influenzae* used to be a common cause prior to vaccination.

In orbital cellulitis, examine the eye for visual acuity, and pupil motility with the swinging torch, looking for a relative afferent pupil defect (RAPD). A RAPD is seen if the optic nerve is compromised and the pupil paradoxically dilates upon shining the light at it in a swinging fashion from one eye to the other. If possible, check colour vision and red desaturation in patients suspected of orbital disease. In such patients, a CT or MRI scan must be obtained by the admitting hospital team and, if this demonstrates a focal collection of pus within the orbit that threatens the optic nerve, this must be surgically drained (usually by nasal endoscopy).

Rarely a rhabdomyosarcoma can present in a child of any age (although more common in 7–9 year old boys) with a red, *rapidly* swollen, proptotic eye, but the skin is *not* hot or tender to touch, as it is in cellulitis. This requires an extremely urgent ophthalmology referral.

Ophthalmia neonatorum

This consists of conjunctivitis within the first month of life, and is a *notifiable disease*. It is associated with maternal genitourinary infection, therefore making referral of both parents to the genitourinary medicine clinic essential. Causative agents include *Chlamydia trachomatis*, herpes simplex, gonococcus, *E. coli*, *Haemophilus* and *Staph. aureus*, and is rarely due to a chemical irritant (e.g. silver nitrate).

- *Gonococcal disease* is particularly hazardous and produces a very purulent discharge between 2 and 4 days of life with marked lid swelling, a haemorrhagic conjunctivitis and pseudomembranes. These peel away from the conjunctiva without excessive bleeding as the epithelium beneath is intact. Treatment is with admission and systemic antibiotics (IV cefotaxime). Frequent cleansing of the eyes to remove the pus is not to be overlooked. Urgent Gram stain of the negative intracellular diplococci is helpful.
- *Chlamydial disease* is the most common cause and presents later (5–14 days) with a more watery mucopurulent discharge. Systemic treatment with erythromycin (25 mg/kg b.d. for 4 weeks) should be given to prevent pneumonitis. Giant follicular conjunctivitis is seen in patients older than 3 months. (In the sexually active young adult, referral to the genitourinary medicine clinic is necessary, and systemic tetracycline is usually safe and effective.)
- *Herpes simplex* causes a non-purulent blepharoconjunctivitis and can lead to keratitis (corneal involvement). An IV antiviral is usually required. (Skin herpetic vesicles are usually seen on the eyelid and, in the non-pyrexial, older child, topical aciclovir five times daily with oral treatment for 1 week is usually sufficient.)
- *E. coli* and *Staph. aureus* infections typically present after 4 days, are less aggressive and can be treated with topical antibiotics.

ALERTS

A child with pyrexia and a sticky eye may have a more serious orbital infection and requires hospital evaluation if suspected. Refer to local ophthalmologist if in any doubt.

Remember neonatal conjunctivitis is a notifiable disease and care should involve the ophthalmologist.

Corneal involvement – ask for specialist advice.

Orbital cellulitis threatening vision with acuity/RAPD, and colour vision.

Spreading facial cellulitis.

In the acutely swollen proptosed red eye, exclude rhabdomyosarcoma.

Congenital glaucoma in the watery eye.

WHO TO TALK TO

(Paediatric) Ophthalmologist.

WHEN TO REFER

Although it is simple to manage a sticky eye, it is strongly recommended that if symptoms persist despite adequate treatment it should be mandatory to take advice from a specialist or refer the patient to hospital.

If the child has pyrexia, or any other sign of complication, it is best to seek advice from an ophthalmologist.

THERAPY

Most *bacterial conjunctivitis* can be treated with topical chloramphenicol four times a day. *Viral conjunctivitis* requires only supportive measures such as artificial tears and cool compresses. *Allergic conjunctivitis* will require topical antihistamines or mast cell stabilisers at least twice daily and oral antihistamines should be considered.

Systemic antibiotics are indicated if the child has a temperature and/or a cellulitis.

In an apyrexial child with *preseptal cellulitis* a 1-week course of oral co-amoxiclav is appropriate. If sinusitis is suspected the dose may be doubled. The child must be followed up daily until there is definite clinical improvement. If the child has a temperature, or is unwell, IV antibiotics and hospital admission are usually required.

Blepharitis is chronic and requires daily lid hygiene for many months. Patients should be advised to use a hot flannel over their eyes for 10 minutes and warm compresses of the eyelids followed by scrubs with either baby shampoo solution (1 part shampoo to 10 parts water) or eye care lid tissues. Chloramphenicol ointment at night, to the eyelash base, is indicated if staphylococcal infection is suspected (indicated by the presence of scales at lash bases).

FOLLOW-UP

Where possible, all patients should be asked to return if symptoms do not improve. Treated bacterial conjunctivitis should be clear by day 5 and viral conjunctivitis may take up to 3 weeks. Any sticky eye that does not respond adequately to treatment requires tertiary evaluation.

KEY POINTS FOR PARENTS

Conjunctivitis is common in children and often self-limiting.

Children can get recurrent styes and chalazions – treatment of any associated blepharitis may be helpful.

Persistent discharge despite adequate treatment needs specialist attention.

In infants under 1 year, a chronic, unilateral, watery discharge is usually due to a non-patent nasolacrimal duct and the vast majority of these spontaneously become patent by the child's first birthday. Vision and ocular development are unaffected.

HEALTH PROMOTION

Conjunctivitis is often self-limiting but can be contagious. Washing hands and avoiding contaminated towels help to prevent spread to the other eye and to other individuals.

Children with bacterial conjunctivitis are contagious and should be excluded from school until the discharge resolves.

Children with viral conjunctivitis are highly contagious and should be excluded from school until the discharge stops and the conjunctiva is white again.

Symptomatic treatment with lubricants may be helpful in patients with allergens.

Warm compresses are helpful to stabilise the tear film and improve comfort in blepharitis-related conditions.

Antibiotics are not useful in resolving non-infected chalazions.

Topical short-term (i.e. for 2 months or less) chloramphenicol is safe and any irritation from it is usually preservative related.

SOURCES

Ophthalmology Teaching Website, University of Toronto – http://eyelearn.med.utoronto.ca

Sheldrick JH, Wilson AD, Vernon SA, Sheldrick CM (1993) Management of ophthalmic disease in general practice. British Journal of General Practice 43: 459–462

Taylor D, Hoyt C (2004) Paediatric ophthalmology and strabismus, 3rd edn. London: Saunders

See also

Chapter 42, Problems with vision; Chapter 44, Sore eyes.

44

SORE EYES

EPIDEMIOLOGY AND AETIOLOGY

In nearly all cases of a sore eye, the eye will be more red than usual. The exception to this is optic neuritis, where the inflammation is usually behind the optic disc and the anterior segment appears normal. In optic nerve disease there is also visual loss (see Chapter 42). It is not uncommon for sinusitis and toothache (the maxillary nerve also supplies the upper jaw) to present with peri-orbital pain.

A red eye is a sign of ocular inflammation and is caused by dilatation of blood vessels in the eye.

Diagnosis may be aided by the differentiation between ciliary and conjunctival injection:

- Ciliary injection involves branches of the anterior ciliary arteries and indicates inflammation of the cornea, iris or ciliary body. The redness is more prominent around the cornea (the limbal area) and the patient is more likely to complain of photophobia.
- Conjunctival injection mainly affects the posterior conjunctival blood vessels. Because these vessels are more superficial than the ciliary arteries, they produce more redness, move with the conjunctiva and constrict with topical vasoconstrictors such as phenylephrine.

PRESENTATION

As above, but may also have other symptoms or signs such as redness, photophobia (dislike of bright lights), blurred or reduced vision, discharge, epiphora (watery eye) and ptosis (due to eyelid swelling).

ASSESSMENT

History

History should explore following areas:

- Duration, discharge, photophobia.
- Recurrence, uni- or bilateral (together or separately?).
- Trauma or foreign body?

- Previous ophthalmic history and contact lens use.
- General well-being with temperature, atopy; enquire about other family members.
- In neonates, delivery details are essential.

Examination

Look at the distribution of any vascular injection of the conjunctiva. Using the direct ophthalmoscope set on high plus lens (+15 or more), a magnified view of the cornea and anterior chamber can be obtained.

Fluorescein staining of the cornea should be determined in all cases of a red sore eye, especially with visual loss or trauma (see 'Diagnostic tests', below). This simple test clearly highlights any epithelial defects, which can have substantial consequences to the vision. The absence of staining should reassure the GP that a corneal ulcer has been excluded.

Optic nerve examination – visual acuity, relative afferent pupil defect (RAPD), fields and colour vision – should be performed in cases of orbital cellulitis or optic neuritis, and is helpful in cases of trauma. A RAPD is seen early in optic nerve disease and can be looked for using a swinging light from eye to eye. Paradoxical pupil dilatation upon light shining into that eye indicates nerve damage.

Diagnostic tests

Fluorescein staining of the cornea with cobalt blue light (found on most ophthalmoscopes) allows removal of excess with repeated blinking and examination under the blue light. A drop of local anaesthetic may facilitate examination but should not be used in the long term in cases of corneal abrasion as it delays epithelial healing.

Photophobia is usually a more prominent feature in cases of keratitis (corneal inflammation), uveitis or intraocular inflammation.

Preauricular (non-tender) lymph nodes in viral conjunctivitis.

DIFFERENTIAL DIAGNOSIS

Conjunctivitis
Lid disease
Preseptal cellulitis
Trauma and subconjunctival haemorrhage
Uveitis
Episcleritis and scleritis
Phlyctenulosis

Conjunctivitis, lid disease, preseptal cellulitis
See Chapter 43, Sticky eye.

Trauma and subconjunctival haemorrhage
Any child with a history of trauma requires a detailed examination, particularly if visual acuity cannot be assessed (too young or in pain).

If there is any doubt, a prompt referral to the ophthalmologist is appropriate.

A subconjunctival haemorrhage is benign and resolves without treatment within 2 weeks. It is important to ensure that there are no associated deeper injuries.

Uveitis (iritis)

Usually presents with a painful, photophobic, red eye. There may be associated epiphora. Magnified examination of the anterior chamber may reveal inflammatory cells. This requires an ophthalmologist's opinion and a referral should be made the same day.

The inflammation responds well to steroid drops (with the child being closely monitored by the ophthalmologist) and cyclopentolate (to diminish the photophobia and make the child more comfortable).

Episcleritis and scleritis

Inflammation of the outer sclera and conjunctiva (episcleritis) is common and presents with a sore eye that has a *segmented* area of redness. In contrast to conjunctivitis there is no discharge (although some may have increased tearing) and the conjunctiva is normal in the unaffected areas (unlike conjunctivitis when it is diffusely involved). It is a benign condition, and treatment with artificial tears and/or non-steroidal anti-inflammatory drops for 1 week is usually sufficient.

Scleritis is more aggressive with pain (particularly at night) and, if anterior, the eye will be pink/red. It requires referral to a paediatric ophthalmologist.

Phlyctenulosis

A non-specific delayed hypersensitivity reaction to bacterial (usually staphylococcal) antigens, phlyctenulosis presents with a photophobic eye and a white nodule surrounded by an area of hyperaemia. Treatment is with steroid eye drops and lid hygiene for any associated blepharitis.

ALERTS

⚠ A child with pyrexia and a sore eye may have a more serious orbital infection and requires hospital evaluation if suspected. Remember neonatal conjunctivitis is a notifiable disease and care should involve the ophthalmologist.

If the cornea is involved, specialist advice should be sought.

Watch out for the following:
- Corneal involvement – ask for specialist advice.
- Orbital cellulitis threatening vision with acuity/RAPD, and colour vision.
- Never treat with steroid eye drops without consulting an ophthalmologist and ensure the child has regular hospital follow-up.

WHO TO TALK TO

(Paediatric) Ophthalmologist.

WHEN TO REFER

If symptoms persist despite adequate treatment it should be mandatory to take advice from a specialist or refer the patient to the local eye service.

Children with a history of collagen vascular disease are more likely to get eye involvement and there should be a low threshold to refer such children, especially as uveitis can be asymptomatic.

An ophthalmologist should evaluate any corneal fluorescein staining.

In cases of trauma always seek advice.

THERAPY

Most *bacterial conjunctivitis* can be treated with topical chloramphenicol four times a day. *Viral conjunctivitis* requires only supportive measures such as artificial tears and cool compresses. *Allergic conjunctivitis* will require topical antihistamines or mast cell stabilisers at least twice daily. Systemic antibiotics are indicated if the child has a temperature and/or a cellulitis.

Blepharitis is chronic and requires daily lid hygiene for many months. Patients should be advised to use a hot flannel over their eyes for 10 minutes and warm compresses of the eyelids followed by scrubs with either baby shampoo solution (1 part shampoo to 10 parts water) or eye care lid tissues. Chloramphenicol ointment is indicated if staphylococcal infection is suspected (presence of scales at lash bases).

Uveitis requires dampening of the inflammation with the use of steroid eye drops in most cases. These should be used only under the supervision of an ophthalmologist who will usually tail the drops off slowly to avoid a rebound inflammation. Photophobia occurs when the iris and uveal tissue are inflamed, and 1% cyclopentolate is helpful in minimising discomfort.

FOLLOW-UP

All patients should be followed up until they are asymptomatic.

Occasionally a child is put on long-term steroid eye drops by the ophthalmologist. The child will need regular monitoring in the eye clinic and this should be encouraged.

KEY POINTS FOR PARENTS

Conjunctivitis is common in children. It is often a self-limiting condition affecting the outer skin layer of the eye only.

Children can get recurrent styes and chalazions – treatment of any associated blepharitis may be helpful.

Steroid eye drops have unpleasant side effects (glaucoma, cataracts) so the child must be monitored in the eye clinic. You can advise the parents to, if possible, place a clean finger over the lower punctum (for 5 minutes) after instilling the drops to minimise systemic absorption.

HEALTH PROMOTION

Conjunctivitis is often self-limiting but can be contagious. Washing hands and avoiding contaminated towels help to prevent spread to the other eye and to other individuals.

Symptomatic treatment with lubricants may be helpful in patients with allergens.

Warm compresses are helpful to stabilise the tear film and improve comfort in blepharitis-related conditions.

SOURCES

Sheldrick JH, Wilson AD, Vernon SA, Sheldrick CM (1993) Management of ophthalmic disease in general practice. British Journal of General Practice 43: 459–462

Taylor D, Hoyt C (2004) Paediatric ophthalmology and strabismus, 3rd edn. London: Saunders

See also

Chapter 42, Problems with vision; Chapter 43, Sticky eyes.

5

45

RUNNY NOSE

Runny nose (rhinorrhoea) is a common paediatric symptom. It is often self-limiting and warrants no treatment except some good nasal hygiene measures.

It is frequently seen with upper respiratory tract infections (URTI).

Nasal mucosal allergy is a common cause of rhinorrhoea in children, which often remains undiagnosed and undertreated.

Other causes of runny nose include non-allergic rhinitis with eosinophilia (NARES), vasomotor rhinitis, bacterial rhinosinusitis, nasal foreign body, CSF rhinorrhoea, choanal atresia, and encephalocele and mucociliary dysfunction.

ASSESSMENT

History

The areas outlined in Box 45.1 should be explored.

Examination

Look for unilateral or bilateral rhinorrhoea, its colour and physical quality.

Presence of midfacial tenderness, oedema, orbital cellulitis and pyrexia need urgent specialist attention.

Nasal mucosal oedema, congestion, inferior turbinate hypertrophy, septal deviation, foreign body or any sign of trauma should be noted.

The throat and ears should be examined for completion.

Itchy nose, runny nose, nasal obstruction and sneezing bouts are suggestive of nasal mucosal allergy. They can present with itchy eyes as in hay fever.

Diagnostic tests

Microbiology culture and sensitivity – for bacterial rhinosinusitis, if persistent and recurrent.

FBC, RAST, skin prick tests, serum IgE and IgA – for allergy, immune deficiency (may be done by some primary care physicians in the community or may require referral to an allergy clinic).

BOX 45.1 Factors in the history of runny nose

- Duration
- Episodic
- Precipitating factors
- Itchiness
- Sneezing
- Nasal blockage
- Olfaction
- Orbital and facial signs
- Trauma
- Asthma
- Eczema
- Atopy
- Immunological disorder

Cause
- Unilateral – foreign body, structural obstruction, CSF leak, sinusitis
- Bilateral – URTI, sinusitis, allergy, NARES, vasomotor rhinitis

Type of discharge
- Watery/mucoid – allergy, vasomotor rhinitis
- Bloody – trauma, bleeding disorder, neoplasm
- Mucopurulent – bacterial infection, foreign body
- Serosanguineous – neoplasm

5

Tests done in the hospital setting
- Coronal CT scan of paranasal sinuses – for sinusitis, orbital cellulitis.
- β_2 Transferrin – for CSF rhinorrhoea.
- Plain x-ray – for metallic foreign body not seen on physical examination.
- Sweat test – in any child with a nasal polyp to exclude cystic fibrosis.
- Ciliary motility – for Kartagener's syndrome.

DIFFERENTIAL DIAGNOSIS

Common
- URTI
- Allergic rhinitis (seasonal/perennial)
- Foreign body (persistent unilateral runny nose)

Uncommon
- CSF rhinorrhoea (traumatic/congenital)
- Choanal atresia
- Encephalocele
- Neoplasia

ALERTS

⚠️
- Unilateral rhinorrhoea
- Copious watery discharge
- Bloody or serosanguineous discharge
- Orbital cellulitis
- CSF leak
- Midfacial pain
- Retro-orbital pain
- Purulent rhinorrhoea unresponsive to oral antibiotics lasting longer than 10 days

WHEN TO REFER

If in doubt seek otolaryngology advice.

Children manifesting serious signs – i.e. acute rhinosinusitis, orbital cellulitis, retro-orbital pain, visual disturbance, headache, high fever, CSF rhinorrhoea, underlying rare systemic disease or suspected neoplasm – should be referred urgently.

THERAPY (Box 45.2)

Education of parents and patients should be a top priority.
Advice on simple nasal hygiene can produce significant benefit.

BOX 45.2 Therapy for runny nose

Prophylaxis (sprays and drops)
- Beclometasone dipropionate
- Budesonide
- Fluticasone propionate
- Mometasone furoate
- Sodium cromoglicate
(Note: Once daily dose)

Symptomatic
- Ipratropium bromide
- Topical antihistamine – azelastine, levocabastine
- Oral antihistamine – cetirizine, desloratadine, levocetirizine
(Note: Avoid sedating antihistamine)

Immunotherapy
- Specific immunotherapy (STA), only in specialist centres

Non-drug treatment
- Normal saline used as nasal wash

Recurrent symptoms of troublesome rhinorrhoea can be controlled with ipratropium bromide (0.03% strength).

Antihistamine and steroid sprays are useful in allergic rhinitis.

Bacterial rhinosinusitis should be treated with culture-derived antibiotics. Co-amoxiclav or erythromycin is a good choice in the absence of bacterial culture, provided there is no previous allergy.

Non-sedating antihistamines (cetirizine hydrochloride or levocetirizine dihydrochloride) are good at controlling symptoms of allergy.

Topical corticosteroids are used mainly for treatment in moderate to severe allergic rhinitis (persistent symptoms >4 weeks, abnormal sleep, problems at school, impairment of daily activities). Special consideration should be given to children receiving steroids in more than one form and in cases of established allergy to steroids.

FOLLOW-UP

Regular follow-up in the community is highly recommended (symptoms lasting >4 weeks) to reduce any chance of undertreatment and missed diagnosis.

KEY POINTS FOR PARENTS

Runny nose is often a self-limiting symptom; persistence warrants accurate diagnosis.

Early identification of signs of potential complications, i.e. orbital and intracranial involvement, will prevent serious morbidities.

Unilateral rhinorrhoea should always be a cause for concern.

HEALTH PROMOTION

Runny nose is common in children and is often harmless. Simple nasal hygiene measures can significantly improve quality of life in patients and produce enormous benefit.

Identification and avoidance of allergen are very effective measures.

Nasal steroid sprays can have systemic side effects, especially if taken simultaneously with other steroid medications.

SUPPORT ORGANISATIONS

British Association of Otorhinolaryngologists – www.entuk.org

46

SORE THROAT AND MOUTH

Sore throat and mouth are usually due to inflammatory or infective causes.

PHARYNGITIS

Pharyngitis (inflammation of the mucosal lining of any part of the pharynx) is more common during cold winter months. It has higher propensity in children above the age of 6 months and is more common in children who go to nursery.

In a healthy child, URTI with or without associated pharyngitis up to eight times a year is considered as a normal range (sore throat, painful swallowing, low grade pyrexia, malaise; usually resolves without antibiotic treatment within a week).

ADENOTONSILLITIS

This is usually of acute onset and of viral aetiology and is treated symptomatically.

Bacterial tonsillitis usually has severe symptoms and requires treatment with antibiotics. Patients will present with dysphagia (difficulty swallowing), odynophagia (pain on swallowing), dysphonia (hoarse voice), pyrexia, dehydration and halitosis (combination of these symptoms if persistent antibiotic treatment will help).

Most cases of tonsillitis and other oropharyngeal infections can be treated effectively within the community but, if undertreated, can lead to various complications, i.e. peritonsillar abscess, parapharyngeal or retropharyngeal abscess, septicaemia, meningitis, acute rheumatic fever and acute glomerulonephritis. Therefore, if bacterial infection is suspected, the child should be treated with antibiotics.

Glandular fever (infectious mononucleosis) is caused by the Epstein–Barr virus (EBV) and is often characterised by generalised cervical lymphadenopathy and tonsillitis.

EPIGLOTTITIS

Epiglottitis, by *Haemophilus influenzae* type B species of bacteria, can be fatal without urgent airway management and vigorous treatment. Although not seen as frequently following the introduction of the Hib vaccine, it still exists and clinicians must always be alert and recognise its symptoms.

It is more common in children between the ages of 2 and 4 years. The onset is often fast (2–6 hours) and the child will typically present with high fever, drooling, sitting in an upright position and having difficulty on inspiration.

No attempt should be made to examine the throat unless there are measures available to secure the airway (i.e. in the hospital environment). These patients warrant urgent hospital transfer.

SORE MOUTH

This is usually caused by dental pathology and ulcerative disorders (e.g. aphthous or herpetic ulcers) with mucosal erosions and ulcerations. Most oral ulcerations are of viral origin and therefore only need symptomatic treatment.

Benzydamine hydrochloride (Difflam) mouthwash is good in temporary control of pain. Local anaesthetic lozenges (benzocaine, lidocaine) may be helpful. Chlorhexidine gluconate (Corsodyl) mouthwash prevents secondary bacterial infection and, therefore, minimises pain.

Children with primary or secondary immunodeficiency are more prone to develop sore throat and mouth.

ASSESSMENT
History
Onset
Duration
Progress
Previous episode
Dysphagia
Odynophagia
Dysphonia
Dehydration
High pyrexia
Halitosis
Malaise/lassitude

Diagnostic tests

In most cases seen in primary care no investigations will be required. However, some very basic baseline tests are useful:

- Baseline tests: FBC (neutrophilic leucocytosis indicates bacterial infection).
- Monospot test (diagnostic for glandular fever), swab and culture (may be performed in primary care).

DIFFERENTIAL DIAGNOSIS

Viral/bacterial tonsillitis
Pharyngitis
Epiglottitis
Pharyngeal space abscess
Herpetic and aphthous oral ulcerations
Dentoalveolar infections (acute periodontitis, dental abscess, etc.)

ALERTS

Acute oropharyngeal infections can endanger the airway, e.g. children presenting with shortness of breath, stertor (snoring noise of upper airway obstruction) or stridor (harsh noise on inspiration and/or expiration due to glottic or subglottic narrowing or obstruction). In children, physiological decompensation takes place fast and therefore needs prompt action.

Many systemic diseases manifest in the oral cavity with mucosal changes, i.e. ulceration, erosion, bulla and change in colour. It is important to look for the underlying cause.

Undertreated/untreated tonsillitis can have serious complications – if there is a suspicion of bacterial tonsillitis it should be treated with antibiotics.

WHEN TO REFER

Most cases are managed in the community and are treated symptomatically. All children with local and systemic complications should be referred.

Any sign (dysphonia, stertor, stridor, tired child and reduced breath sounds) of potential airway compromise should be picked up early and the child referred to an otolaryngologist.

Children with recurrent oral ulceration and/or persistent sore mouth will benefit from seeing an oral medicine/oral pathology consultant.

THERAPY

Corsodyl mouth wash, Difflam spray, appropriate oral antibiotics (co-amoxiclav, erythromycin) can be used as required by the individual case, in the community setting.

FOLLOW-UP

Every patient should be followed up until a diagnosis is made or hospital referral has been arranged.

KEY POINTS FOR PARENTS

Most cases of sore throat and mouth are self-limiting and symptomatic treatment will often suffice.

Any child with unresolved sore throat despite adequate treatment needs specialist attention.

Potential cases of airway compromise and rare serious disease will not be missed if one is vigilant.

SUPPORT ORGANISATIONS

British Association of Otorhinolaryngologists – www.entuk.org
British Dental Health Foundation – www.dentalhealth.org.uk

5

47

EARACHE

Earache is a very common symptom in children. This can often be transient with spontaneous recovery. *Acute otitis media following upper respiratory tract infection (URTI) and Eustachian tube dysfunction are more common types of ear pathology.*

Children presenting with otalgia (pain in the ear) require complete assessment and management of pain based on a working diagnosis. Examination of the pinna, the peri-auricular area, external auditory canal and tympanic membrane (TM) should help to establish any otological cause of otalgia. *In the presence of a normal ear, complete head and neck examination is mandatory.*

Referred otalgia is a not uncommon presentation. Commonest cause of referred otalgia in children is tonsillitis.

ASSESSMENT

History

History should explore the following areas:

Duration
Recurrence
URTI
Nasal obstruction
Rhinitis
Sinusitis
Trauma
Painful swallowing
Pyrexia
Otorrhoea
Deafness
ENT surgery, i.e. grommet
Foreign body

Examination
Complete examination of the ear, nose and throat is essential.
Diagnosis can be often achieved based on history, but examination is still
necessary.

Diagnostic tests
In recurrent otalgia without obvious physical sign, consider hearing test
and tympanogram.
Take microbiology swab for culture and sensitivity in the presence of
otorrhoea.

DIFFERENTIAL DIAGNOSIS
See Table 47.1.

Table 47.1   Differential diagnosis of earache

Otological causes	Non-otological causes
Acute otitis media with effusion	URTI
Chronic otitis media with acute exacerbation	Tonsillitis
Otitis externa	Dental pathology
Eustachian tube dysfunction	Recurrent oral ulceration
Perichondritis	Glandular fever
Furunculosis	Sialadenitis
Acute mastoiditis	Rhinitis/sinusitis
Herpes zoster	Post-tonsillectomy
	Temporomandibular joint pain
	Rare: Nasopharyngeal tumour

5

ALERTS

Complications of otitis media can be potentially life
threatening.
Otalgia with otorrhoea should be treated until healthy tympanic
membrane is seen and the patient is asymptomatic.
Clinicians should have very low thresholds for referral to a
paediatric otolaryngologist.
Watch out for the following complications:

- Acute mastoiditis
- Spreading facial cellulitis
- Facial paralysis
- Intracranial complications, e.g. meningitis

Remember that some patients may present primarily with any of
these complications if acute otitis media has not been treated
adequately.

WHEN TO REFER

If symptoms persist despite adequate treatment it should be mandatory to take advice from a specialist or consider hospital referral.

If the child has high grade pyrexia, headache, cranial nerve involvement and drowsiness, consider urgent ENT review.

THERAPY

Some middle ear infections will resolve spontaneously. However, persistent middle ear infection with earache (>1 week) will resolve faster with a short course of antibiotic.

If there is otorrhoea indicating TM perforation, ear drops (antibiotic + steroid, e.g. dexamethasone) are much more effective.

Otitis externa is rare in younger children. It is best treated with aural toilet and ear dressings when unresponsive to ear drops.

All patients should be advised to keep their ears dry.

Pain, in these conditions, can be controlled with paracetamol, ibuprofen or codeine.

FOLLOW-UP

All patients should be followed up until they are asymptomatic and ENT examination is normal.

KEY POINTS FOR PARENTS

Earache is common in children and often self-limiting.

Children can get earache from other common diseases of the nose and throat.

Persistent earache despite adequate treatment needs specialist attention.

Earache with discharge, fever, headache and drowsiness needs urgent specialist attention at the hospital.

KEY POINTS FOR CLINICIANS

Earache is often self-limiting.

Symptomatic treatment with NSAIDs will usually suffice.

Middle ear infection can be treated with oral antibiotics. In the presence of otorrhoea, antibiotic ear drops give better results, e.g. dexamethasone (Sofradex), hydrocortisone (Gentisone), etc.

It is safe to give a short course of ear drops (10 days) in the presence of a perforated TM.

All patients with discharging ears should be followed up until normal TM is seen on examination.

Early discussion with an ENT specialist or referral is highly recommended if symptoms persist or complications develop.

SUPPORT ORGANISATIONS

British Association of Otorhinolaryngologists – www.entuk.org

48

PROBLEMS WITH DENTAL AND FACIAL SWELLINGS

Orofacial swellings in children are frequently of dental origin and inflammatory in nature. Epidermoid, dermoid, odontogenic and non-odontogenic cysts form another important category.

Good history taking and thorough examination of the oral cavity and face are essential.

Diagnosis is often made without any special tests. Uncommon things are rare but should always be borne in mind.

ASSESSMENT

It is important to do a thorough examination of the oral cavity, oropharynx, head and neck. Good history will often lead to a diagnosis.

All patients with swellings on the neck or face should have their oral cavity examined

History
Chronological
Surface – colour, texture
Size/site/shape
Pain before or after appearance of swelling
Painless (these swellings are often non-inflammatory)
Discharge
Change in size (slow/fast)
Tenderness
Fluctuant
Consistency
Number
Recurrent
Past medical history – systemic disease, drugs, trauma

Examination
Signs to look for include:

- orbital complications (cellulitis) of sinusitis – need urgent coronal CT scan of paranasal sinuses in a hospital setting

- any swelling persisting for more than 2 weeks without any sign of resolution.

Note: Most diagnoses can be made with a good history and thorough examination.

Sites of dental and facial swellings are outlined in Box 48.1.

BOX 48.1 Sites of dental and facial swellings

Dental swellings
- Floor of the mouth – mucocele, ranula, abscess, haemangioma, lymphangioma, torus mandibularis
- Cheek – bite, parotid papilla, haemangioma, fibroepithelial polyp, mucocele
- Palate – unerrupted tooth, cysts, torus palatinus, uvular swelling (viral URTI)
- Periodontium (gum) – abscess, cysts, unerrupted tooth, phenytoin/ciclosporin hypertrophy
- Tongue – angioedema, haemangioma, lymphangioma, fibrous epulis
- Oropharynx – tonsils (hypertrophy, inflammation, infection, retention cyst), retropharyngeal abscess

Facial swellings
- Skin – epidermoid and dermoid cysts
- Lips – haemangioma, lymphangioma, angioedema, mucocele, herpetic stomatitis
- Midface – peri-apical abscess (upper canine), odontogenic/non-odontogenic cysts, fibrous dysplasia
- Eyelids – orbital cellulitis, meibomian cyst (chalazion), dacrocystitis (medial canthus), haematoma
- Nose – dermoid cyst (on nasal bridge)
- Forehead – osteoma, frontal sinusitis, sebaceous cyst
- Preauricular – parotid pathology (mumps), sebaceous cyst, infected preauricular sinus
- Pinna – perichondritis, haematoma, chondrodermatitis, cysts

ALERTS

⚠️ Any swelling on the face of acute onset with systemic illness, not resolving with antibiotic treatment, needs specialist advice.

Suspected inflammatory swelling persisting for more than 1 week after adequate treatment needs specialist review.

Remember that oropharyngeal swelling, e.g. tonsillitis with complications, can endanger the airway.

Retropharyngeal abscess following oropharyngeal infection or trauma is associated with dysphagia. This condition is rare but must not be missed.

Swelling of the floor of the mouth, e.g. large dental abscess, can also complicate the airway.

Orbital cellulitis from rhinosinusitis is a medical emergency as it can cause loss of vision, and therefore warrants urgent ENT/Ophthalmology referral.

WHEN TO REFER

Inflammatory swelling persisting after adequate observation and treatment (1 week).

Periorbital cellulitis (urgent referral) – only those following rhinosinusitis.

Needs special investigations, i.e. CT, MRI, endoscope.

Needs dental treatment.

Vision/airway compromise.

If in doubt and unable to make a working diagnosis.

THERAPY

Most inflammatory and infective conditions respond to NSAIDs and oral antibiotics, e.g. co-amoxiclav (Augmentin), erythromycin (if required). *Any other form of medical treatment should be provided by the specialist after an accurate diagnosis.*

In potential airway compromise, slow IV dexamethasone can be life saving along with basic airway management.

Do not attempt to treat orbital cellulitis in the community setting.

FOLLOW-UP

All patients should be followed up until cured or referral has been made.

5

HEALTH PROMOTION

Treatment of dental pathology provides an excellent opportunity to teach children oral hygiene measures.

All patients with oral and dental pathology should be strongly advised to see their dental practitioner regularly; this will prevent recurrence of some problems.

SUPPORT ORGANISATIONS

British Association of Otorhinolaryngologists – www.entuk.org
British Dental Health Foundation – www.dentalhealth.org.uk

49

HEADACHE

DEFINITION

Idiopathic headache is a pain disorder: the pain and associated features are not due to an underlying disease.

Pain is an unpleasant sensory and emotional experience associated with actual or potential tissue damage or described in terms of such damage.
International Association for the Study of Pain (Merskey 1979).

The International Headache Society has published operational diagnostic criteria for migraine and tension-type headaches (which lie on the spectrum of idiopathic headaches).

EPIDEMIOLOGY AND AETIOLOGY

All children have occasional headaches.

Sometimes headache is a way of communicating distress (see definition of pain above).

About 10% of prepubertal children have had migraine, rising to 20% of female adolescents. Family history is common but of no diagnostic use.

Symptomatic headache is usually due to an obvious cause, e.g. an upper respiratory tract infection or head injury.

A serious potentially treatable cause, e.g. a brain tumour, may be expected in 1% of referrals to hospital clinics and in 10% of Emergency Department presentations. These cases usually have warning symptoms and signs.

PRESENTATION

Think what it is that leads this family to present at this time with these headaches:

- How are they impacting on the child's and the family's activities and participation?
- What family health experiences and beliefs frame the presentation, e.g. a close family history of brain tumour or cerebral aneurysm?

- Is there anything happening in the school or home environment that needs to be taken into consideration?

ASSESSMENT

History
Ask about:

- the pain (site, severity), associated features (e.g. difficulty with balance, vomiting, collapse), impact
- stress, especially at school, at home, with hobbies
- past medical history
- drug history
- migraine aura symptoms, e.g. affecting vision, and how long these last
- triggering factors, e.g. particular food types.

Severity
Migraine tension-type headache spectrum can be graded by impairment:

- *Mild*: Continues with normal activities.
- *Moderate*: Reduces activity/exertion.
- *Severe*: Unable to do anything except lie still and quiet or sleep.

Warning symptoms
Single/first severe headache ('first and worse').
Accelerating course – every few months, then weeks, then days.
Change in usual headache for worse over weeks or days.
Mainly from sleep or awakening.
Worse lying down, bending over or coughing.
Vomiting from sleep or awakening.
Confusion or personality change.

Examination
Measure BP and head circumference (plot on centile chart).
Look in fundi, look for a new focal neurological deficit, e.g. of cranial nerves or head tilt, ataxia, gait abnormality.
Look for signs of intercurrent illness – fever, upper respiratory tract infection, sinusitis (percussion).

Warning signs
Confusion or personality change
Large head circumference
Papilloedema
VI nerve palsy
Head tilt
Head nodding
Cerebellar ataxia
Focal neurological deficit

DIAGNOSIS

Helped by prospective headache diary:

- Migraine/migranous features:
  - paroxysmal, well in between
  - 1–48 hours
  - unilateral or bilateral: frontal/temporal
  - banging or pulsating
  - moderate or severe
  - worse with routine exertion
  - nausea or vomiting or photo-/phonophobia
- Episodic tension-type headache features:
  - <15/month
  - 30 minutes to 7 days
  - pressing or tight
  - mild or moderate
  - bilateral
  - not worse with routine exertion
- Chronic daily headache features:
  - ≥15/month
  - analgesia-associated headache (e.g. transformed migraine)
  - chronic tension-type headache (can occur with migraine)
  - new persistent daily headache – consider raised intracranial pressure, carbon monoxide toxicity, other symptomatic headaches, depression, general fatigue.

WHO TO TALK TO

School liaison through school nurse or community paediatrician.

Child headache clinic or programme if available, otherwise general paediatrician in hospital or community setting, or paediatric neurologist, use or develop local pathway.

Sometimes Child and Adolescent Mental Health Services can help.

WHEN TO REFER

Children with warning symptoms and signs, especially in combination.

Treatment failed.

Reassurance failed.

Associated with complex symptoms/impairments, e.g. general fatigue, social or school withdrawal, depression.

> **ALERTS**
>
> ⚠ Urgent brain imaging with CT or MRI will occasionally be indicated by the warning symptoms and signs, especially if in combination, or where reassurance has failed.
> For mild symptoms without warning symptoms, vision should be tested.

THERAPY

Migraine tension-type headache spectrum
- Education, explanation and reassurance.
- Lifestyle advice: ensure adequate
  - rest and relaxation
  - sleep
  - hydration
  - food.
- Identify and address depression or other psychological factors.
- Avoid triggering factors such as particular food types, e.g. chocolate, cheese, bananas.

Rescue medication
- Oral, sublingual/buccal, nasal, rectal, subcutaneous routes.
- Only up to 2 or 3 days/week (to avoid analgesia-associated headache):
  - paracetamol, paracetamol–antiemetic combinations
  - ibuprofen, diclofenac
  - triptans (consider referral to more experienced paediatrician/paediatric neurologist or headache clinic/programme for this).

Daily preventative medication
- Consider for frequent migraine, e.g. ≥4/month, but generally not effective in chronic daily headache:
  - pizotifen
  - beta blockers, e.g. propranolol (avoid with current asthma).
- Consider referral to more experienced paediatrician/paediatric neurologist or headache clinic/programme for other options including antiepileptic drugs, amitriptyline, calcium antagonists.

FOLLOW-UP

Use headache diary.
Empower child/family to take control of migraine or tension-type headache.
Review fairly frequently if diagnosis uncertain.
More support needed for chronic daily headache.
Recommend stick-on carbon monoxide detectors for the boiler.

KEY POINTS FOR PARENTS

Migraine and tension-type headaches are common.
Most patients with headache do not need brain imaging.

HEALTH PROMOTION

Avoid frequent analgesia use if prone to migraine.
See lifestyle advice (above).

SUPPORT ORGANISATIONS

Contact a Family
    209–211 City Road
    London EC1V 1JN
    Tel: 020 7608 8700
    www.cafamily.org.uk

SOURCES

British Association for the Study of Headache – www.bash.org.uk
    A useful evidenced-linked guideline.
Merskey H (1979) Pain terms: a list with definitions and notes on usage
    recommended by the IASP subcommittee on taxonomy. Pain 6: 249–252
The International Headache Society (IHS) – www.i-h-s.org

5

50

SEIZURES AND FUNNY TURNS

DEFINITION

Seizure is a paroxysmal abnormality of motor, sensory, autonomic and/or cognitive function due to transient brain dysfunction.

Mechanisms are syncopal (anoxic), epileptic, brain stem (hydrocephalic, coning), basal ganglia, emotional (psychogenic non-epileptic) or undetermined.

PRESENTATION

Convulsions

- A motor seizure or ictus (attack) with tonic or dystonic spasm (stiffening), clonic or myoclonic (jerking) and/or hypermotor (thrashing) activity.
- Mechanisms are as for seizure (see above).
- Convulsions may be falsely assumed to be epileptic seizures, either from the history or when witnessed, and it should be remembered that convulsive syncope is more common.

Transient loss of consciousness (T-LOC)

- Causes include syncopes (including those due to arrhythmias), epilepsies, hydrocephalic attacks, sleep attacks, various other neurological disorders, emotional attacks and unexplained attacks.

Unresponsive stares

- Causes include epilepsies with absence seizures or focal seizures (complex partial seizures), 'day dreaming', preoccupation/inattention, syncope (rarely).
- Unresponsive stares may be thought as possibly epileptic by teachers but absence seizures are only occasionally picked up this way.

Alarming aggressive outbursts

- These may be suspected of being epileptic seizures but almost never are, although they may be related to ongoing epileptic activity.

Correct diagnosis is especially difficult in children with brain injury, e.g. cerebral palsy, or other neurodevelopmental disorders, or if they have learning difficulties or autistic spectrum disorders.

ASSESSMENT

History

Past medical, developmental, family and social history are important but a witness account of what the child was doing just before, during and after the seizure is the most important.

It is in eliciting and interpreting this history that epilepsy experts differ from less experienced doctors.

Provocation such as venepuncture, standing up having their hair combed or a sudden knock to the back of the head suggests syncope rather than an epileptic seizure.

Examination

A general and neurological examination will be needed but diagnosis is 95% history.

Examine the skin for clues to a neurocutaneous syndrome, measure and plot the head circumference, look in the fundi, look for a focal neurological deficit, observe the gait. Assess the regularity of the pulse (sinus arrhythmia is usually normal), examine the heart and take the BP.

In older children consider a lying and standing BP and pulse (BP should rise slightly on standing, but heart rate should not rise by 30 bpm or more or exceed 120 bpm).

Diagnosis

This can be straightforward but is more often difficult and may not be possible until more seizures have occurred, the history is reviewed or the condition has evolved.

Ictal home video recordings are very helpful, especially when reviewed by an expert.

Diagnostic tests

These can be requested in primary care but this depends on the experience of the clinician.

- A standard ECG for convulsive seizures, e.g. for long QT syndromes.
- A standard EEG is helpful if absence seizures are suspected (has reasonably high sensitivity and specificity for absence epilepsies).
- An EEG is *not helpful* in other situations of diagnostic uncertainty.
- There is a high rate of non-specific abnormalities, and epileptiform discharges will be found in 2–5% of normal children and in 25–75% of children with neurodevelopmental disorders, e.g. autistic spectrum, cerebral palsy.

- Brain imaging, usually requested after referral from primary care (MRI is generally better and safer than CT scan) may be indicated by other clues on history or examination.
- Blood tests: Check a stick test blood glucose if convulsion is ongoing or recent and the child is still postictal. Other bloods may be indicated by other clues. FBC and U&E are indicated for frequent or troublesome T-LOC (transient loss of consciousness).

WHO TO TALK TO

In various settings a false diagnosis of epilepsy has been reported to be between 5 and 40%.

It may be better to have a local network and systematic multidisciplinary approach to children with suspected epilepsies.

The concentration of diagnostic expertise among a smaller number of epilepsy-trained community- and hospital-based paediatricians, linked to a regional centre of expertise, e.g. with paediatric neurologists and paediatric epilepsy clinical nurse specialists, may help.

In children, epilepsy should be diagnosed by a paediatrician with appropriate training, experience and continuing professional development and who is not working in isolation. The referral can then be made from primary care to this paediatrician.

WHEN TO REFER

All children with seizures/funny turns starting in infancy should be referred to a paediatric epilepsy specialist or programme.

Older children where epilepsy or other potentially serious disorders are considered a possibility should also be referred to an appropriate paediatrician or programme.

A clear clinical diagnosis of a sleep disorder may be made in primary care but extreme or unusual cases should be referred.

Older school-aged children with a good history of vasovagal syncope can be managed in primary care, but should be referred if attacks are very frequent or troublesome.

See also
Chapter 52, Syncope.

51

EPILEPTIC SEIZURES AND EPILEPSIES

DEFINITIONS

- *Epileptic seizure*: A paroxysmal abnormality of motor, sensory, autonomic and/or cognitive function due to transient dysfunction of cerebral cortical neuronal electrical activity (typically excessive and/or hypersynchronous), of which there are many clinical, electrical and pathological varieties (see below).
- *Epilepsies*: A group of brain disorders defined by recurrent, unprovoked*, epileptic seizures, which include many categories and syndromes (see below).

Types of clinical seizure (ictal semiology)

- *Motor seizures* include tonic, spasm, dystonic, myoclonic, tonic–clonic and/or atonic.
- *Automatisms* include oro-alimentary, mimetic (e.g. fear), manual/pedal, hyperkinetic, hypokinetic (e.g. as in an unresponsive stare and/or motor arrest), dysphasic, dyspraxic, gelastic and/or interactive.
- *Sensory seizures/auras* include somatosensory, visual, auditory, olfactory, gustatory, epigastric and/or autonomic.
- *Experiential seizures* include affective, mnemonic, hallucinations, illusions, dyscognitive and/or autonomic.

These may all occur in isolation, synchronous combinations and/or in sequence. Motor arrest with an unresponsive stare and no ictal memory may be an absence seizure or a type of complex partial seizure.

*'Unprovoked' excludes from the concept of the epilepsies acute symptomatic epileptic seizures due to injury or insult to a normal brain. Recurrent epileptic seizures triggered by photic stimulation are not normal and constitute a photosensitive epilepsy. Recurrent febrile convulsions constitute a borderline, epilepsy-related syndrome.

Types of electroclinical seizure

These depend on observed or assumed ictal onset EEG.

- *Generalized onset seizures* include absence seizures and primarily generalised tonic–clonic seizures (GTCS).
- *Focal seizures*, usefully designated by (observed or more often assumed) cerebral cortical origin, e.g. Rolandic (facial motor with salivation), temporal lobe, frontal lobe (many clinical patterns).
- *Complex partial seizures* are focal seizures with loss of responsiveness and ictal memory ± motor components ± automatisms.

Epilepsies

Epilepsy types can be categorised, even if an epilepsy syndrome has not yet been diagnosed, including:

- *Idiopathic generalised epilepsies* (brain otherwise normal), e.g. childhood absence epilepsy (CAE), juvenile absence epilepsy, juvenile myoclonic epilepsy (JME), GTCS on awakening.
- *Idiopathic focal epilepsies* (benign partial epilepsies), e.g. benign Rolandic epilepsy (BRE).
- *Epileptic encephalopathies* (includes some symptomatic and 'probably symptomatic' generalised epilepsies), e.g. West syndrome/infantile spasms.
- *Symptomatic focal epilepsies*, typically due to focal cortical structural abnormality, e.g. arising from the mesial temporal lobe due to mesial temporal sclerosis.
- *Febrile convulsions* ('febrile seizures') are an age-related idiopathic 'benign' seizure disorder seen mainly in preschool children, affecting about 3%. Convulsions occur with a rising temperature, often in a previously well child. Associated upper respiratory tract infections are common. 30% have a recurrence but only a few percent later develop recurrent unprovoked afebrile epileptic seizures (epilepsies). The risk is greater if prolonged, focal, repeated within 24 hours: associated with later mesial temporal lobe epilepsies; first convulsion under 6 months or over 5 years, high total number (>3): associated with later generalised epilepsies, e.g. CAE.

EPIDEMIOLOGY AND AETIOLOGY

- *Cumulative incidence*: The risk of experiencing an epileptic seizure is time dependent: 10% of people can be expected to have at least one and 4% to develop an epilepsy if they live to 90 years of age.
- *Incidence*: Proportion of a population developing a new epilepsy each year is highest in early childhood: 150/100,000/year in infants, dropping to 50/100,000/year in teenagers.
- *Point prevalence* of epilepsies rises with age from 3/1000 preschool to 5/1000 in teenagers to 8/1000 (almost 1%) in the total population. Remission and death make the prevalence less than the cumulative incidence.

Idiopathic epilepsies are not due to other diseases: they are mostly due to chance and the interaction of a few susceptibility alleles ('epilepsy genes').

Symptomatic and 'probably symptomatic' epilepsies may also be genetic or partly genetic or acquired, e.g. due to cortical damage or malformation from almost any cause.

As an epilepsy can share the same aetiology in a child as cerebral palsy and/or developmental delay and/or autism, epilepsies are more common in children with these brain disorders.

ASSESSMENT

Diagnostic tests

- *ECG* should be done in all children with convulsions in case convulsive syncope due to a cardiac arrhythmia is the correct diagnosis (see below). An ECG channel should be included in any EEG recordings.
- *EEG* is an essential tool in the categorisation of epilepsies and can diagnose absence seizures. If seizures generally happen in sleep then a sleep EEG may be more informative than a standard awake recording. A 24–48 hour ambulatory EEG includes normal sleep at home and can capture ictal events if they are happening most days. Formal inpatient 5-day video-EEG ('video-telemetry') is very resource costly but can be helpful in more specialist hands.
- *MRI* of the brain is usually not urgent but is needed in all cases apart from those with easy-to-manage, typical idiopathic generalised epilepsies (IGEs), e.g. CAE, JME or BRE.

Ictal video recordings, e.g. at home or school, are always diagnostically helpful.

DIFFERENTIAL DIAGNOSIS

There is a huge differential diagnosis for epileptic seizures with convulsions or unresponsive stares, a few more of which are discussed below.

- *Day dreaming* is a useful term for non-epileptic lapses in concentration and attention with delayed or absent response to a parent's or teacher's vocalization. Children will usually respond to touch and the episodes do not interrupt ongoing function such as talking, chewing, running, etc. Interictal and ictal EEGs show no generalised spike wave.
- *Infantile gratification* (infantile masturbation) typically occurs in preschool or primary school-aged girls who sit and rock rhythmically, eyes glazed over and staring, as if in a world of their own.
- *Emotional attacks* (psychogenic non-epileptic attacks/pseudoseizures/pseudosyncope):
  - Can present with episodes of collapse or swoon or convulsions that may be described in similar terms to syncope or epileptic seizures.

 – May have an epilepsy as well.
 – May have post-traumatic stress disorder or, in many cases, no particular underlying psychiatric disorder.
 – Reassurance, support and a search for stress, e.g. related to specific learning difficulties or peer group dynamics, may be helpful.

WHO TO TALK TO

The diagnosis of epilepsy is difficult and paediatricians should work in networks linked to paediatric epilepsy specialists, specialist nurses and investigative facilities.

WHEN TO REFER

Share difficult cases and, as above, children under 1 year of age with local paediatric epilepsy specialists.

THERAPY

Antiepileptic drug (AED) treatments can be used as rescue treatment, prehospital, by family, carers, ambulance crew, and in hospital for acute epileptic seizures and convulsive status epilepticus.

Rectal diazepam (~0.5 mg/kg) or buccal midazolam (~0.5 mg/kg) are effective.

The family or carers should be taught when and how to use rescue treatment, backed up with written information, if the child is at risk of convulsive status epilepticus.

AEDs can be used intermittently for clusters of seizures, particularly clobazam or acetazolamide.

AEDs can be used short term to reduce the immediate risk of acute symptomatic epileptic seizures, e.g. phenobarbital or phenytoin for acute epileptic seizures with severe acquired brain injury.

Regular AED therapy may be used if the risk of further seizures and their impact or effects merit daily drug treatment, after discussion of treatment goals with the child and family.

It is vital *not* to use carbamazepine, oxcarbazepine, phenytoin, tiagabine or vigabatrin for CAE and similar IGEs as they usually make absence, myoclonic and atonic generalised seizures worse.

Clobazam, lamotrigine, levetiracetam, topiramate and valproate have a broad spectrum; carbamazepine and gabapentin are mainly used for focal epilepsies. Ethosuximide is mainly used for absence seizures.

Choice will be determined by likely benefit and the likelihood and nature of potential adverse effects. These are affected by the age and sex of the child, associated disorders, seizure types, epilepsy syndrome or category and aetiology.

AED doses start low and are built up, if needs be, to maximum tolerated dose or a relatively high dose or plasma concentration.

Typically, at first, we will hope for seizure freedom, in which case the AED can be withdrawn over a few weeks after 1 or 2 years.

About 30% of AEDs are not that effective; other AEDs are introduced and fail; untolerated AEDs are withdrawn.

For basic drug information, see *Medicines for Children* or the *British National Formulary For children.*

The ketogenic diet can be effective and safe for some children with intractable epilepsies, as can vagal nerve stimulation.

Paediatric epilepsy surgery is highly effective in well-selected children, e.g. hemispherectomy or equivalent disconnection works well, with little or no additional impairment in children with hemiplegia and focal epilepsy due to damage or disease restricted to one hemisphere. Temporal lobectomy is also highly effective and well tolerated in selected cases.

Referral for assessment to a paediatric epilepsy surgery programme should be by the treating paediatrician in potentially suitable cases.

FOLLOW-UP

This may be shared with a paediatric epilepsy specialist depending on the case.

Paediatric clinical nurse specialists in epilepsy can also contribute to the child's follow-up.

Visits will be more frequent when seizures are very frequent and troublesome or there are other important medical issues.

Routine blood tests or AED levels are not generally indicated in well children with epilepsies.

KEY POINTS FOR PARENTS

Epilepsies are common, and most patients are otherwise normal.

Most epilepsies respond well to medication.

Intractable epilepsies, especially if symptomatic, are associated or can even cause developmental, learning, emotional and behavioural disabilities.

AEDs are usually well tolerated, but a few people do experience adverse effects.

ALERT

⚠ Combinations of multiple ineffective or only marginally effective AEDs are likely to cause significant adverse effects and should be avoided if possible.

Effective treatment for convulsive generalised epileptic seizures, e.g. longer than 5 or 10 minutes, and convulsive status epilepticus prevents further disability and can be given in the community prehospital.

SUPPORT FOR THE FAMILY

Discuss the aims/goals of investigations, treatments and follow-up with the child and family.

Support the information given with generic written material and individualised copy clinic letters.

Involvement of a clinical nurse specialist will be very helpful, especially in reviewing information and understanding, and liaising with nurseries and schools.

NICE (www.nice.org.uk) and SIGN (www.sign.ac.uk) have developed evidenced-based guidelines for adults and children with epilepsies.

SOURCES

British Medical Association and the Royal Pharmaceutical Society of Great Britain. British National Formulary. London: BMA/RPSGB. Online. Available: www.bnf.org.uk

Royal College of Paediatrics and Child Health and the Neonatal and Paediatric Pharmacists Group (2003) Medicines for Children. London: RCPCH Publications

National Institute for Clinical Excellence (2004) Diagnosis and management of epilepsy in adults and children. London: NICE. Online. Available: www.nice.org.uk

Royal College of Paediatrics and Child Health and the Neonatal and Paediatric Pharmacists Group (2003) Medicines for children. London: RCPCH Publications

Scottish Intercollegiate Guidelines Network (2004) Diagnosis and management of epilepsies in children. Edinburgh: SIGN. Online. Available: www.sign.ac.uk

SYNCOPE

- Often dismissed as trivial.
- Severe syncope can be very distressing and, if frequent, can be handicapping.
- Convulsive syncope can be easily misdiagnosed as an epileptic seizure and, if due to heart disease such as an arrhythmia, e.g. a prolonged QT syndrome, it can be life threatening.

DEFINITIONS

- *Syncope*: Arrest of cortical cerebral activity with loss of consciousness due to transient impairment of cortical and/or brain stem oxygenated blood supply.
- *Neurally mediated syncope* (NMS) or *reflex syncope* results from transient systemic hypotension or circulatory arrest caused by the autonomic nervous system, typically with an increase in parasympathetic vagal activity slowing or stopping the heart for 6–30 seconds, and a reduction in sympathetic activity with consequent vasodilatation and a fall in vascular resistance. The heart, vasculature and autonomic nerves are normal.
- *Vasovagal syncope* is the common, familiar variety of NMS. Investigation and treatment may be indicated if there is diagnostic doubt or the syncopies are severe and frequent or disabling.
- *Reflex asystolic syncope* (RAS), starting in toddlers, is an almost purely vagal variety; it can present with *reflex anoxic seizures*:
  - The young child is surprised, e.g. by a bump to the back of the head, or is upset/frustrated. They stop breathing, go stiff and can jerk. The transient circulatory arrest makes them look dead, grey/white/blue around the lips. After 6–30 seconds they breathe, come round, then usually fall into a postictal sleep. RAS can look like expiratory apnoea syncope (EAS; blue breath-holding spells, see below), bad behaviour, epilepsy and, at the time, sudden death.
  - Information and support can be provided by the support group STARS.

- RAS is not dangerous but can be handicapping if severe and frequent.
- In such cases referral for investigation and therapy to a paediatrician, paediatric neurologist or paediatric cardiologist with an interest locally should be considered.
- *Expiratory apnoea syncope*
  - Being unable to 'catch your breath' (expiratory apnoea, 'breath-holding') is a normal part of crying.
  - In some toddlers this is so marked that reduced venous return, shunting and hypoxia produce syncope and sometimes a reflex anoxic seizure, which can look like RAS.
  - The breath is not held deliberately in inspiration. This is not a sign of a naughty or wilful child or of a weak or anxious parent.
  - This is not dangerous but, if frequent and disabling, RAS or other differential diagnoses should be considered.
- Imposed *upper airway obstruction* is a rare and potentially fatal cause of convulsive syncope that can look like an epileptic seizure in an infant.
- *Prolonged QT syndromes* and other arrhythmias can also produce convulsive syncope easily mistaken for epilepsy. Convulsions or transient loss of consciousness on *exertion* and in *sleep* (associated with a tachycardia) or sudden death can occur.
- *Fainting lark* or 'mess trick' is common in secondary school children and young people. One in a group or in turn will crouch, hyperventilate, then stand up suddenly, inducing a syncope or convulsive syncope.
- *Adolescent stretch syncope* (less common) is self-induced where susceptible people learn to induce syncope by stretching their neck up and back, impeding vertebral artery flow to the brain stem.

Sleep disorders

- *Benign neonatal sleep myoclonus* presents as multifocal or massive generalised jerks in sleeping babies. Ictal (sleep) EEG confirms they are not epileptic.
- *Rhythmic movement disorder* usually starts in infancy as rocking, rolling, yawing or head-banging in bed, both as the child goes off to sleep and at times (of partial arousal) through the night. The sometimes violent banging can wake up the whole family. Padding the headboard to reduce the noise can help.
- *Parasomnias*, such as sleep walking, sleep talking, and especially confusional arousals or night terrors, are sometimes mistaken for epileptic seizures.

SUPPORT ORGANISATIONS

Syncope Trust And Reflex anoxic Seizures (STARS)
PO BOX 175
Stratford upon Avon
Warwickshire CV37 8YD
Helpline: 0800 028 6362
Email: Trudie@stars.org.uk
www.stars.org.uk

SOURCES

British Medical Association and the Royal Pharmaceutical Society of Great Britain.
British National Formulary. London: BMA/RPSGB. Online. Available:
www.bnf.org.uk

5

FEVER

DEFINITION

Fever is a controlled increase in body temperature. It is the body's normal response to infection.

Pyrexia of unknown origin (PUO) is said to occur when a child has been resident in hospital with a documented fever of unknown cause for >1 week.

Unfortunately, there is no agreed consensus on what degree of temperature constitutes a 'fever'. However, most clinicians use a cut-off of 38°C or more.

EPIDEMIOLOGY AND AETIOLOGY

Febrile episodes in children are common. Most are self-limiting viral infections that do not require investigation or treatment.

Young children will have an average of six respiratory infections with fever per year.

ASSESSMENT

History

Systems enquiry for symptoms of specific infections such as coryza, cough, diarrhoea, vomiting, abdominal pain, headache, irritability.

Antibiotics in the course of the illness (if so, consider partially treated infection).

Symptoms suggesting serious infection particularly in younger children – lethargy, irritability, disinterest in playing, poor eye contact/recognition of parents.

Past history: information on immunisation status, foreign travel, previous serious infections, immune disorder or other disorders which increase the risk of infection (e.g. sickle cell disease) should be sought.

Examination

Overall assessment of whether the child appears well or unwell.

Rash (blanching or non-blanching).

ENT examination.
Lymphadenopathy.
Bulging fontanelle in an infant
Signs of meningism.
Full examination of cardiovascular, respiratory and abdominal systems for
localising signs and perfusion.

DIFFERENTIAL DIAGNOSIS

● *Infection*: Bacterial (e.g. pneumonia), viral (e.g. upper respiratory tract
infection), parasitic, fungal.
● *Malignancy*: e.g. neuroblastoma, lymphoma.
● *Autoimmune disorders*: Systemic onset juvenile chronic arthritis (JCA),
systemic lupus erythematosus (SLE).
● *Other*: Kawasaki disease, factitious fever, drug reaction, central line
infection, inflammatory bowel disease, post-immunisation.

THERAPY

Distinguishing children with serious bacterial illness (SBI) from those with
self-limiting viral illness is a challenge for even the most experienced
paediatrician.

<3 months

Infants in this age group are particularly at risk of SBI as they have poorly
developed immune mechanisms and present with non-specific signs
such as poor feeding. Fever may be the only manifestation of a serious
illness such as pneumonia or meningitis. However, most infections in
this age group are due to viral illnesses but differentiating bacterial
from viral can be extremely difficult.
Low threshold for a full septic screen including CSF, urine, chest x-ray,
FBC, blood culture and C-reactive protein.
Treatment: Broad spectrum IV antibiotic (see Table 53.1).

>3 months (no source of infection identified)

Investigations: Since urinary tract infection (UTI) can often present in a
non-specific fashion, it is useful to collect a urine specimen.
Carers should be advised about appropriate use of antipyretics and be
given advice regarding the expected length of illness and in particular
to seek further medical attention if they feel there is deterioration.
If positive urine microscopy or nitrites on dip testing, treat as a UTI (see
Table 53.1); otherwise no antibiotic treatment needed.

>3 months (source of infection identified)

History and examination will guide investigations of the suspected source,
e.g. chest x-ray if pneumonia suspected, lumbar puncture for
meningitis (*Note*: only if there are no contraindications).

Table 53.1 Therapy for fever

Diagnosis	Likely organism (if bacterial)	Antibiotic regimen
<3 months	Group B streptococci, *Escherichia coli, Listeria*	Check local regimen
>3 months (suspected sepsis but no obvious focus)	*Streptococcus pneumoniae, Neisseria meningitidis, Haemophilus influenzae type b* (now rare)	Broad spectrum antibiotic such as ceftriaxone IV
UTI	*E. coli, Klebsiella*	Cephalosporin
Pneumonia	*S. pneumoniae*	Penicillin (amoxicillin if using oral route)
Meningitis	*N. meningitidis, S. pneumoniae*	Broad spectrum antibiotic such as ceftriaxone IV until organism identified and sensitivities available

Any child who appears unwell at presentation should have blood taken for culture and be treated with a broad spectrum IV antibiotic immediately (see Table 53.1).

PUO

These children will need a period of inpatient assessment to monitor and document the fever and investigate.

Investigations: The following would be appropriate to commence investigation although they are by no means a definitive list:

FBC + film
C-reactive protein
Blood culture
ESR
Urine and stool culture
Mantoux test
Serum for acute and convalescent serology
Autoimmune screen
Imaging, e.g. chest x-ray, abdominal ultrasound

General management of fever

Antipyretics such as paracetamol and ibuprofen (which can be used in combination) will help to control the fever. This is particularly important in children with a history of febrile fits. Parents should be warned that some children will still go on to develop a febrile fit despite regular antipyretics, and be reassured that this is the disease process, not a failing on their part.

Tepid sponging with cold water is not now recommended; however, it is important to ensure the child is not wrapped in too many layers of clothes.

WHEN TO REFER

Any infant <3 months.
Older infants or children who are systemically unwell.
Focus of infection requires IV antibiotics.
Child has PUO.

KEY POINTS FOR PARENTS

Appropriate use of antipyretics (paracetamol and ibuprofen).

5

HEART MURMUR

Most cardiac problems are congenital in origin. They commonly present as murmurs. Management is confounded by a significant proportion of cardiac pathology remaining asymptomatic with minimal signs on examination. The vast majority of murmurs over the age of 1 year are attributable to 'innocent murmurs'. Early diagnosis of pathological murmur is desirable to prevent later serious complications. Antenatal screening will identify only a small proportion of congenital problems.

PRESENTATION

Symptoms (infancy)

Signs of central cyanosis, especially during feeding, are a cause for immediate concern. Symptoms of heart failure (prolonged feeding >30 minutes, persistent tachypnoea and associated failure to thrive) warrant immediate referral.

Symptoms (beyond infancy)

Above 1 year of age, most cardiac pathology may remain asymptomatic, with children rarely presenting with heart failure. Infective endocarditis and sudden death secondary to hypertrophic obstructive cardiomyopathy are recognised in teenagers and young adults.

Signs (causes for immediate concern)

Under 1 year of age

General inspection (sweaty), short of breath, pale, cyanosed.

The presence of any heart murmur (see Table 54.1) is of concern and those under 6 months of age require a paediatric cardiology referral and ultrasound.

Identify the position of the apex (to exclude dextrocardia).

Establish the presence of femoral pulses (absent or diminished in coarctation of the aorta).

Hepatosplenomegaly greater than 2 cm below the costal margin indicates hyperexpansion of the lungs or heart failure with lymphatic congestion.

Over 1 year of age

Infants can present with a murmur (30–75%), with or without symptoms of shortness of breath, prolonged feeding (>30 minutes) and increased infections. These symptoms are a sign of pulmonary oedema and may be associated with sweatiness and, in more chronic cases, failure to thrive.

In rare cases, sudden weight gain secondary to fluid retention is recognised as a sign of heart failure.

Cyanosis, especially when crying or feeding, warrants immediate referral.

ASSESSMENT

Examination

Under 1 year of age

Do they appear sweaty, pale or cyanosed?

Identify the position of the apex as dextrocardia will have a right-sided apex, associated with more complicated cardiac pathology.

Always check for the presence of femoral pulses.

Document any significant hepatosplenomegaly and the presence of costal recession.

Over 1 year of age

Cyanotic murmurs would hopefully have been identified in the younger age group above, though children born in countries with less rigorous screening programmes may present with Fallot's tetralogy and other complex malformations.

Acyanotic lesions – ventriculoseptal defects (VSDs), atrioseptal defects (ASDs), etc. – usually remain asymptomatic; however, they can rarely present with signs of pulmonary oedema as shortness of breath on exertion and poor weight gain.

VSDs cause increased turbulence of blood. Small holes cause more turbulence and hence louder murmurs than large VSDs or ASDs (see Table 54.1).

Parents should be advised that an ECG and echo are the only definitive tools for defining the presence or absence of pathology. A combination of other signs (e.g. cyanosis or absent femoral pulses) will, of course, increase the likelihood of pathology.

Table 54.1 Innocent and pathological murmurs

Innocent	Pathological
No thrills	Thrills, loud murmur (greater than 3/6)
Soft, variation with posture	No variation of posture
Localised praecordium	Radiates to back or neck
Ejection systolic	Pansystolic
Venous hum is continuous	Diastolic

Diagnostic tests

- *Blood pressure* (BP) measurements in all four limbs (there will be a discrepancy in BP between all four limbs in coarctation of the aorta). This is associated with diminished or absent femoral pulses. A four-limb BP is easier to perform on children under the age of 1 and if attempted in older children will require appropriately sized blood pressure cuffs. Measurements are made over the thighs.
- *ECG*: Used to identify disorders of cardiac rhythm and cardiac chamber enlargement. Right bundle branch block is associated with atrial septal defects.
- *Chest x-ray*: Used substantially less following the introduction of echo.
- *Echocardiogram*: The resolution of cardiograms has improved substantially over the last few years, especially in combination with Doppler. This is the definitive tool.

DIFFERENTIAL DIAGNOSIS

Listening areas for common paediatric heart murmurs are outlined in Table 54.2.

Still's murmur, an innocent murmur, is vastly more common than any pathological murmur heard over the age of 1 year. Referral is often associated with significant parental anxiety, and explanation for the need for diagnostic evaluation has to be carefully handled.

Acute bacterial endocarditis can present with a changing murmur, though this problem is extremely rare in the UK. These children have pre-existing cardiac pathology (either recognised or unrecognised) and present with pyrexia of unknown origin (see Chapter 53).

WHO TO TALK TO

Paediatric cardiologist.

Table 54.2 Listening areas for common paediatric heart murmurs

Area	Murmur
Upper right sternal border	Aortic stenosis, venous hum
Upper left sternal border	Pulmonary stenosis, pulmonary flow murmurs, atrial septal defect, patent ductus arteriosus
Lower right sternal border	Tricuspid valve regurgitation
Lower left sternal border	Innocent murmur, ventricular septal defect, hypertrophic cardiomyopathy, subaortic stenosis
Apex	Mitral valve regurgitation

WHEN TO REFER

If symptomatic.
If cyanosed.
If features of pathological murmur (see above and Table 53.1).
Failure to thrive.
Increased respiratory symptoms.

THERAPY

Heart failure is treated with diuretics (furosemide and potassium-sparing diuretics) while awaiting urgent cardiac opinion.

Cyanosis warrants immediate referral for cardiac opinion depending upon the underlying pathology.

Treatment can vary from immediate surgical correction or shunts through observation of the child with later correction beyond the neonatal period.

FOLLOW-UP

Murmurs *below* 1 year of age require referral for echocardiogram, given the high incidence of cardiac pathology. Centres without specialist facilities may have alternative arrangements, requiring follow-up by a nominated paediatrician as defined within their protocols.

Murmurs *above* 1 year of age are most commonly due to Still's murmur and hence innocent. An asymptomatic child can be reviewed at 3 months provided nothing abnormal is detected on examination beyond the isolated murmur.

A clinician has to advise the parents regarding the need for antibiotic prophylaxis with dental treatment if the murmur is felt not to be innocent. This depends upon the clinician's level of confidence around judging that the murmur is innocent.

See also
Chapter 53, Fever.

5

BLOOD PRESSURE – GUIDELINES ON MEASUREMENT

DEFINITION

The main aim of blood pressure (BP) measurement is to detect hypertension or the predisposition to hypertension, i.e. pre-hypertension. Normal BP is defined as systolic or diastolic BP above the 90th centile for sex, age and height; hypertension is systolic or diastolic BP above the 95th centile; pre-hypertension is systolic or diastolic BP between the 90th and 95th centiles.

The National Heart, Lung and Blood Institute Task Force (National Institutes of Health, US) has produced current standards.

Successive surveys confirm obesity-related rise in BP in the young, and also an increase likely to reflect other lifestyle changes such as diet and reduced exercise.

Elevated BP in adolescence predicts adult hypertension and an increased risk of heart disease and stroke.

EPIDEMIOLOGY AND AETIOLOGY

Primary or essential
- Genetics, diet, obesity, stress

Secondary
- Renal/renovascular (75%) – chronic pyelonephritis
- Cardiac (15%) – coarctation, vasculitis
- Endocrine (5%) – adrenal disorders, phaeochromocytoma
- Other (5%) – raised intracranial pressure, neuroblastoma

PRESENTATION

Hypertension is usually asymptomatic and detection depends on planned surveillance or coincidental health events.

ASSESSMENT

History
Family history of hypertension-related problems.

Examination
Serial BP measurements with ambulatory values if equivocal.
Height, weight and BMI.
BP measurement in both arms and both legs for aortic coarctation.
Cardiovascular examination.
Abnormal skin pigmentation, cushingoid features, abdominal masses.

Blood pressure technique
The sphygmomanometer, using appropriate cuff width (approximately two-thirds upper arm length), is suitable for older children. The emergence of the first Korotkoff sound indicates systolic pressure; muffling before disappearance indicates the diastolic. Oscillometric (Dinamap) devices are effective if used properly. Abnormal values should be confirmed by repeat readings and potentially by ambulatory methods.

When to measure
BP measurement is not a component of routine child health surveillance. It should, however, be incorporated in late childhood and adolescent healthcare when there is a family history of hypertension, early heart attacks or strokes. It is also appropriate to the management of obesity.
Secondary hypertension seldom produces direct symptoms. Recognition depends on BP measurement being part of the assessment of all ill children but especially those with:

- headaches, visual disturbance and other CNS symptoms
- renal disease
- cardiac disease
- growth and endocrine disorders (e.g. adrenal)
- severe or uncommon illness patterns.

Diagnostic tests
Urinalysis.
Plasma electrolytes, urea and creatinine.

DIFFERENTIAL DIAGNOSIS
See above.

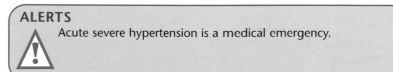

ALERTS

Acute severe hypertension is a medical emergency.

WHO TO TALK TO
Paediatrician/paediatric nephrologist.

WHEN TO REFER

Three issues to be discussed:

- Does this child have hypertension, i.e. serial values above the 95th centile?
- Is it primary or secondary?
- What is the appropriate management plan – dietary or drug based?

SOURCES

Munter P, He J, Cutler JA et al (2004) Trends in blood pressure among children and adolescents. Journal of the American Medical Association 291: 2107–2113. Online. Available: http://jama.ama-assn.org

National Institutes of Health (NIH) – www.nih.gov

Ramsay LE, Williams B, Johnston GD et al (1999) Guidelines for management of hypertension: report of the third working party of the British Hypertension Society. Journal of Human Hypertension 13: 569–592. Online. Available: www.bhsoc.org

DIFFICULTIES WITH BREATHING

DEFINITION

No standard definition exists but it usually refers to a child who either has the sensation of or is actually unable to get enough air. The term may also refer to any child with 'an unusual pattern of breathing'. Mothers may describe this in different ways by using terms such as 'noisy', 'fast' or 'interrupted' (World Health Organization 1995). The child may present with a variety of clinical signs.

EPIDEMIOLOGY AND AETIOLOGY

Most children have between four and six episodes of respiratory infection per year (World Health Organization 1995). Despite a reduction in the mortality rate for children with respiratory illness from 16.5% in 1971 to 8.5% in 1995 (Office of Population Census and Surveys 1995), the hospital admission rate for children with asthma rose by 13% in children aged 0–4 years from 1962 to 1985 (Strachan & Anderson 1992).

PRESENTATION

Respiratory illness remains the commonest reason for children to be seen in primary care. Most are self-limiting upper respiratory infections. Children with a breathing difficulty account for 30% of children presenting to the Emergency Department with a medical problem (Armon et al 2001). Children may present with mild, moderate or severe symptoms (see Table 56.1), some of whom may require urgent attention and resuscitation.

ASSESSMENT

History

Date of onset of symptoms.

History of increased work of breathing described as 'breathing fast', 'drawing-in the chest', 'noisy breathing in'.

271

Table 56.1 Assessment of severity of breathing difficulty

| | Breathing difficulty | | |
	Mild	Moderate	Severe
Oxygen saturation in air	>95%	92–95%	<92%
Chest wall in-drawing	None/mild	Moderate	Severe
Nasal flaring	Absent	May be present	Present
Grunting	Absent	Absent	Present
Apnoea/pausing	None	Absent	Present
Feeding history	Normal	Approximately half of normal intake	Less than half of normal intake
Behaviour	Normal	Irritable	Lethargic Unresponsive Flaccid Decreased level of consciousness Inconsolable

Adapted from WHO (1995).

Description of clinical signs such as runny nose, simple cough, productive cough, barking cough, stridor, wheeze.

Signs of more severe breathing difficulty – pausing or absence of breathing; decreased fluid intake; change in behaviour such as lethargy, drowsiness, agitated, flaccid and unresponsive.

Presence or absence of fever.

Contact history, family history, travel, choking.

Past medical history, in particular presence of allergies or previous history of respiratory disease.

Examination

Initial assessment to identify preterminal signs, or signs requiring urgent attention – exhaustion, bradycardia, silent chest, apnoea, agitation and cyanosis.

Look for signs of increased work of breathing – increased respiratory rate, chest in-drawing, nasal flaring, tracheal tug, use of accessory muscles and grunting.

Assess severity (Table 56.1).

Look for presence of stridor, stertor, wheeze or cough. Admit if severe distress, complicating factors or symptoms of serious illness.

Diagnostic tests

Dependent on differential diagnosis.

In most instances the diagnosis is based on the history and clinical examination. In some instances additional tests may need to be performed (e.g. blood tests or chest x-rays) but these should be used rationally and appropriately (Lakhanpaul et al 2003).

DIFFERENTIAL DIAGNOSIS

Presence of stridor or stertor

If barking cough and not toxic, consider croup and treat with steroids. If signs of respiratory failure, needs urgent attention in hospital.

If barking cough and toxic, consider bacterial tracheitis. Needs urgent attention in hospital.

Other causes of stridor include epiglottitis (the drooling child) and foreign body aspiration. Stertor may be caused by enlarged tonsils. Both require urgent referral to hospital.

Presence of wheeze

If history of paroxysmal cough or choking, consider foreign body aspiration.

If age <2 years, cough with inspiratory crackles and wheeze on examination, consider British Thoracic Society guidelines for asthma (see 'Sources' below).

Cough

If accompanied by wheeze or stridor, see above.

If cough with breathing difficulty, consider community acquired pneumonia.

5

ALERTS

Signs of respiratory failure or preterminal signs.

Complicating factors such as presence of co-morbidity, social factors.

Signs indicating serious distress.

Toxic or drooling.

Child may present with breathing difficulty in the presence of other serious illness.

WHO TO TALK TO

For advice for children with mild to moderate disease, referrals and advice can be taken from community paediatricians, hospital paediatricians and those at the interface, i.e. 'ambulatory' paediatricians. Specialist nurses can provide advice for non-acute problems.

Immediate referral to the emergency services may be required for a small percentage of children.

WHEN TO REFER

Children with moderate to severe illness.

Consider referral for children who cannot be easily managed at home or in whom there is concern that their condition could deteriorate, e.g. infants under 2 months of age, those with a co-morbidity and those for whom there are social concerns.

THERAPY

Dependent on diagnosis. See guidelines in 'Sources', below.

FOLLOW-UP

Most children with minor common childhood illnesses will not require follow-up.

For more serious diseases, follow-up for identification or management of sequelae to the illness will be required. Consideration for follow-up by community clinics, specialist health visitors, specialist nurses and general practitioners should be made

KEY POINTS FOR PARENTS

On discharge of the child the following advice should be given:

- Encourage the child to drink plenty and often.
- Check the child's breathing and colour.
- Give the child the medication prescribed by the doctor (if any).

The child may continue to have mild respiratory symptoms but should be taken to see a doctor or taken back to the hospital if:

- the child is struggling to breathe or getting very tired
- the child is too breathless to talk or the baby is grunting
- the child changes colour, becomes pale grey, white or blue around the lips.
- there are concerns that the child is getting worse.

HEALTH PROMOTION

Families should be given advice about the risks to children regarding objects that they can swallow or choke on.

Risks related to passive inhalation of smoke and respiratory disease.

Risks to children who smoke themselves.

Advice regarding importance of immunisation.

ADDITIONAL POINTS

Parents should be made aware of symptoms which are commonly present after a respiratory illness but which can be managed at home.

SOURCES

Armon K, Stephenson T, Gabriel V et al (2001) Determining the common medical presenting problems to an accident and emergency department. Archives of Disease in Childhood 84: 390–392

British Thoracic Society (2005) The BTS/SIGN guideline on asthma management, November 2005 Update. Online. Available: www.brit-thoracic.org.uk/pdf/paediatriccap.pdf

Lakhanpaul M, Armon K, Eccleston P et al (2003) An evidence-based guideline for the management of children presenting with acute breathing difficulty. Online. Available: www.nottingham.ac.uk/paediatric-guideline/breathingguideline.pdf

Strachan DP, Anderson HR (1992) Trends in hospital admission rates for asthma in children. British Medical Journal 304(6830): 819–820

World Health Organization (1995) Management of acute respiratory infections in children. Geneva: WHO

5

RECURRENT ABDOMINAL PAIN

DEFINITION

Recurrent abdominal pain (RAP) can be defined as pain occurring on at least three occasions over a period of 3 months and interfering with normal activities.

EPIDEMIOLOGY AND AETIOLOGY

Prevalence of around 10% in an unselected group of children; >10% had organic pathology. Table 57.1 outlines the basis of common, less common and uncommon episodes of gastrointestinal and extragastrointestinal pain.

Table 57.1

Prevalence	Gastrointestinal	Extragastrointestinal
Common	Functional abdominal pain Abdominal migraine Constipation Irritable bowel syndrome Mesenteric adenitis	Renal pain Pneumonia Diabetes mellitus
Less common but important	Inflammatory bowel disease Coeliac disease Gastritis Malabsorption (including fructose and lactose intolerance)	Sickle cell disease Porphyria Epilepsy Referred from spine, ovaries, testes, pelvis
Uncommon	Pancreatitis Hepatitis	

ASSESSMENT
History
Frequency, timing and location of pain (periumbilical less likely to be organic).

Associated vomiting (including bile and/or blood).

Diarrhoea (including blood and/or mucus).

Constipation.

Systemic symptoms (fever, rash, arthralgia).

Weight loss.

Anorexia.

Family history of gastrointestinal (GI) symptoms.

Examination
Growth parameters are crucial.

Check – clubbing, mouth ulcers, anus, skin rashes, site of maximal tenderness and radiation, guarding, percussion tenderness, masses, bowel sounds.

Diagnostic tests
- *First line* (if causes such as constipation, irritable bowel or abdominal migraine are not considered to be the cause):
  - urine culture; stool culture, microscopy and sensitivity; FBC, ESR, CRP; renal function; liver function; coeliac serology (check with local laboratory what these are).
- *Second line* (after referral from primary care and only if first line investigations are abnormnal or suggested by history):
  - endoscopy, upper and lower GI contrast studies, pH study, abdominal USS, *Helicobacter pylori* investigations.

Specific conditions
- *Inflammatory bowel disease*: Colitis (either Crohn's or ulcerative) presents with diarrhoea and bloody stools *but* Crohn's of small intestine can comprise abdominal pain, anorexia and systemic symptoms only. Unlikely to have normal first line investigations (usually raised CRP and ESR). Treatment will be decided by gastroenterologist.
- *Coeliac disease*: RAP may be the only complaint but is usually associated with other symptoms and weight loss. Abnormal coeliac serology should have endoscopy and biopsy. If found to be positive for coeliac, a dietitian should be involved to advise on a gluten-free diet.
- *Constipation*: A common cause of RAP in childhood. History should suggest it – *beware* overflow diarrhoea. Commonest cause of abdominal mass in childhood (see Chapter 60 for management).
- *Helicobacter pylori*: Those with new onset of epigastric pain, worse on lying down or eating, should be referred to a paediatrician for an

endoscopy and *H. pylori* investigation. Treatment will be prescribed according to the findings, i.e. antacids ± antibiotics.

- *Irritable bowel syndrome*: Increasingly common, especially in adolescence. Abdominal pain associated with frequent and loose stools and/or constipation/mucus; abdominal distension but no weight loss. Can be treated with antispasmodics but should try to focus on managing the pain, avoiding illness behaviour and overinvestigation. Consider triggering factors.
- *Functional abdominal pain*: Genuine pain caused by dysmotility or visceral hypersensitivity. Typical features include periumbilical pain, age 4–14 years, more common in girls, no relationship to food or other activities, interrupts normal activity, clustering of episodes, no associated symptoms (diarrhoea, vomiting, weight loss).
- *Abdominal migraine*: Episodic RAP, associated with nausea or vomiting, associated pallor, periumbilical; attacks last at least 1 hour, complete resolution of symptoms in between. There is little evidence that medical interventions help. If medical intervention is to be considered, referral to a paediatrician beforehand is suggested. Dietary manipulation can be tried first.

Malabsorption

- *Fructose intolerance and lactose intolerance* can cause symptoms of RAP, diarrhoea and anorexia; history may not be clearly associated with precipitants but a food diary may be helpful. First line investigations are normal. Trial of dietary exclusion may be useful.
- *Mesenteric adenitis*: Frequent episodes may lead to RAP. Associated with viral symptoms; symptom-free between episodes. Often have shotty (small nodes that feel like buckshot under the skin) cervical lymphadenopathy.

WHO TO TALK TO

General or community paediatrician.

Gastroenterologist if initial investigations reveal inflammatory bowel disease or malabsorption.

WHEN TO REFER

Significant illness behaviour, especially time off school; associated symptoms (diarrhoea/vomiting); weight loss or failure to thrive (FTT); abnormal examination; abnormal first line investigations; parental anxiety.

Some primary care physicians may wish to refer if they do not consider the problem to be of a 'simple' nature and may wish for first line investigations to be performed by a paediatrician.

ADDITIONAL POINTS

RAP is common in childhood.

Take a full history, looking for associated symptoms.

Weight loss or FTT should be taken seriously.

Aim to make a positive diagnosis (either of organic disease or functional abdominal pain or abdominal migraine).

Do not overinvestigate. First line investigations can be reassuring for the child, parents and doctor. Only go on to second line if the history is suggestive or the first line tests are abnormal.

See also

Chapter 60, Soiling and constipation.

5

ACUTE ABDOMINAL PAIN

EPIDEMIOLOGY

Abdominal pain is one of the most common reasons why the paediatric surgeon is called upon to review a child in the Emergency Department or on the medical wards. Most children referred to the Emergency Department with abdominal pain are usually referred to exclude a diagnosis of appendicitis. There is, however, a wide range of other causes of abdominal pain in children who need immediate resuscitation and/or surgical intervention as does the patient with appendicitis.

PRESENTATION

The child with abdominal pain can be easily divided into one of two groups:

- *Group 1*: no other associated symptoms and looking well despite the pain.
- *Group 2*: other symptoms present (e.g. vomiting), usually with the child looking unwell and in need of fluid and electrolyte resuscitation.

ASSESSMENT

History

The key to establishing the diagnosis of the child presenting with abdominal pain is the history and to a lesser extent the examination findings, as in >90% of cases a diagnosis can be made on the history alone.

Children in Group 1

The child with an isolated finding of abdominal pain is usually a well child and warrants little if any investigations if, after a careful history and examination, little else is revealed. Most such cases are termed 'non-specific abdominal pain' which usually settles within 24–48 hours of presentation. In cases where doubt exists, a period of admission for observation is recommended as it also reassures parents and avoids the impression that is occasionally held by some parents that the child's symptoms are being ignored.

All such children should have a urinalysis performed to exclude a urinary tract infection, especially in the child less than 5 years of age whose only complaint in the presence of a urinary tract infection may be vague abdominal discomfort.

Many children presenting with vague, non-specific abdominal pain may also have relevant social issues which need to be addressed and may not be picked up unless one pays attention to the social history and family circumstances, e.g. recently divorced parents or the presence of bullying at school. Be thorough with history-taking, especially with children who present repeatedly (see Chapter 57).

Children in Group 2

The following are features which must be elicited early on in the history in order not to miss important diagnoses:

- *The presence of bilious vomiting*: Children vomit for a wide range of reasons from mild head injury to gastroenteritis. *Bilious vomiting, however, must never be ignored.* In a previously well child it is a worrying finding as the diagnosis is malrotation, with or without volvulus, until proven otherwise. In the presence of mid-gut volvulus, almost the entire small intestine can be lost to ischaemic gangrene if the condition is not recognised and treated early.

  The other circumstance in which bilious vomiting is important is in children who have had previous surgery, e.g. the child with a history of gastroschisis who is at an increased risk of adhesive obstruction.
- *Urinary symptoms such as frequency and dysuria*: These children must *never* be started on antibiotics – not even trimethoprim – until a proper urine sample is obtained and sent off for microbiological analysis. The same rule applies if the child has had a urinary infection in the past – *obtain a sample before starting antibiotics.*
- *Systemic findings – fever, generalised malaise, anorexia*: The presence of fever in children must not be ignored and every effort must be made to find a cause.
- *Refusal to feed*: Children with abdominal pain who are not drinking fluids can rapidly become dehydrated and are best admitted rather than being managed at home.
- *Refusal/reluctance to move*: This is a useful finding in young children with peritonitis. A 2 year old who gradually is no longer interested in climbing and running about is indeed a sick child! A useful piece of history that is usually obtained, if sought, is the observation that the child appears to be quite comfortable in a parent's arms, but as soon as any attempt is made at movement, e.g. to transfer the child or the parent changes position (no matter how carefully), the child cries out in pain. In these situations one is most certainly encountering a child who has peritonitis, the most common cause being acute appendicitis.

- *Screaming episodes during which the child is inconsolable*: This finding may or may not be associated with the passage of 'redcurrant jelly' stool (blood-stained stool), and is usually seen in cases of intussusception. A significant number of children with intussusception, however, present at an advanced stage and are no longer having 'screaming attacks' but are quiet, lethargic and in hypovolaemic shock.

Examination
Significant findings on examination include the following.
- *Involuntary guarding* – a sign of peritoneal irritation. Beware the child who guards voluntarily. This may occur as a protective mechanism, e.g. because the hand of the examiner is cold or the child is anticipating pain. Overcome these challenges by ensuring your hands are always warm and dry prior to examining the child, informing the child of what you intend to do and your intention to be gentle, and then try to distract the child either with a toy or conversation depending on the child's age.
- *Abdominal distension* – especially in the presence of constipation, failure to pass flatus and/or vomiting.
- *Abdominal scars* – the astute physician will not fail to observe the presence of scars on the abdominal wall which may point to the cause of obstructive symptoms with associated abdominal pain, e.g. adhesive obstruction. Pay attention to the umbilicus – children with previous repair/reduction of gastroschisis can have very neat umbilical scars.

Diagnostic tests
There are very few investigations which the child will need prior to being referred to the paediatric surgical unit.

- *Urinalysis* (in all children): This simple investigation will provide many useful hints to aid in establishing the diagnosis. The presence of white blood cells and red blood cells is very common in appendicitis/peritonitis and is due to associated bladder irritation. Ketones may also be present, their severity indicating how dehydrated the child is. If, however, nitrates are also present, a diagnosis of urinary tract infection must be entertained and an appropriate sample of urine sent for microscopy, culture and sensitivity.

The following investigations may be arranged on referral of a child with abdominal pain:

- Serum inflammatory markers (CRP)
- FBC
- Urea, creatinine and electrolytes
- Plain abdominal x-ray
- Abdominal ultrasound
- Upper GI contrast study – the investigation of choice in a previously well child presenting with bilious vomiting.

DIFFERENTIAL DIAGNOSIS

- *Malrotation with or without volvulus*: This is one of the most serious causes of abdominal pain in children which is associated with significant preventable morbidity and mortality. A delay in presentation and/or establishing the diagnosis can result in the child losing a significant portion of the gut in the presence of volvulus. Any age group may be affected.
- *Intussusception*: The most affected group is children weaned off milk onto solids – usually around 6–10 months old.
- *Appendicitis*: Cases of appendicitis can usually be distinguished from those of gastroenteritis with regard to when diarrhoea and vomiting occur in relation to the pain. The child with appendicitis is usually noted to first develop pain, then vomiting, with diarrhoea developing later if there is inflammation extending into the pelvis: [Pain → Vomiting → Diarrhoea]

In cases of gastroenteritis, however, diarrhoea, vomiting and abdominal pain are likely to occur simultaneously.

- *Urinary tract infection*: It is essential that all children presenting with abdominal pain have a urinalysis.
- *Urological pathology*: Children with a palpable bladder and/or urinary symptoms need specialist, multidisciplinary care. Refer these children early. Examples include cases of late presentation of posterior urethral valves or spina bifida occulta.
- *Constipation*: An increasingly common cause of abdominal pain in all age groups.
- *Pelvic/gynaecological pathology*: These differentials are especially important in adolescent girls and include cases of ovarian masses/cysts, mid-cycle menstrual pain and pelvic inflammatory disease.
- *Pulmonary pathology*: It is not unusual for children with pneumonias – especially of the lower lobes – to present with abdominal pain.

> **ALERTS**
> ⚠ The presence of bilious vomiting in a previously well child.
> A child who is in hypovolaemic shock – these children can deteriorate quite rapidly and are also more likely to succumb to septic shock.

WHO TO TALK TO

Advice for children with abdominal pain referrals can be taken from the paediatric surgical registrars in tertiary referral centres. In district hospitals where there is no Paediatric Surgical Department, the paediatricians are usually happy to make an initial assessment and refer if needed.

WHEN TO REFER

- *All children with bilious vomiting and abdominal pain:* This calls for an emergency transfer to the nearest paediatric surgical centre.
- *Obese children with abdominal pain:* It can be difficult to examine these children at initial presentation and a period of observation as an inpatient is usually recommended.
- *Children with a palpable abdominal mass:* Before discharging children with abdominal masses a diagnosis must be confidently and accurately made and clear-cut plans *must* be in place for follow-up. It is inappropriate for these children to be managed in the GP surgery or clinic on initial presentation.
- *Peritonitis:* All children with abdominal pain with signs of peritonitis or in cases where doubt exists as to the presence of peritonitis.

FOLLOW-UP

The surgical team will indicate (usually in writing) when they no longer wish to follow the child up in clinic and are happy to discharge back to your care.

KEY POINTS FOR PARENTS

Parents and carers must be aware that children whose posture and/or gait changes with associated abdominal pain must be seen as soon as possible and not be monitored at home.

Bilious vomiting or 'green sick' is never normal, especially if the child was previously well or has had abdominal surgery in the past.

HEALTH PROMOTION

In cases of doubt it is always better to admit the child for a period of observation.

SOURCES

National Guideline Clearinghouse (USA) – www.guideline.gov.

See also

Chapter 57, Recurrent abdominal pain – medical approach.

ENURESIS

DEFINTION

An involuntary discharge of urine, regularly, during sleep, over 5 years of age without neurological or urological cause.

EPIDEMIOLOGY AND AETIOLOGY

1 in 5 children at age 5; 15% of boys and 9% of girls age 7; 1% at age 16.
Causes: Genetic predisposition; stressful life events; physiological – nocturnal polyuria, small functional bladder capacity, decreased arousal response to a full bladder.

PRESENTATION

Up to 50% of parents do not seek help; children often very embarrassed.

ASSESSMENT

History

Developmental delay? Behaviour problems? Social history? Family history of enuresis?
Daytime urgency and/or frequency?
Enuresis: How often in the week? More than once a night? How soon after bedtime? Does child wake?
Parents' response to wet nights: Is child lifted? Routine in the morning? Impact on the family? Responsibility for wet beds? Use of nappies?
Bedtime? Sleeping arrangements?
Where is toilet? Fear of the dark?

Examination

Height and weight.
Abdominal examination and genitalia.
Lower limb reflexes.
Spine.
Blood pressure.

Diagnostic tests
Urinanalysis, exclude urinary tract infection (UTI).

DIFFERENTIAL DIAGNOSIS
UTI.
Genitourinary pathology.
Child abuse.

> **ALERTS**
>
> ⚠ Children with UTIs, renal impairment, hypertension – *essential to check BP.*

WHO TO TALK TO
School nurse may manage treatment with alarms if organic cause excluded.
Community paediatrician.
Paediatric nephrologist.

WHEN TO REFER
Children with daytime urinary problems.
Treatment failures.
Concerns over family dynamics.

THERAPY
Not indicated for children under 5 or 6 years other than star chart to encourage and reward progress.
Alarms effective and safe, but require time and parental commitment – two-thirds will improve and 45% stay dry.
Desmopressin relieves symptoms, but no evidence that it provides a cure – use for short term (e.g. holidays) or initial 3-month trial.
Interval training programmes for children with low functional bladder capacity are best carried out by specialist nurses or paediatricians.
Imipramine not recommended because of serious adverse effects.

FOLLOW-UP
Regular follow-up and support are essential.
Monitor and reward progress towards dryness.
Six weeks of dry nights before discharge.

KEY POINTS FOR PARENTS AND CHILDREN
Parents need to understand this is a developmental problem, not bad behaviour.

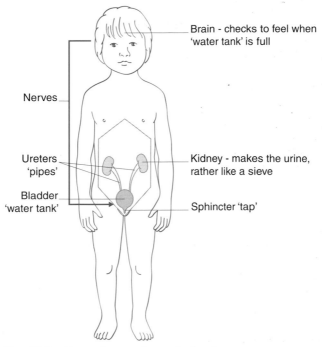

Fig. 59.1 Enuresis – anatomy for beginners.

Tolerant attitude combined with praise for success are important.
Parents and children need to be given explanations about the anatomy (Fig. 59.1) and physiology of micturition and sleep.

HEALTH PROMOTION

Some children may also need guidance in other areas of daily living such as washing, dressing, general organisation. It is important to emphasise individual responsibility and empower the child as much as possible
Emphasise good fluid intake during the day and not fluid restriction.

SUPPORT ORGANISATIONS

Parents may also have enuresis and need help. Information is available from:

Education and Resources for Improving Childhood Continence (ERIC)
    34 Old School House
    Britannia Road
    Kingswood
    Bristol BS15 8DB
    Tel: 0117 960 3060
    www.enuresis.org.uk

SOURCES

Bosson S, Lyth N (2003) Nocturnal enuresis. Clinical Evidence 9: 407–413

Centre for Reviews and Dissemination (2003) Treating nocturnal enuresis in children. Effective Health Care Bulletin 8(2). York: Centre for Reviews and Dissemination

Drug and Therapeutics Bulletin (DTB) Reviews (2004) Management of bedwetting in children. DTB 42(5): 33–37

See also

Chapter 55, Blood pressure – guidelines on measurement.

SOILING AND CONSTIPATION

DEFINITION

Constipation is associated with infrequent defecation (usually less than once a week), bulky and firm stools that are difficult to evacuate. It can present as faecal soiling. The latter is due to leakage of faecal matter from the rectum and sigmoid colon around the impacted faecal mass in the rectum.

Encopresis is a different entity where faecal soiling is due not to constipation or any neurological deficit but is of psychogenic origin.

EPIDEMIOLOGY AND AETIOLOGY

Constipation associated with or without soiling is a very common childhood problem. It can amount to 25% of referrals to paediatric gastroenterology. In surgical or medical conditions, constipation starts immediately after birth. Common causes are:

- dietary factors – lack of fluids and fibre
- holding back – behavioural problems and faulty toilet training
- emotional environment not conducive to child, at home (birth of sibling etc.) or school (bullying)
- intercurrent illness requiring bed rest, narcotic analgesics or associated with episodes of dehydration and loss of appetite
- surgical – Hirschsprung's disease, anorectal malformation, lower spinal lesions
- medical – hypothyroidism, disorders of calcium metabolism.

PRESENTATION

Severe constipation can present as pain at defecation, bleeding per rectum, abdominal pain or rectal prolapse.

Chronic constipation can present as soiling, abdominal mass or distension.

ASSESSMENT

History

A history of passage of meconium is very important. In term babies, 95% pass meconium within 24 hours of birth and 98% pass within 48 hours. Meconium passage is often delayed in preterm infants. A history of delayed passage of meconium should alert to Hirschsprung's disease (HSCR), as should a family history of HSCR. It is important to recognise HSCR as omission can lead to enterocolitis which still has high morbidity and mortality.

A history of passage of toothpaste-like stools suggests anal stenosis which could be associated with anterior ectopic anus – anus located anterior to its normal position. In classic constipation the history dates back to 6 months of age onwards.

Dietary or emotional factors cause passage of hard stool that tears the sensitive anal lining causing an anal fissure. This makes further acts of defecation painful and starts a vicious cycle of pain, holding back and pain leading to constipation.

It is important to take a history of any intercurrent illness and toilet training, and endeavours should be made to elicit any behavioural and emotional issues.

Examination

General physical examination to rule out any significant medical problems such as hypothyroidism.

Examination of the abdomen may reveal a hard faecal mass. These masses are felt along the line of the colon, especially sigmoid.

Gentle inspection of the anal region can reveal soiling or fissure. It may be possible to see anterior ectopic anus, commonly associated with anal stenosis.

Careful examination of the spinal region is essential to diagnose some children with spinal dysraphism and spinal cord lipomas.

Digital examination is a very sensitive issue and should only be performed after detailed discussion and explanation to parents and child and only if both are willing. It is done to rule out anal stenosis and any rare presacral lesion. In neonates and infants with HSCR, withdrawal of the finger is associated with gush of faeces. Never perform digital examination in acute constipation because of pain associated with underlying fissure.

Diagnostic tests

Plain x-ray is sometimes performed to see faecal loading.

Other investigations such as anorectal manometry to document anal pressures and recto-inhibitory reflex, rectal biopsy to rule out HSCR and bowel transit studies for slow transit constipation (STC) are carried out in tertiary referral centres depending upon local expertise and facilities.

If there is suspicion of hypothyroidism, blood should be sent for thyroid hormone (T3 and T4) and thyroid stimulating hormone (TSH) assay.

DIFFERENTIAL DIAGNOSIS

It is essential to distinguish constipation leading to soiling from encopresis and soiling due to a neurological or anatomical problem.

WHO TO TALK TO

After a good history and physical examination (which rule out any surgical and medical causes of constipation), one is left with non-organic constipation, the majority of which can be dealt with in general practice and community paediatric settings initially.

WHEN TO REFER

Constipation associated with a history of delayed passage of meconium (? Hirschsprung's disease) and passage of toothpaste-like stools (? anal stenosis) are absolute indications for referral to a paediatric surgeon.

History and examination suggestive of hypothyroidism requires a paediatric endocrinology opinion.

THERAPY

Acute constipation (usually in a 6- to 8-month-old) is the easiest to treat. A good explanation of the pathophysiology, and dietary advice along with simple laxatives such as lactulose to break the cycle of 'pain–constipation–pain', are helpful in the majority. In certain cases one can use Microlax enemas as a short-term measure to break the same cycle. Dietary advice involves reduction in the volume of cow's milk so that there is more room for water, juice and high-fibre foods.

Chronic constipation can sometimes be difficult to treat. Treatment can be prolonged and there can be several setbacks. The rationale is to treat megarectum – empty the rectum and keep it empty so that the normal rectal dimensions are attained. This restores normal rectal tone and its sensory and motor functions. Treatment involves the following.

1. A simple and clear-cut explanation of the problem to child and carers. Knowledge allays fears and anxiety and enhances compliance and cooperation of both child and carers – a must in the management of this challenging problem.
2. Dietary advice – high fibre diet and plenty of fluids.
3. Behavioural treatment to establish regular bowel habit. This can be a challenge as megarectum associated with a lack of sensation can suppress the urge to defecate in spite of a reasonable volume of stool in the rectum.

4. A combination of stool softeners (lactulose) and stimulant laxatives (Senokot). Try explaining the mode of action and reason for the laxatives as this improves compliance. Enemas are sometimes necessary to help in making a good start but should be discouraged in the long run.

FOLLOW-UP

The results of acute constipation treatment are excellent. Good follow-up is essential so that the precipitating factors are kept under check and laxatives are gradually weaned off.

Chronic constipation needs a longer follow-up. As a rough guide it takes one-third of the time from presentation to onset of constipation to get better, e.g. if the history of constipation is of 3 years' duration it takes 1 year to get better.

KEY POINTS FOR PARENTS

Acute constipation in children has an excellent prognosis.

Chronic constipation with soiling can be a challenge to treat. It needs active cooperation from the child and carers to achieve good results. Enemas help in ultra-short term, laxatives in short term; dietary and lifestyle changes bring lifelong relief.

HEALTH PROMOTION

Dietary advice for increased intake of fibres and fluids.

ADDITIONAL POINTS

Always keep in mind the possibility of Hirschsprung's disease in any child with constipation and never forget to take a meconium history.

61

LUMPS AND BUMPS

There are a variety of cutaneous and subcutaneous lesions which can present as lumps and bumps in the body; the most common are covered in this chapter.

EPIDEMIOLOGY AND AETIOLOGY

The common lumps and bumps in children are vascular malformations, lymphatic malformations, dermoid cysts, pilomatrixoma, naevus sebaceous, keloids and hypertrophic scars, ganglia, neurofibromatosis, fibromatosis, lipomas and soft tissue sarcomas. The list is long, but those missing from this list are very rare.

- *Vascular malformations:* One of the commonest swellings in childhood. They can present as isolated congenital lesions or as part of a syndrome with multisystem involvement.
- *Lymphatic malformations:* Small nodular lesions to large cystic hygromas on the face, neck or anterior chest wall or abdominal wall. They are prone to infections which require aggressive antibiotic treatment. Well-defined lesions can be excised without any danger to surrounding important structures, and leaving an acceptable scar are treated with surgical excision. Those not suitable for operative intervention are treated with aspiration followed by injection of bleomycin or OK432 (a sterile streptococcus extract). This creates a sterile inflammation which can obliterate the lymphangioma. Recurrence is common in both modalities and some surgeons leave them to involute.
- *Dermoid cysts*: Commonly occur in the region of the head and neck. External angular dermoids are the most common. They are usually deep and can be under the pericranium and hence fixed. In midline dermoids (especially in the region of nasal bridge) a deep intracranial extension is possible.
- *Pilomatrixoma*: Common in younger children and can be on the face, neck or upper extremities. They are hard, non-tender and irregular in shape, and appear white or yellowish through the skin. If they are found in multiple locations, suspect Gardner's syndrome with multiple polyposis.

5

293

- *Naevus sebaceous*: Present at birth and appear as yellowish, slightly raised lesions, usually on the face or scalp. They have a likelihood of developing into basal cell carcinoma in adulthood and hence should be excised in an elective manner in childhood.
- *Keloids and hypertrophic scars*: Children can produce thick raised scars from a surgeon's incision or injuries. These scars take 1–2 years before they involute to become pale and flat. Locations that are more susceptible to hypertrophic scars are earlobes, sternum and deltoid region. Afro-Caribbean and Asian communities are more susceptible.

  Keloids tend to grow beyond the margins of the original wound. They can be itchy and can cause contractures when in flexural locations. Management is challenging. A detailed explanation of the pathophysiology and natural history should be given to the patients and their carers. Treatment modalities comprise injection of steroids into the lesions, pressure with custom-made elasticated garments and use of silicone gel sheeting.
- *Ganglia*: These can arise from tendon sheaths and may be uncomfortable. Treatment modalities comprise excision or aspiration followed by corticosteroid injections and splintage.
- *Neurofibromatosis*: This is an autosomal dominant condition which affects 1 in 3000 children and presents as neurofibromas with café-au-lait pigmented spots. The plexiform lesions of the nerve trunks may be quite disfiguring.
- *Fibromatosis*: This self-limiting idiopathic proliferation of fibroblasts tends to occur in digits, palms and abdominal wall. They are non-malignant but recur locally and hence need a wide surgical excision and prolonged follow-up.
- *Lipomas*: Lipomas are rare in children, unlike adults.
- *Soft tissue sarcomas*: These lesions need an early diagnosis. They constitute 6–8% of all malignancies in childhood. The commonest are rhabdomyosarcomas. The diagnosis is established on incision or excision biopsy. Treatment involves surgery, chemotherapy and sometimes radiotherapy. In certain cases reconstructive surgery is required in the long term.

PRESENTATION

They present as lumps which can be painful.

ASSESSMENT

History

A good history can go a long way to clinch the diagnosis. Always remember that findings at the time of examination may not coincide with those when the lump was first noticed. Ask questions to elicit:

- When was the lump first noticed?
- How did it come to notice?

- What were the initial symptoms?
- Have the symptoms and signs changed since appearance?
- Any fluctuation in size or disappearance?
- Any previous history of lumps?
- What does the child or the carer think about the aetiology?

Examination

Always examine the whole patient before you examine the lump. On local examination the location of the lump must be ascertained in exact anatomical terms. Other points include:

- status of the overlying skin – colour and texture
- temperature – use the dorsal surface of the fingers to ascertain if the lump is hot
- tenderness – always ask about the painful part of the lump and approach it last and watch the child's facial reactions while eliciting this sign
- size, shape and symmetry – remembering the lump has three dimensions: surface (smooth or irregular), edge, consistency, fluctuation, fluid thrill, translucency, pulsatility, compressibility, bruits, reducibility, relationship to surrounding structures.

Never forget to palpate the lymph nodes in the draining territory and look for the state of local tissues.

5

Diagnostic tests

Depend on the differential diagnosis being entertained on the basis of history and physical examination.

DIFFERENTIAL DIAGNOSIS

This is different for each lump and bump.

> **ALERTS**
> A lump which is rapidly or slowly but steadily increasing in size.
> A lump which appears infected or inflammatory.

WHO TO TALK TO

Paediatric surgeon.

WHEN TO REFER

Urgent if malignancy or complication is suspected.

THERAPY

Depends on the status of the individual lump.

FOLLOW-UP

In paediatric surgical services.

KEY POINTS FOR PARENTS

Most soft tissue swellings are benign; however, they should be treated seriously as they can be malignant. Early diagnosis improves the outlook of malignant lumps.

HEALTH PROMOTION

All lumps and bumps require medical assessment.

ADDITIONAL POINTS

Soft tissue sarcomas constitute 6–8% of malignant tumours in children. Early diagnosis improves prognosis.

VOMITING

DEFINITION

Vomiting is the body's response to noxious stimuli in the gastrointestinal tract or from systemic disturbance. It must be distinguished from posseting, which is the regurgitation of small amounts of feed by babies who are otherwise well with no weight loss.

EPIDEMIOLOGY AND AETIOLOGY

Viral gastroenteritis is the commonest cause of vomiting in childhood.

ASSESSMENT

History

Vomits – number, size, projectile, bilious or non-bilious, presence of blood, relation to feeds, exacerbated by positioning, e.g. worse on lying flat suggests gastro-oesophageal reflux (GOR).

Associated symptoms to suggest infection – diarrhoea, fever, abdominal pain, headache, cough.

Relation to food ingestion, in particular cow's milk or egg.

Is there a history of recurrent episodes of severe vomiting with periods of being well in between?

Enquire about school and social history.

Examination

Hydration status, growth, systems examination for signs of infection, head circumference and neurological examination (signs of raised intracranial pressure); abdominal examination, particularly for distension, tenderness, pyloric mass, peristaltic waves or mass suggesting intussusception.

Diagnostic tests

Investigations (can be arranged with the hospital or child can be referred to a paediatrician first):

- *Uncomplicated GOR*: No investigations or treatment.
- Barium swallow.

5

- *Pyloric stenosis*: Test feed ± abdominal ultrasound, electrolytes and blood gas; hypochloraemic hypokalaemic metabolic alkalosis is highly suggestive.
- *Surgical causes*: Abdominal x-ray to look for signs of bowel obstruction ± barium studies.

Other investigations will be guided by the history and examination, e.g. toxicology screen for suspected ingestion, exclusion diet if food intolerance.

DIFFERENTIAL DIAGNOSIS

<1 year

The commonest causes are viral infections, e.g. gastroenteritis and upper respiratory tract infection, and GOR. The vast majority of babies with GOR are thriving and grow out of the tendency to vomit in the first year of life as they assume a more upright position and solids are introduced.

- *Pyloric stenosis*: Consider in a baby 1–4 months with projectile vomits and weight loss.
- *Cow's milk protein intolerance*: Often a history of associated diarrhoea, atopic tendency and facial wheals.
- *Surgical*: Intussusception, malrotation (think of a surgical cause if bilious vomiting present).

Other rarer causes that may present in infants who are not thriving include metabolic disease, renal disease, raised intracranial pressure and accidental ingestion.

>1 year

In a minority of infants and children, GOR will be symptomatic with weight loss, iron deficiency anaemia, aspiration pneumonia and irritability.
Surgical and rarer causes above still apply.
Also consider cyclical vomiting (sometimes called abdominal migraine), psychogenic vomiting, ingestion (deliberate or prescription drugs), gastro-intestinal disorders such as coeliac disease, Crohn's disease and migraine.
Most common cause is still a viral illness.

> **ALERTS**
>
> ⚠ - *Signs of raised intracranial pressure in infants*: Bulging fontanelle, separated sutures, vomiting and lethargy.
> - *Signs of raised intracranial pressure in children*: Vomiting, headache, change in behaviour, progressively decreased consciousness, lethargy, neurological deficits and seizures.

THERAPY

Most children with vomiting secondary to viral illnesses can be rehydrated with small amounts of fluid regularly (see www.pier.co.uk). Intravenous fluids are required in severe cases.

- *Uncomplicated GOR*: Reassurance, no treatment needed.
- *Symptomatic GOR*: Medical treatment is sufficient in most cases with feed thickeners and medications such as ranitidine. Occasionally surgical treatment is required.

Most vomiting in children is self-limiting and does not require treatment with antiemetics. They may be indicated in migraine and cyclical vomiting.

WHEN TO REFER

Any child unable to maintain hydration, with bilious vomiting or other symptoms or signs to suggest a surgical cause for the vomiting or in children who are failing to thrive. If raised intracranial pressure is suspected.

KEY POINTS FOR PARENTS

Maintain hydration by giving the child fluids little and often.

SOURCES

Armon K, Stephenson T, Eccleston P, Werneke U, Baumer H (2001) An evidence and consensus based guideline for acute diarrhoea management. Archives of Disease in Childhood 85: 132–142
Paediatric Information and Education Resource (PIER) – www.pier.org.uk

5

63

DIARRHOEA

DEFINITION

Diarrhoea is defined as a change in bowel habit for the individual child resulting in substantially more frequent and/or looser stools.

Chronic diarrhoea is persistence of diarrhoea for >2 weeks.

EPIDEMIOLOGY AND AETIOLOGY

Diarrhoea caused by acute infective gastroenteritis is one of the commonest diseases of childhood, accounting for 15% of medical attendances to the Emergency Department.

In the developed world the aetiology is most often viral.

ASSESSMENT

History

What is the normal stool pattern and how has it changed?

Enquire specifically about frequency, volume, colour of stool, presence of mucus, blood (inflammatory bowel disease (IBD), haemolytic uraemic syndrome (HUS), infective diarrhoea, e.g. Campylobacter) or vegetable matter (toddler diarrhoea), and nocturnal diarrhoea (IBD).

If acute diarrhoea, how much fluid has the child taken over the last 24 hours? What is the urine output (number of wet nappies)?

Is the child passing large lumps of stool in between the 'diarrhoea', suggesting constipation with overflow?

Was the onset of diarrhoea associated with weaning (coeliac disease) or is it exacerbated by certain foodstuffs (allergy)?

Are there associated symptoms such as vomiting, cough or irritability suggesting a systemic infection?

Is there a history of weight loss, poor appetite or abdominal pain?

History of foreign travel?

Examination

General examination – height, weight, signs of infection, hydration (see Chapter 62), mouth ulcers or clubbing (IBD), abdominal examination, perianal area.

Diagnostic tests

Stool sample for microbiology, culture and sensitivity if there is a history suggestive of food poisoning, recent travel abroad, bloody diarrhoea or chronic diarrhoea (also send for ova, parasites and cysts).

Send stool for reducing substances if secondary lactose intolerance is suspected.

Urea and electrolytes are only indicated when hypernatraemic dehydration is suspected or in severe dehydration when IV fluids are indicated.

In chronic diarrhoea the investigations will be determined by the most likely underlying cause.

DIFFERENTIAL DIAGNOSIS

- *Infection*: Acute viral gastroenteritis (diarrhoea with or without vomiting); also consider non-enteral infections such as urinary tract infection, meningitis.
- *Surgical causes*: appendicitis, intussusception.
- *Malabsorption*: cystic fibrosis, coeliac disease.
- *Systemic illness*: e.g. immunodeficiency.
- *Dietary disturbance*: cow's milk protein intolerance, secondary lactose intolerance.
- *Inflammation*: ulcerative colitis, Crohn's disease.
- *Miscellaneous*: Constipation with overflow, child abuse (fabricated or induced illness), antibiotic associated, irritable bowel syndrome, toddler diarrhoea, HUS.

5

ALERTS

Although viral gastroenteritis is the commonest cause of acute diarrhoea in children, the great majority of infections in children can present with a history of loose stools. Always consider other infections, e.g. urinary tract infection, meningitis, pneumonia.

Be alerted if the patient/carer reports blood in the stools.

WHEN TO REFER

Acute diarrhoea.

Any child with signs of dehydration (consider referring children who are not dehydrated but at high risk such as <6 months or >8 stools per day).

Any child in whom the diarrhoea suggests a more serious underlying illness such as appendicitis or meningitis.

Diarrhoea from birth strongly suggests underling pathology and the child should be referred and investigated.

Chronic diarrhoea warrants referral as should diarrhoea in any child who is failing to thrive.

THERAPY

There is no place in acute diarrhoea for the use of antidiarrhoeal agents such as loperamide – they do not work and have serious side effects.

Give oral rehydration solution if the diarrhoea is associated with vomiting and dehydration (see Chapter 62). If there is no vomiting or dehydration, continue normal diet and encourage larger volumes of fluid (normal fluid or oral rehydration solution). Treat any suspected underlying infection.

Treatment of chronic diarrhoea will depend on the underlying diagnosis, e.g. gluten-free diet for coeliac disease.

HEALTH PROMOTION

Parents should be educated that the commonest cause of acute diarrhoea is viral gastroenteritis which is a self-limiting disease. Antidiarrhoeals are not indicated.

The diarrhoea may go on for 7–10 days (a much longer illness than in adults). Seek medical advice if >14 days or concerns about dehydration.

SOURCES

Armon K, Stephenson T, Eccleston P, Werneke U, Baumer H (2001) An evidence and consensus based guideline for acute diarrhoea management. Archives of Disease in Childhood 85: 132–142

Paediatric Information and Education Resource (PIER) – www.pier.org.uk

See also
Chapter 62, Vomiting.

64

PENILE PROBLEMS AND CIRCUMCISION

PHIMOSIS

DEFINITION

There is no specific definition for phimosis that is universally accepted, leading to considerable controversy for circumcision. For practical purposes, phimosis can be defined as a non-retractile foreskin that causes problems in voiding.

EPIDEMIOLOGY AND AETIOLOGY

Most common causes are:

- *Developmental*: The inner epithelium of the prepuce and glans penis are stratified squamous and are fused to each other at birth. The foreskin is retractable at birth in only 4% of boys but becomes progressively retractable. It is retractable in 20% of males by 6 months of age, and 90% by the age of 3 years. It is very important to highlight this fact to the parents.
- *Balanitis Xerotica Obliterans* (BXO; scarred, thickened foreskin): This disorder is rare in those under 5 years of age and is an absolute indication for circumcision. The exact aetiology of BXO is unknown but is presumed to be of autoimmune pathology.

PRESENTATION

The most common complaint is inability to retract the foreskin. Other complaints are ballooning of the foreskin at the time of micturition and frequent episodes of redness of the foreskin called posthitis (the latter mostly settling on its own or after a prescription of local antibiotics by the GP). These episodes of redness can be associated with dysuria.

Balanoposthitis is a condition in which foreskin inflammation involves the glans penis.

ASSESSMENT

History

Redness of the foreskin is quite common but infection (manifesting in the form of pus discharge and redness and tenderness of the penile shaft – balanoposthitis) is very rare. It is important to distinguish between the two as the former requires reassurance while the latter requires a Paediatric Surgical opinion.

Examination

It is quite possible to tear the foreskin during clinical examination. This upsets the child and the family and hampers non-medical management, which is gentle retraction of the foreskin. Always ask the child to retract the foreskin, if possible, as they are very unlikely to pull it hard enough to tear it.

During examination look for any signs of scars and thickening of the foreskin to suggest BXO, which is an absolute indication for circumcision. When in doubt, take an opinion from a Paediatric Surgeon. It is very rare to see BXO in boys less than 5 years of age.

Diagnostic tests

The only diagnostic test is to see the child pass urine in front of you during the clinical visit.

ALERTS

⚠ Be careful of BXO; when in doubt, take a Paediatric Surgical opinion.

WHO TO TALK TO

Paediatric Surgeon when there is any suspicion of BXO.

WHEN TO REFER

Suspected BXO.
Non-retractile foreskin in a boy >12 years old.

THERAPY

For routine physiological phimosis, it is very important to explain to the parents and the child the pathophysiology and natural history of non-retractile foreskin. Recommend 1% hydrocortisone ointment to be applied locally once a day followed by gentle stretch, preferably by the child.

The main thing is to stress to the child and the family that they should neither expect dramatic results nor aim for them. The latter can cause tears in the foreskin which heals with scarring and leads to worsening of the problem.

FOLLOW-UP

Six-monthly to begin with, then depending on progress.
Inability to retract the foreskin after the age of 12 warrants a Paediatric
Surgical opinion.

KEY POINTS FOR PARENTS

It is very common to have a non-retractable foreskin. It is not medically
significant in the majority of cases.

HEALTH PROMOTION

Cleaning the glans and local hygiene can be explained at the time of first
and subsequent visits.

ADDITIONAL POINTS

It is important not to miss the diagnosis of BXO as conservative management
can lead to progressive disease which can subsequently involve the meatus
and anterior urethra, the management of which is a surgical challenge.

PARAPHIMOSIS

DEFINITION

Paraphimosis is a condition in which the retracted foreskin cannot be
returned to its normal position due to prepucial tightness. This results
in oedema of the glans penis due to lymphatic congestion, leading to a
swollen and painful penile tip.

EPIDEMIOLOGY AND AETIOLOGY

Paraphimosis is a relatively uncommon condition and the underlying
cause is phimosis.

PRESENTATION

The most common complaint is painful swelling of the foreskin and glans
penis.

ASSESSMENT

History

There is a history to suggest phimosis (as explained above) in some children.

Examination

Close inspection confirms the diagnosis. The key diagnostic feature is that
the whole glans with meatus at the tip is visible.

Diagnostic tests

A good history and clinical inspection are all that are required to make this diagnosis.

DIFFERENTIAL DIAGNOSIS

Balanoposthitis is the main differential diagnosis.

It is important to distinguish between paraphimosis and balanoposthitis as the former requires antibiotics and reassurance, whereas the latter requires an urgent paediatric surgical opinion.

> **ALERTS**
>
> ⚠ Immediate Paediatric Surgical referral. Transport the child in a fasting state.

WHO TO TALK TO

Paediatric Surgeon.

WHEN TO REFER

Immediately.

Keep the child fasting as some paraphimoses need to go to the operating theatre for reduction under general anaesthesia.

THERAPY

On very rare occasions, where the history is short, and the child is old enough and cooperative enough, the doctor can gently compress the oedema and reduce the paraphimosis without an anaesthetic. Local anaesthetic (e.g. EMLA) cream can be a useful adjunct.

Most children will need to be treated in the operating theatre where the compression to reduce the oedema is followed by reduction of paraphimosis. In certain circumstances a dorsal slit is required to release the tight band to achieve reduction.

Circumcision is never performed in the acute stage and may not be required in the majority of children in the long run. However, Paediatric Surgical follow-up is essential for all children with paraphimosis.

FOLLOW-UP

Paediatric Surgical.

KEY POINTS FOR PARENTS

Not all paraphimoses will require circumcision.

HEALTH PROMOTION

Cleaning the glans and local hygiene can be explained at the time of subsequent visits.

ADDITIONAL POINTS

When in doubt in distinguishing paraphimosis from balanoposthitis, take a Paediatric Surgical opinion.

CIRCUMCISION

The majority of circumcisions are performed for religious reasons in Muslim and Jewish communities. Circumcision is a controversial subject in Paediatrics. There is ongoing debate whether neonatal circumcision prevents urinary tract infections or carcinoma of the penis. This is an operation which has complications in the form of bleeding and infection. Removal of excessive foreskin can lead to lifelong sexual dysfunction.

The only absolute indications are BXO and recurrent urinary tract infections in a male child, especially in association with upper renal tract abnormality, e.g. duplex system.

Phimosis is a relative indication in those above 12 years, as some can benefit. Open technique under general anaesthesia is the safest approach.

5

65

VAGINAL DISCHARGE

DEFINITION

Vulvovaginitis is the inflammation and excoriation of the labia majora, labia minora, clitoris or introitus with a vaginal discharge.

EPIDEMIOLOGY AND AETIOLOGY

Most common gynaecological complaint in the prepubertal girl.

- *Common causes*: Poor hygiene (e.g. faecal contamination of the vulva from wiping from the anus forward), constipation with soiling, use of local irritants (e.g. bubble bath), dermatitis, foreign body, bacterial infections arising from a previous respiratory or skin infection, a sexually transmitted infection or a threadworm infection.
- *Rare causes*: Crohn's disease, pelvic abscess, tumours.

The introitus in non-oestrogenised genitalia has a reduced protective cover, making the genitalia more susceptible to infection.

PRESENTATION

Genital pain
Pruritus
Dysuria
Frequency of micturition
Vaginal discharge
Vaginal bleeding

ASSESSMENT

History

When did the symptoms start?
What are the symptoms?
Is there vaginal discharge? If so, ask amount, colour, odour, bleeding.
Any preceding infections/illnesses?
Any other symptoms, e.g. frequency, anal pruritus?

Use of bubble bath, oils, etc.
History of enuresis, constipation, soiling?
Type of underwear?
How does the child clean herself after going to the toilet?
What treatments have been tried?
Does the child have a dermatological disorder?
Does anyone else have similar symptoms?
Ask about the possibility of a foreign body.
Any concerns about sexual interference?

Examination
Height and weight (centiles).
General appearance and demeanour.
Skin condition including injuries.
Pubertal stage.
Abdominal, genital and anal examination.

Diagnostic tests
Swabs of discharge, vulva, posterior fourchette or transhymenal from the posterior vaginal wall for microscopy, culture and sensitivity, Chlamydia and gonococcus and a Gram stain.
Urinalysis to exclude urinary tract infection.
'Sellotape' test for threadworms (although has a relatively low yield).

DIFFERENTIAL DIAGNOSIS
Oestrogen deficiency
Poor hygiene
Infection
Bacterial, fungal, viral infestation
Threadworms
Lichen sclerosus
Local irritants
Constipation with soiling
Dermatitis
Foreign body
Child sexual abuse (CSA)
Anatomical anomalies
Rare causes include Crohn's disease with a fistula, pelvic abscess, tumours.

ALERTS
Children who are sexually abused are generally coerced into secrecy and therefore a high level of suspicion may be required to recognise the problem.

WHO TO TALK TO

Doctor on call for CSA to arrange examination with a colposcope.

Dermatologist if child has a dermatological disorder which is unresponsive to standard treatments.

Gynaecologist.

Reference to local child protection guidelines for local policies and contacts.

Health visitor, social services, the named or designated doctor for child protection if abuse is suspected.

WHEN TO REFER

Any concerns about CSA.

Presence of a sexually transmitted infection suggesting sexual abuse.

Treatment failures.

Concerns over family dynamics.

For examination under anaesthetic if:

- recurrent vaginal discharge resistant to treatment
- offensive, bloody vaginal discharge
- possibility of a foreign body
- foreign body found but irretrievable
- uncooperative child.

THERAPY

Dependent on cause.

Advice on hygiene and irritant avoidance.

Topical or oral antibiotic use dependent on swab results if a pure or dominant growth of a pathogen is identified.

If anal pruritus is a symptom, empirical treatment with mebendazole of both the child (over 2 years) and the family.

FOLLOW-UP

Follow-up of swab results.

Until symptoms resolve.

KEY POINTS FOR PARENTS AND CHILDREN

Encourage wiping bottom from front to back, regular washing, avoiding local irritants (e.g. bubble bath, perfumed soaps).

Wearing of cotton underwear rather than synthetic fibres.

HEALTH PROMOTION

As above.

SOURCES

Joishy M, Ashtekar CS, Jain A, Gonsalves R (2005) Do we need to treat vulvovaginitis in prepubertal girls? British Medical Journal 330: 186–188

Thomas AJ (2004) Beneath the surface. Archives of Disease in Childhood – Education and Practice 89: ep15–ep22

Thomas AJ, Forster G, Robinson A, Rogstad K (2003) National guideline for the management of suspected sexually transmitted infections in children and young people. Archives of Disease in Childhood 88: 303–311

5

66

NAPKIN RASHES

DEFINITION

Napkin dermatitis is an irritant contact dermatitis caused by prolonged
  contact with wet napkins.
Bacterial conversion of the urine to ammonia causes an alkaline irritant.
Usually spares the skin folds as they are less exposed to urine.

EPIDEMIOLOGY AND AETIOLOGY

Common in babies, toddlers and children wearing napkins.
Causes: prolonged contact with wet napkin, poor hygiene and rarely
  immunological disorders.

PRESENTATION

Widespread erythema ± ulcerated lesions.

ASSESSMENT

History
Infants in nappies
Type of nappies worn, e.g. disposable, terry towelling.
Frequency of change of nappy.
Cleaning agents, e.g. soap and water, wipes.
Use of creams.
Use of bubble bath, soaps, etc. in the bath.
Frequency of bathing.
Any skin conditions, e.g. eczema.
General health, e.g. diarrhoea, faltering growth.
Family history of skin conditions, e.g. psoriasis.

Children out of nappies
Type of underwear, tights or trousers (cotton or synthetic).
History of enuresis or constipation.
Ability to wipe themselves.
Skin conditions.
General health, e.g. faltering growth.
Family history of skin conditions, e.g. psoriasis.

Examination
Height and weight (centiles).
Full examination for signs of ill health or neglect.
Signs of skin conditions, e.g. eczema, psoriasis.
Signs of infection, e.g. oral thrush.

Diagnostic tests
Swab for microscopy, culture and sensitivity if infection suspected.
Urine dipstick for glucose in the older child with thrush.

DIFFERENTIAL DIAGNOSIS

Candidiasis (thrush)
Commonly superimposed on a napkin rash.
Small satellite erosions/pustules on a background of erythema.
Concentrates in the skin folds.

Seborrhoeic dermatitis
Erythematous, greasy, yellow lesions in the napkin area, behind the ears,
   on the scalp (cradle cap), forehead and eyelids.
No treatment needed in mild cases, topical hydrocortisone is otherwise
   effective.

Bacterial skin infections (e.g. staphylococcal, scalded skin syndrome, streptococcal)
Involves skin folds touching each other, e.g. labia majora.
Erythematous rash with a clear, serous discharge ± ulceration.
Think about child abuse, neglect, child sexual abuse (CSA).

Napkin psoriasis (sebopsoriasis)
Form of psoriasis.
Occurs in the first 3 months of life.
Non-specific napkin dermatitis suddenly becoming more severe and
   extensive with bright, well-demarcated erythema involving most of the
   napkin area including the folds.
Lesions resembling psoriasis erupt elsewhere, usually first on the face,
   scalp and neck fold, the axillae and finally trunk and limbs.
On the scalp may appear similar to seborrhoea.
Should be considered in any child who responds poorly to conventional
   measures, particularly if lesions have well-defined margins and appear
   fairly fixed in position.

THERAPY

Mild rashes – simple measures are effective:

- Frequent nappy change.
- Careful washing at each change of napkin.

- Protective cream, e.g. zinc/castor oil, white soft paraffin/liquid paraffin (50/50).
- Disposable napkins generally protect against this disorder, providing they are changed regularᵒly.
- Avoid bubble bath, soaps.
- Wearing cotton underwear and loose clothes.
- Careful wiping of perineum after toileting.
- Treatment of enuresis and constipation.

More severe rashes require additional measures:

- Leave the area exposed to the air.
- Creams such as metanium are useful for helping the skin to heal quickly (can be purchased over-the-counter).
- Treat secondary infections, e.g. nystatin for thrush, flucloxacillin for staphylococcal and amoxicillin for streptococcal infections.
- Napkin psoriasis often clears up quickly with hydrocortisone and anticandidal agents for the flexural areas and a weak hydrocortisone elsewhere.

WHO TO TALK TO

Health visitor.
General practitioner.
Paediatrician.

FOLLOW-UP

Nil needed unless a recurrent problem.

KEY POINTS FOR PARENTS

Napkin rashes can occur in young children even if their nappies are changed regularly and there is a good level of hygiene.

HEALTH PROMOTION

Regular nappy changes should be reinforced, with careful washing of the napkin area and the use of barrier creams in babies and children susceptible to napkin rash.
Avoidance of bubble bath, strongly scented soaps.
Wearing cotton underwear.
Wearing loose, cotton clothing in hot weather.

SOURCES

Campbell AGM, McIntosh N (eds) (1998) Forfar and Arneil's textbook of pediatrics, 5th edn. New York: Churchill Livingstone

67

LIMP AND GAIT PROBLEMS

DEFINITION

Limp and gait problems are difficulties with normal walking on level ground.

EPIDEMIOLOGY AND AETIOLOGY

Abnormal gait can result from disorders affecting several levels of the nervous system or are manifestations of orthopaedic disorders.

During early childhood (1–3 years), a painful limp can be caused by septic arthritis, osteomyelitis, juvenile arthritis, trauma, transient synovitis or intervertebral discitis. A painless limp can be caused by developmental dysplasia of the hip (DDH) or cerebral palsy.

In children aged 3–10 years, additional causes for a painful limp include acute Perthes disease, while a painless limp can be caused by chronic Perthes disease or muscular dystrophy.

In adolescents and young adults, painful limp can be caused by septic arthritis, osteomyelitis, juvenile arthritis, trauma or acute slipped capital femoral epiphysis, while a painless limp can be caused by chronic slipped upper femoral epiphysis, DDH or neuromuscular disorders.

ASSESSMENT

History

Onset of problems
Acute or chronic
Any recent infections
Systemically unwell
Association with pain, paraesthesia
Family history
History of trauma
Developmental milestones
Weakness
Bowel and bladder function

Examination

General examination – general well-being, joint examination, muscle tone, power and reflexes, tenderness.

Gait examination depends on the child's age and ability to cooperate:

- In younger children examination is opportunistic and best done by observation during play. In older children, gait is best observed when walking at a steady pace and turning around, as well as walking on heels, on toes, and 'walking on a tightrope'.
- Romberg's sign is tested to determine maintenance of balance, by standing erect with feet together, first with eyes open and then with eyes closed.
- Normal gait has a stance phase (60%) and a swing phase (40%) on the same limb. The stance phase is when the foot is on the ground and the swing phase is when the foot is off the ground. In limping, the stance phase and the stride length are shortened (antalgic gait). In painless limping, associated with neuromuscular disorders, there is a normal stance phase but a persistent trunk sway (Trendelenburg gait; Fig. 67.1). If this is bilateral, it causes a waddling gait.
- A painful knee causes limitation of knee flexion, a shortened stance phase and elevation of the pelvis during swing phase.

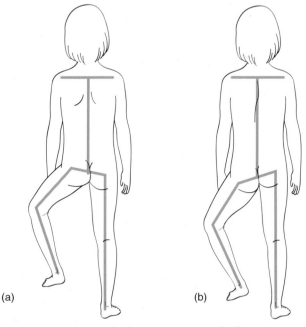

(a) (b)

Fig. 67.1 (a) Negative Trendelenburg test (normal); (b) positive Trendelenburg test (weakness of gluteus medius muscle).

- Poor dorsiflexion of the foot causes increased knee flexion for clearance of the foot, resulting in steppage gait.

Diagnostic tests

Based on clinical findings. Tests to consider include FBC, inflammatory markers such as ESR and CRP, blood culture, autoantibody screen including rheumatoid factor (RF) and antinuclear antibody (ANA), x-ray, and computed tomography and magnetic resonance imaging (CT/MRI) scan.
FBC and inflammatory markers might be helpful, if indicated, prior to referral.

DIFFERENTIAL DIAGNOSIS

Septic arthritis
Osteomyelitis
Juvenile arthritis
Trauma
Transient synovitis
Intervertebral discitis
Developmental dysplasia of the hip
Cerebral palsy
Perthes disease
Muscular dystrophy
Acute slipped capital femoral epiphysis
Chronic slipped upper femoral epiphysis

5

> ## ALERTS
> ⚠ Child abuse, suspicion of septic arthritis or osteomyelitis.
> Hysterical disorders of gait produce a bizarre gait, unlike any evoked by organic disease.

WHO TO TALK TO

Community paediatrician
Paediatric rheumatologist
Physiotherapist
Occupational therapist
Paediatric neurologist
Orthopaedic surgeon for possible surgical management

WHEN TO REFER

Acute onset of painful limp needs to be referred immediately for appropriate evaluation and management; a painless limp needs to be evaluated for neurological or orthopaedic problems.
Infants not yet walking or with an abnormal gait by 2 years of age should be referred for a medical review and/or to a community paediatrician for assessment.

THERAPY

A toddler's gait needs reassurance.

In septic arthritis/osteomyelitis, it is imperative to treat with IV antibiotics.

FOLLOW-UP

Determined by cause.

KEY POINTS FOR PARENTS

There are wide variations in gait – a toddler's gait is veryinconsistent and also depends on when the child started to walk. Additionally, a toddler's gait is very broad based and does not include the reciprocal arm swing.

Barefoot walking helps to develop the small muscles of the foot. Encourage children to spend time barefoot where it is safe.

Make sure the child's shoes fit well.

HEALTH PROMOTION

Active lifestyle should be encouraged.

If necessary, encourage usage of appropriate support for mobility and aids to prevent long-term disuse atrophy of muscle groups.

SUPPORT ORGANISATIONS

Arthritis Research Campaign – www.arc.org.uk
  Includes leaflets for children, teenagers, parents and teachers.
Chartered Society of Physiotherapy –
  www.csp.org.uk/director/physiotherapyexplained.cfm
  The A–Z of conditions section has brief explanations on pain, gait, fractures and juvenile arthritis.
HemiHelp – www.hemihelp.org.uk
  Information and support for children and young people with hemiplegia.
National Library for Health: Musculoskeletal Specialist Library –
  http://libraries.nelh.nhs.uk/musculoskeletal
NHS Direct's Health Encyclopaedia –
  www.nhsdirect.nhs.uk/alphaindex.asp
Virtual Children's Hospital –
  www.vh.org/navigation/vh/topics/pediatric_patient_
  bones__joints_and_muscles.html
  For information on Osgood–Schlatter's disease, Perthes disease, arthritis, fractures, sprains.

68

LEG PAIN – BONES AND JOINTS

DEFINITION
Leg pain involves any pain in the legs.

EPIDEMIOLOGY AND AETIOLOGY
Leg pain is a common symptom.

It may be challenging to distinguish between bone, muscle, joint or referred pain as the causes change with age:

- In children <2 years old, transient synovitis, septic arthritis/osteomyelitis, hypermobility, discitis, trauma, child abuse, neoplasias (including leukaemias and metastatic disease), juvenile arthritis and referred pain
- In childhood, additional causes include muscle cramps, sickle cell pain crisis, neoplasia (including primary bone tumours), Legg–Calve–Perthes disease, Henoch–Schönlein purpura, collagen vascular diseases (systemic lupus erythematosus, dermatomyositis, sarcoid), rheumatic fever, Caffey's disease, psychological/behavioural, non-specific limb pain such as 'growing pains'
- In adolescence, slipped upper femoral epiphysis (SUFE), Osgood–Schlatter's disease, osteochondritis and rickets can all present with leg pain.

ASSESSMENT
History
General health.

Family history of disease.

Onset of pain, its severity, duration and associated symptoms such as limp, refusal to bear weight, physical activity, fever and rash.

A history of recent upper respiratory infection or trauma is important.

Examination
A close physical examination of the entire affected limb and areas proximal to the affected site (looking for sources of referred pain) such as the lower abdomen, pelvis and spine is important.

Inspection for swelling and erythema should be done with palpation of muscle and bone and notation of localised heat. Additionally, range of motion of all joints should be noted (including hypermobile joints).

Neuromuscular examination including gait should be assessed. A general physical examination for signs of systemic infection is also indicated.

Diagnostic tests

Based on clinical findings. Tests to consider include FBC, differential count and blood film, inflammatory markers, blood culture, auto-antibody screen including rheumatoid factor (RF) and antinuclear antibody (ANA), LFTs, bone chemistry, x-ray, bone scan and computed tomography (CT) scan.

FBC and inflammatory markers might be helpful, if indicated, prior to referral.

> **ALERTS**
> ⚠ Child abuse, suspicion of septic arthritis or osteomyelitis, child systemically unwell (? malignancy).

WHO TO TALK TO

Paediatric rheumatologist.
Physiotherapist.
Occupational therapist.
Orthopaedic surgeon for possible surgical management.

WHEN TO REFER

If the child is systemically unwell; has persistent stiffness, pain or swelling over joints; suspected non-accidental injury.

THERAPY

Most children usually have a self-limited, localised disease process such as transient synovitis or trauma. These can be treated with conservative management, including thermotherapy and pain relief. More complicated orthopaedic disease such as Legg–Perthes and SUFE need orthopaedic management.

If an infectious disease is suspected, appropriate antibiotics should be administered.

Systemic diseases such as connective tissue disease and neoplasias require a team approach to evaluation and management.

KEY POINTS FOR PARENTS

Growing pain often presents as leg pain. This usually presents as recurrent pain during the night, with the child being well otherwise. Massaging the legs, hot water bottles and simple analgesics can be helpful.

HEALTH PROMOTION

Preserve active lifestyle.

SUPPORT ORGANISATIONS

Arthritis Research Campaign – www.arc.org.uk
  Includes leaflets for children, teenagers, parents and teachers.
Chartered Society of Physiotherapy –
  www.csp.org.uk/director/physiotherapyexplained.cfm
  The A–Z of conditions section has brief explanations on pain, gait, fractures and juvenile arthritis.
HemiHelp – www.hemihelp.org.uk
  Information and support for children and young people with hemiplegia.
Hypermobility Syndrome Association – www.hypermobility.org
  Hypermobility and managing chronic pain.
National Library for Health: Musculoskeletal Specialist Library –
  http://libraries.nelh.nhs.uk/musculoskeletal
NHS Direct's Health Encyclopaedia –
  www.nhsdirect.nhs.uk/alphaindex.asp
Pain Concern – www.painconcern.org.uk
  Information and support for pain sufferers.
Perthes Association (osteochondritis) – www.perthes.org.uk
Virtual Children's Hospital – www.vh.org/navigation/vh/topics/
  pediatric_patient_bones__joints_and_muscles.html
  For information on Osgood–Schlatter's disease, Perthes disease, arthritis, fractures, sprains.

5

69

BACK PAIN

DEFINITION

Back pain is common in children, particularly during adolescence. Whereas a medical cause needs to be sought in some cases, most occur as a result of a variety of mechanical factors, including poor posture, inappropriate forms of exercise and carrying heavy schoolbags.

EPIDEMIOLOGY AND AETIOLOGY

50% of children of secondary school age.
Uncommon <5 years old.
Causes – musculoskeletal, psychological, obesity, poor posture, sedentary lifestyle, discitis, spondylolysis, Scheuermann's kyphosis, tumour.

PRESENTATION

Only 2% of children with back pain present to doctors. Most children have fleeting musculoskeletal pain.

ASSESSMENT

History

Description of pain – site, radiation, frequency, severity.
Disabling effects on schooling, sleep, sport, etc.
Presence of fever, weight loss, muscle weakness, paraesthesia.
Loss of bladder or bowel control.
Background lifestyle history and experience of pain within the family.

Examination

Posture and gait
Tenderness
Scoliosis
Range of spinal movement
Lower limb reflexes
Abdominal palpation

Diagnostic tests
- FBC and ESR
- Spinal x-ray
- Bone scan
- Magnetic resonance imaging

All the above can be ordered in secondary care if needed.

DIFFERENTIAL DIAGNOSIS
Discitis.
Spondylolysis.
Scheuermann's kyphosis.
Tumours (osteoid osteoma).

> **ALERTS**
> Fever, weight loss, radiation to lower limbs, weakness or paraesthesia, sphincter involvement – age <5 years.

WHO TO TALK TO
Parents to identify background issues.
School nurse to address environmental issues (backpacks, desk height, etc.).
Physiotherapy and occupational therapy.

WHEN TO REFER
Pain lasting >1 week and pain in children <5 years old.
Presence of fever and localised tenderness suggests discitis.
Abnormal lower limb neurology/sphincter disturbance should prompt urgent review to exclude spinal cord compression.
Pain that interferes with the activities of daily living should be taken seriously – the child may need input from the multidisciplinary team to prevent further disability.

THERAPY
Physiotherapy – posture, backpacks, physical exercise.
Occupational therapy – seating, desks, activities of daily living.
Avoid bed rest.
Non-steroidal anti-inflammatory drugs (NSAIDs) and heat for pain relief.

KEY POINTS FOR PARENTS

Prevention is the key:

- avoid sedentary lifestyle
- think about posture
- distribute load evenly in backpacks (use both shoulder straps ± waist support)
- adjust the height of desks and chairs to avoid unnecessary stretching.

HEALTH PROMOTION

Maintain an active lifestyle.
Avoid obesity.
Maintain good posture.

ADDITIONAL POINTS

Parents may also suffer with chronic back pain, which needs managing.

SUPPORT ORGANISATIONS

BackCare (The Charity for Healthier Backs) – www.backcare.org.uk
Chartered Society of Physiotherapy
  14 Bedford Row
  London WC1R 4ED
  www.csp.org.uk

SOURCES

Trombly CA, Radomski MV (eds) (2002) Occupational therapy for physical dysfunction, 5th edn. Philadelphia: Lippincott Williams and Wilkins

70

SWOLLEN JOINTS

DEFINITION

Transient or persistent swelling of one or more peripheral joints, often but not always associated with pain.

EPIDEMIOLOGY AND AETIOLOGY

Joint swelling could be a presenting symptom of a variety of conditions. A large number of children are seen with transient synovitis, reactive arthritis or postinfectious arthritis but these benign conditions should only be diagnosed after exclusion of more serious conditions such as septic arthritis and malignancy. Trauma and haemarthrosis are other conditions to be considered in the differential diagnosis of acute monoarthritis.

Multiple swollen joints can result from viral infections, leukaemia, rheumatic fever and rheumatological conditions. A diagnosis of juvenile idiopathic arthritis (JIA) can be made in a child under the age of 16 years who has had persistent arthritis for more than 6 weeks when other causes of arthritis have been excluded.

Joint swelling could be part of a multisystem vasculitis or connective tissue disease.

PRESENTATION

It is important to differentiate the well child with a swollen joint from the ill child. The latter needs prompt hospital review to consider infection. Swelling with associated pain is more likely to present early, whereas the well child with a swollen joint may not come to medical attention until there is functional loss.

Tuberculosis should always be considered even in children with no obvious risk factors or known contacts.

ASSESSMENT

History

- *Mode of onset*: Acute or chronic.
- *Duration*: Hours, days or weeks.
- *Preceding illness*: Upper respiratory tract infections, diarrhoea, trauma, rash, fever and bleeding tendency.
- *Number of joints involved*: Mono- or polyarthritis.
- *Associated features*: Pain, loss of function, disability, muscle wasting.
- *Family history*: Arthritis, inflammatory bowel disease, psoriasis and iritis.

Examination

- *General and systemic examination*: Rash, anaemia, lymphadenopathy, hepatosplenomegaly, conjunctivitis.
- *Affected joints*: Swelling, redness, tenderness, warmth, range of movement, deformity, bony tenderness, muscle wasting, effusion, synovial thickening, overgrowth of the affected limb.
- *Other joints*: Screening examination.

Diagnostic tests

Depend on the presentation.

- *Acute painful and swollen joints*: Children should be referred urgently for investigation – FBC, CRP, ESR, blood film, blood culture, plain x-ray, joint aspiration for culture, MRI, bone marrow aspiration.
- *Joint swelling of long duration*: These investigations can be initiated in the community while awaiting a specialist opinion – FBC, ESR, antinuclear antibody (ANA), rheumatoid factor (RF).

DIFFERENTIAL DIAGNOSIS

Septic arthritis.
Transient synovitis associated with viral infections.
Postinfectious arthritis associated with enteric infections.
Accidental or non-accidental trauma.
Malignancy – leukaemia, neuroblastoma.
Juvenile idiopathic arthritis.
Vasculitis – systemic lupus erythematosus (SLE) and Henoch–Schönlein purpura (HSP).

ALERTS

- Pain
- Fever
- Red and hot joint
- Severe bone pain
- Foreign travel
- Partially or un-immunised child
- Tuberculosis contact

WHO TO TALK TO

Orthopaedic surgeon for joint aspiration.
Paediatric rheumatologist.
Radiologist for appropriate investigations.
Physiotherapist.

WHEN TO REFER

Acutely unwell children with joint swelling of short duration should be referred urgently to a paediatrician to rule out the possibility of septic arthritis or malignancy.
Joint swelling in a well child with no self-limiting and precipitating cause.
Associated rash, anaemia or weight loss or other systemic features

THERAPY

Antibiotics for septic arthritis.
Orthopaedic management for trauma.
Multidisciplinary care under the direction of a paediatric rheumatologist for JIA.
Non-steroidal anti-inflammatory drugs (NSAIDs) and analgesia for pain.
Physiotherapy.
Oral or subcutaneous methotrexate for JIA

FOLLOW-UP

Slit-lamp examination of the eye to exclude chronic iritis.
Early follow-up to confirm that joint swelling secondary to benign causes, e.g. transient synovitis, postinfective arthritis, is getting better.
Specialist nurse input to achieve self-management skills.
Regular multidisciplinary paediatric rheumatology follow-up if a chronic rheumatological condition is diagnosed.

KEY POINTS FOR PARENTS

To gain knowledge about chronic conditions such as JIA and to help the child understand their condition.
To help the child to take control of their treatment.

HEALTH PROMOTION

Preserve active lifestyle.
Maintain positive body image.
Prevention of mental health problems.

SUPPORT ORGANISATIONS

Arthritis Research Campaign – www.arc.org.uk

Children's Chronic Arthritis Association – www.ccaa.org.uk

Choices for Families of Children with Arthritis –
www.kidswitharthritis.org

NICE Appraisal No. 35: Guidance on the use of etanercept for the
treatment of juvenile idiopathic arthritis – www.nice.org.uk/pdf/
JIA-PDF.pdf

SECTION

6

CHILD HEALTH PROMOTION PROGRAMME

PRECONCEPTION AND ANTENATAL SCREENING

Table 71.1 Screening activities during early pregnancy

Gestational age	Recommended screening tests	Comments
Preconception		Folic acid prophylaxis of neural tube defects
8–12 weeks	Rubella, VDRL, HIV, hepatitis B, blood group, Rhesus antibody, full blood count, red cell alloantibodies Screening for haemoglobinopathy in high prevalence areas	
11–13 weeks	Ultrasound scan (USS)	For dates and to confirm number of fetuses
	USS for nuchal translucency (NT)	For women >35 years Positive in 80% of babies with Down's syndrome
16–18 weeks	Triple test: alphafetoprotein (AFP), human chorionic gonadotrophin (HCG) and estriol (uE3)	Triple test detection rate of Down's syndrome 64%; false-positive rate 5%
	Quadruple test: as above + inhibin A	Quadruple test detection rate 70%; false-positive rate 5%
18–20 weeks	Detailed USS	For fetal anomalies

HIV, human immunodeficiency virus; VDRL, Venereal Disease Research Laboratory slide test.

6

SOURCES

National Institute for Clinical Excellence (2003) Routine care for the healthy pregnant woman. London: NICE. Online. Available: www.nice.org.uk/page.aspx?o=89310

NEONATAL REVIEW

PURPOSE

- To reassure parents that their baby is healthy.
- To detect congenital abnormalities.
- To provide health promotion advice.

The review is carried out by a doctor or midwife with appropriate training and is ideally done before discharge from hospital. It should be performed by 72 hours of age and ideally within the first 48 hours.
Babies discharged early from hospital should be examined by a GP.
The review has three components:

- Parental interview:
  - pregnancy and birth details
  - family history: vision, hearing or hip problems.
- Physical examination:
  - weight
  - head circumference
  - centile plotting
  - heart and pulses
  - genitalia
  - hips
  - spine
  - tone and head control
  - eyes for red reflex.
- Health promotion advice:
  - promotion of breast feeding
  - vitamin K to prevent haemorrhagic disease of the newborn (breast-fed babies will require additional doses at 1 week and 4 weeks of age)
  - accident prevention (see Chapter 77)
  - prevention of SIDS, i.e. sleeping position, avoidance of smoking
  - avoidance of shaking
  - immunisations as appropriate, e.g. BCG, hepatitis B
  - seek medical advice if jaundice persists beyond 2 weeks of age.

6

NEWBORN HEARING SCREENING

The purpose of this screen is to detect children with congenital sensorineural deafness at the earliest possible opportunity. Early detection has been shown to improve outcome in terms of language development and educational progress.

In some areas this will be done selectively for babies felt to be at increased risk, i.e. those who:

- have a family history of sensorineural deafness
- have been admitted to the neonatal unit.

In many areas all babies are being screened in the early neonatal period (universal neonatal hearing screening).

Otoacoustic emissions (OAE) is a test performed prior to discharge, followed by auditory brain stem responses for those babies who fail OAE. Automated otoacoustic emissions are acoustic responses produced by the cochlea and detected with a sensitive microphone placed in the ear canal. The OAE test screens auditory pathways as far as the cochlea and is very sensitive.

Auditory brain stem response audiometry involves computer analysis of EEG signals produced in response to a series of clicks. This test screens the auditory pathways as far as the brain stem.

NEONATAL SCREENING

Screening for inherited metabolic disease (Guthrie test)

This heel-prick test is carried out around 6 days of age, usually by the midwife.

Conditions screened for include:

- phenylketonuria (PKU) (phenylalanine levels raised)
- congenital hypothyroidism (TSH raised)
- cystic fibrosis (immune reactive trypsin raised).

Screening for haemoglobinopathies

All babies are screened for thalassaemia and sickle cell disease in the neonatal period using the Guthrie blood spot card.

SOURCES

Hall DMB, Elliman D (eds) (2003) Health for all children, 4th edn. Oxford: Oxford University Press

See also

Chapter 77, Child health promotion and accident prevention.

73

HIP EXAMINATION – SCREENING FOR DEVELOPMENTAL DYSPLASIA OF THE HIP

DEFINITION

The term developmental dysplasia of the hip (DDH) covers congenital dislocation of the hip (CDH), subluxation and instability of the hip, including poorly developed joints that may not actually dislocate and abnormalities determined after birth.

Effective screening resulting in early diagnosis and treatment reduces the need for surgical intervention. If left untreated, CDH results in a limp and early osteoarthritis.

EPIDEMIOLOGY AND AETIOLOGY

Major risk factors

Any of these factors increase the risk of hip dysplasia and should prompt re-examination or ultrasound:

- Positive family history (10% are unstable). There is a higher incidence in some ethnic groups, e.g. Lapps and North American Indians; DDH is almost unknown in Chinese and Africans.
- Breech presentation at end of pregnancy (5% are unstable).

Minor risk factors

Congenital deformities of the feet.
Talipes or pes calcaneovalgus.
Oligohydramnios or large baby.
Hypermobility syndromes.
First-born females.

Prevalence

1 in 5 newborns will have some evidence of neonatal laxity at birth, but the true incidence of dislocation is between 1 and 2 per 1000 live births.

ASSESSMENT

The baby's hips should be examined at regular intervals as recommended in the 4th edition of *Health for all Children*, as follows.

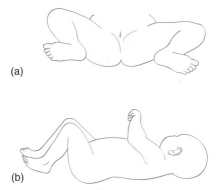

Fig. 73.1 (a) Limited abduction in flexion; (b) apparent shortening and knees flexed.

Neonatal examination
GP examination at 4–8 weeks.

In some areas a further examination is done at the time of the second or third immunisation, between 3 and 5 months of age.

Also at any age if a parent is concerned about their baby's hips or legs.

HISTORY
Enquire about the birth and family history.

If the parent has any concerns about the baby's hips or legs, do *not* ignore these, but refer for ultrasound to exclude DDH.

Examination
The baby should be warm and quiet.

Abnormal physical signs should prompt immediate referral for ultrasound/ x-ray and referral to a paediatric orthopaedic surgeon if either shows a hip abnormality.

- Observe the baby at rest – are the leg(s) held in adduction, does one leg look shorter?
- Examine for limited abduction in flexion – tight adductors may indicate a hip at risk of subluxing/dislocating (Fig. 73.1a).
- Look for apparent shortening of the femur by flexing the knees together in adduction (Fig. 73.1b).
- Examine the hips using the Ortolani and Barlow manoeuvres.

Some babies may have a hip that clicks. This by itself is not diagnostic of DDH but these babies should be referred for ultrasound as 1% have hip dysplasia.

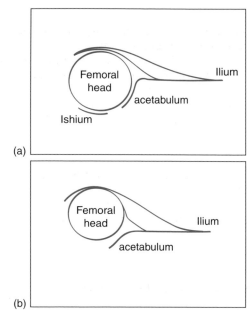

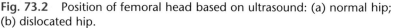

Fig. 73.2 Position of femoral head based on ultrasound: (a) normal hip; (b) dislocated hip.

Diagnostic tests
Ultrasound up to 6–8 months of age (Fig. 73.2).
X-ray 6–8 months and older.

DIFFERENTIAL DIAGNOSIS
Tight adductors may be an early sign of a neurological problem, part of the moulded baby syndrome of plagiocephaly, mild scoliosis and limited abduction, or physiological.

WHEN TO REFER
If DDH is suspected, refer immediately for ultrasound if the baby is <6 months; x-ray if >6 months.

If either of the above is positive, refer immediately for an urgent orthopaedic opinion.

(Some areas/countries ultrasound every baby's hips within a few weeks of birth; others have an 'at-risk' screening policy and all babies with major risk factors are referred for ultrasound.)

THERAPY

Observation of stable hip(s) with mild dysplasia shown on ultrasound; monitor development with repeat scans.

Abduction splinting for hip(s) that are subluxing or unstable.

Examination under anaesthetic (EUA) – arthrogram ± adductor tenotomy, hips that are subluxing or unstable, or not reducing.

Major bony surgery for irreducible hips or later to correct the leg position.

For details of treatment of DDH, refer to orthopaedic texts.

FOLLOW-UP

Routine community screening for all those that have not required orthopaedic referral.

Listen to parents, and take their concerns about their baby's hips or legs seriously. It is better to refer for an ultrasound or x-ray than miss a dislocated hip.

KEY POINTS FOR PARENTS

Make parents aware of the screening programme.

When you examine the baby's hips, explain what you are looking for and encourage the parent to report any concerns to their GP or health visitor.

SOURCES

Department of Health and Social Services (1986) Screening for the detection of congenital dislocation of the hip. London: DHSS

Hall DMB, Elliman D (eds) (2003) Health for all children, 4th edn. Oxford: Oxford University Press

6

BIRTH VISIT

In the UK a birth visit is carried out by the health visitor. The timing of the visit is negotiated between health visitor and midwife, at a point when midwifery involvement is ending. This would usually be between 14 and 28 days of age.

The focus of this review is largely health promotion for both mother and baby. The family's circumstances and needs are reviewed in order to make an initial plan with them for future care. It is an opportunity to identify situations that might be considered as 'high risk'.

ASSESSMENT

Mother

Mental health and well-being.
Family support.
Breast feeding support.

Baby

Feeding and weight gain.
Avoiding sudden infant death syndrome.
Accident prevention (see Chapter 77 and Table 77.2).
Recognition and management of illness.
Advice about immunisation.
Hip check may be performed.

SOURCES

Hall DMB, Elliman D (eds) (2003) Health for all children, 4th edn. Oxford: Oxford University Press

See also

Chapter 77, Child health promotion and accident prevention.

6-WEEK REVIEW AND OTHER PRESCHOOL REVIEWS

6-WEEK REVIEW

This review is carried out by a GP or other appropriately trained person. It may be completed as early as 4 weeks of age but the optimum time is at 6–8 weeks of age. The purpose of the review is to:

- establish the baby is healthy and growing appropriately
- offer health promotion advice.

In some practices this review is combined with the first immunisations at 8 weeks of age.

PARENTAL INTERVIEW

Enquire about family history of vision, hearing or hip problems.
Ask about any feeding difficulties.
Check infant has had a neonatal hearing test if appropriate.
Check developmental milestones, e.g. smiling, socialisation, visual fixation, vocalisation.
Parental health.
Any other concerns?

PHYSICAL EXAMINATION

Weight
Length
Head circumference
Centile plotting
Heart and pulses
Genitalia
Hips
Spine
Tone and head control
Eyes for red reflex
Visual fixation

Any significant abnormalities detected at this examination, e.g. heart murmur, hip problem, undescended testes, should be referred on to secondary care services for further advice.

HEALTH PROMOTION

For breast-fed babies, check three doses of vitamin K have been given.
Advice about avoiding weaning before 6 months of age.
Accident prevention (see Chapter 77).
Prevention of sudden infant death syndrome.
Avoidance of shaking.
Recognition and management of illness.
Advice about immunisations (medical authorisation of infant's fitness to commence immunisation course may be obtained at this stage if necessary).

The 4th edition of *Health for all Children* (see 'Sources', below) does not recommend screening by physical examination between the 6–8 week review and school entry. However, in some areas, other reviews are done and may include the following.

3–4 MONTH REVIEW

This review is usually performed by the health visitor or a member of the health visiting team, e.g. nursery nurse. While largely based around health promotion topics, weight measurement and a hip examination may also be done.
Topics for discussion include:

- weaning advice
- accident prevention
- advising against use of baby walkers
- awareness of future developmental milestones
- promotion of language and social development
- maternal mental health.

8–12 MONTH REVIEW

This review is usually done by a health visitor and may include:

- review of gross motor development
- measurement of growth – height, weight and head circumference
- parental observation of or history of eye problems, e.g. squint
- health promotion and anticipatory guidance around a range of issues including:

- speech and language development
- discontinuing bottles and dummies
- play and behaviour
- nutrition – moving on to family food, drinking from a cup, finger foods
- safety and accident prevention
- dental hygiene
- anticipatory guidance around child development – to include stimulation, play, behaviour management and local resources. Inform parents about the developmental progression of their child so that they know what to expect and can contact the health visitor if they have concerns.

If areas of concern are identified, a programme of care/planned intervention may be needed.

SOURCES
Hall DMB, Elliman D (eds) (2003) Health for all children, 4th edn. Oxford: Oxford University Press

See also
Chapter 77, Child health promotion and accident prevention.

76

SCHOOL ENTRY REVIEW

PURPOSE
- To introduce the school nurse and school health service.
- To ensure that there are no outstanding issues, e.g. incomplete immunisations.
- To screen for growth, vision and hearing concerns.
- To provide health promotion advice relevant to age group.

The review should be carried out in the child's first year at school. It contains both screening and health promotion elements. Routine medical examination of all children is not recommended.

Screening
- Height and weight.
- Visual acuity, using Snellen or logMAR charts. Each eye is tested separately. Refer to an orthoptist or optometrist if vision is found to be 6/12 or greater, or 6/9 or greater in a child with other difficulties.
- Hearing, using pure tone audiometry, sometimes known as the sweep test.

Health promotion
- Healthy eating
- Safety in the sun
- Dental care
- Stranger awareness
- Accident prevention

The 4th edition of *Health for all Children* (see 'Sources', below) recommends no further routine reviews be done after school entry. There is insufficient evidence to support the continuation of school medical examinations by either doctor or school nurse.

However, the school health service remains very much involved with the emphasis on health promotion and support for children with either special educational needs or specific medical needs.

Health service professionals who work with children also have a statutory duty to contribute to the assessment and provide advice to the local education authority (LEA) about children with special educational needs.

SOURCES

Hall DMB, Elliman D (eds) (2003) Health for all children, 4th edn. Oxford: Oxford University Press

See also

Chapter 92, Special medical needs in education; Chapter 93, Special educational needs; Chapter 94, Checklist for advice to local education authorities.

6

CHILD HEALTH PROMOTION AND ACCIDENT PREVENTION

CHILD HEALTH PROMOTION

People's patterns of behaviour are often set in early life and influence their health throughout their lives. Infancy, childhood and young adulthood are critical stages in the development of habits that will affect people's health in later years.

Department of Health (2004a)

Health promotion is not solely the role of health services. Increasingly, other agencies such as education and voluntary bodies are becoming involved and are making a valuable contribution to improving children's health in the long term (Table 77.1).

For problems such as obesity, interventions involving the child's wider social context, i.e. family, school and local environment, are likely to be more successful than those targeted at individuals alone.

ACCIDENT PREVENTION

Prevention of injuries is one of the key objectives of the White Paper *Saving Lives: Our Healthier Nation* (DH 1999).

A national target has been set 'to reduce death rates from accidents by at least one-fifth and to reduce rates of serious injury from accidents by at least one-tenth by 2010' (Table 77.2).

Table 77.1 Child health promotion: infancy to secondary schooling

Age range	Health promotion issues	Recommendations	Key personnel and sources of information
Less than 1 year	Maternal and foetal nutrition Maternal smoking cessation Prevention of SIDS Breast feeding and healthy eating Dental care Sun safety Passive smoking (see below) Accident prevention Immunisations	**Mother:** • Periconceptual folic acid reduces incidence of neural tube defects • Healthy eating during pregnancy • Stop smoking – deleterious effects on foetal growth, lung function, increased risk of stillbirth and SIDS • Breast feeding – optimum nutrition for first 4–6 months of life, reduced risk of infections and allergy **Infant:** • Prevention of SIDS by sleeping supine, using blankets not duvet, correct room temperature, caution about bed sharing. Care of the Next Infant (CONI) programme for families who have suffered a previous cot death • Weaning at 4–6 months. Do not add extra salt or sugar to food • Prevention of dental caries by avoiding sugary drinks or acidic drinks such as fruit juice	Personnel: • Midwife • Health visitor • SureStart Resources: • *Birth to Five* (DH 2004b) • Foundation for the Study of Infant Deaths – www.sids.org.uk/fsid • *Successful Breastfeeding* (Royal College of Midwives 2002) • BDA *Food for the Growing Years* – www.bda.uk.com/Downloads/paedgroupform.pdf

continued

Table 77.1 Child health promotion: infancy to secondary schooling—cont'd

Age range	Health promotion issues	Recommendations	Key personnel and sources of information
		• Prevention of sunburn by use of high factor sun lotions and covering up • Reduced exposure to cigarette smoke. Passive smoking doubles risk of wheezing, croup and ear infections and tonsillitis • Accident prevention (see Table 77.2) • Immunisations (see Ch. 78)	
1–4 years	Prevention of obesity – healthy eating, regular exercise Dental care Sun safety Passive smoking Accident prevention Immunisations	• Balanced diet, including five portions of fruit and vegetables a day (also reduces incidence of some cancers) Avoidance of high fat, high sugar foods Encourage regular exercise of 1 hour per day Reduce TV advertising of high fat, high sugar foods to children • Prevention of dental caries by avoiding sugary drinks or acidic drinks such as fruit juice • Prevention of sunburn by use of high factor sun lotions and covering up	Personnel: • Health visitor • SureStart • Preschool settings, e.g. School Fruit & Vegetable Scheme for 4–6 year olds Resources: • *Birth to Five* (DH 2004b) • BDA *Food for the Growing Years* – www.bda.uk. com/Downloads/ paedgroupform. pdf • *Management of Obesity in Children and Young People* (SIGN 2003)

continued

Table 77.1 Child health promotion: infancy to secondary schooling—cont'd

Age range	Health promotion issues	Recommendations	Key personnel and sources of information
		• Reduced exposure to cigarette smoke; passive smoking doubles risk of wheezing, croup and ear infections and tonsillitis • Accident prevention (see Table 77.2) • Immunisations (see Ch. 78)	For parents: • www.yourover-weightchild.org – website by parents for parents • Media advertising – '5 a day' TV adverts • Giving up smoking – local support groups, helplines, GP, TV advertising – www.givingup smoking.co.uk
Primary school age	Prevention of obesity – healthy eating, regular exercise Dental care Sun safety Active and passive smoking Healthy personal relationships Alcohol and substance misuse Accident prevention Immunisations	• Raise awareness of importance of diet and exercise through National Curriculum Balanced diet, including five portions of fruit and vegetables a day (also reduces incidence of some cancers) Avoidance of high fat, high sugar foods Encourage regular exercise of 1 hour per day Encourage breakfast clubs, cookery clubs, remove vending machines	Schools: • National Healthy Schools Standard (NHSS) – www.wiredfor health.gov.uk (see also Ch. 29) • School Fruit & Vegetable Scheme for 4–6 year olds • *National Smile Week* dental health promotion in schools and elsewhere – www.dental health.org.uk • Health professionals:

6

continued

Table 77.1   Child health promotion: infancy to secondary schooling—cont'd

Age range	Health promotion issues	Recommendations	Key personnel and sources of information
		Reduce TV advertising of high fat, high sugar foods to children • Prevention of dental caries by avoiding sugary drinks or acidic drinks such as fruit juice • Prevention of sunburn by use of high factor sun lotions and covering up • Reduced exposure to cigarette smoke; passive smoking doubles risk of wheezing, croup and ear infections and tonsillitis Health promotion in schools about not starting smoking Encourage role models, e.g. parents to quit smoking • Education about sex and relationships • Accident prevention (see Table 77.2) • Immunisations (see Ch. 78)	• BDA *Food for the School Years* – www.bda.uk.com/Downloads/paedgroupform.pdf For parents: • www.yourover weightchild.org • Media advertising – '5 a day' TV adverts • www.giving upsmoking.co.uk
Secondary school age	Prevention of obesity – healthy eating, regular exercise Smoking Alcohol and substance misuse Sexual health –	• Teaching about the importance of diet and exercise Balanced diet, including five portions of fruit and vegetables a day (also reduces	Schools: • NHSS Parents and young people: • www.yourover weightchild.org • Media – '5 a day' TV adverts

continued

Table 77.1 Child health promotion: infancy to secondary schooling—cont'd

Age range	Health promotion issues	Recommendations	Key personnel and sources of information
	contraception and prevention of sexually transmitted infections (STIs) Dental care Sun safety Accident prevention Immunisations	incidence of some cancers) Avoidance of high fat, high sugar foods Encourage regular exercise Reduce TV advertising of high fat, high sugar foods to children • Education about smoking Encourage role models, e.g. parents to quit smoking • Issue of dependency on drugs and alcohol form part of curriculum Advice about safe alcohol intake • Raise awareness of STIs and their long-term consequences • Education about sex and relationships • Prevention of dental caries by avoiding sugary drinks or acidic drinks such as fruit juice. • Prevention of sunburn by use of high factor sun lotions and covering up. • Accident prevention (see Table 77.2) • Immunisations (see Ch. 78)	• www.wiredfor health.gov.uk • www.ruthin king.co.uk • www.teenage healthfreak.com • www.giving upsmoking.co.uk Government: • Teenage Pregnancy Unit and SureStart Plus.

BDA, British Dietetic Association; SIDS, sudden infant death syndrome; SIGN, Scottish Intercollegiate Guidelines Network.

Table 77.2 Accident prevention: infancy to secondary schooling

Age range	Common accidents	Means of prevention	Personnel involved
Less than 1 year	Falls-from beds, tables, baby walkers	Advice about avoidance and suitable alternatives, e.g. playpen	Health visitor, SureStart worker Advice given at all routine reviews in first year Emergency Department staff
	Injuries in motor vehicles	Use of car seat	As above
	Burns and scalds from, e.g. carrying infant at same time as hot drink	Advice about avoidance Fireguard for mobile babies Smoke alarm	As above Also Fire and Rescue Service
	Choking/suffocation	Avoid toys with small removable parts Avoid pillows and duvets in cots	As above
1–4 years	Falls, e.g. down stairs, from windows	Advice about stair gates, window locks	Health visitor, SureStart worker, nursery school staff Emergency Department staff
	Poisoning, e.g. detergents, medicine	Advice about cupboard locks, bottles with child proof caps Dispose of unwanted medicines	As above
	Drowning, e.g. child left alone in bath or in pond or pool	Parental education Fences around ponds/pool Teach children to swim	As above
	Burns and scalds, e.g. from hot liquids, open fires	Fireguards, smoke alarms, coiled flexes on electrical appliances, stair gates across kitchen doorways	As above. Fire and Rescue Service

continued

Table 77.2 Accident prevention: infancy to secondary schooling—cont'd

Age range	Common accidents	Means of prevention	Personnel involved
	Choking/suffocation	Avoid toys with small removable parts Avoid peanuts Keep plastic bags out of reach	As above
	Road traffic injuries, e.g. in cars, bicycles or pedestrian	Car seats, seatbelts, cycle helmets Traffic calming measures, e.g. speed bumps	As above. Government and local authority staff Police
5–16 years	Road traffic injuries as described above	As above	As above
	Sporting injuries	Parent and child education Warming up prior to exercise	Parents School staff Emergency Department staff GP

SOURCES

Department of Health (1999) Saving lives: our healthier nation. Cm 4386. London: TSO

Department of Health (2004a) Choosing health. London: TSO, Ch. 3

Department of Health (2004b) Birth to five. London: TSO

Polnay L (ed.) (2002) Community paediatrics, 3rd edn. Edinburgh: Churchill Livingstone

Royal College of Midwives (2002) Successful breastfeeding, 3rd edn. Edinburgh: Churchill Livingstone

Scottish Intercollegiate Guidelines Network (2003) Management of obesity in children and young people. Edinburgh: SIGN. Online. Available: www.sign.ac.uk/guidelines/fulltext/69/index.html

See also

Chapter 29, Nutritional issues – preschool years and older children; Chapter 78, Immunisation.

78

IMMUNISATION

Table 78.1 The UK immunisation schedule

Age	Immunisations required	Live/inactivated
Birth	BCG and/or hepatitis B (see immunisation for selected patient groups below)	BCG is live
2 months	DtaP/IPV/HiB and pneumococcal vaccine	All inactivated
3 months	DtaP/IPV/HiB, meningitis C vaccine	All inactivated
4 months	DtaP/IPV/HiB, meningitis C and pneumococcal vaccine	All inactivated
12 months	Hib/men C combined vaccine	
13 months	MMR and pneumococcal vaccine	MMR is live
$3\frac{1}{2}$ to 5 years	DTaP/IPV or dTaP/IPV MMR	MMR is live
14 to 16 years	Td/IPV	All inactivated

Notes
1. D = full dose diphtheria, d = low dose diphtheria
2. All vaccines except BCG are given intramuscularly. The incidence of local reactions is less if vaccine is given intramuscularly rather than subcutaneously. Vaccine should be given subcutaneously in children with bleeding disorders. BCG is given intradermally.

CONTRAINDICATIONS
- **All vaccines**. Anaphylaxis (to a previous dose or to a specific component) or an acutely unwell child are absolute contraindications to immunisation with all vaccines.
- **Live vaccines**. Live vaccines should not be given to children who are immunocompromised i.e. those with immunodeficiency, malignancy, HIV, those undergoing chemotherapy or children on high doses of oral steroids for prolonged periods (2 mg/kg/day for more than

1 week or 1 mg/kg/day for 1 month or for adults, 40 mg per day for more than a week).

Where possible immunisation may proceed when treatment is complete and once immunity has returned to normal (usually about 3 months after treatment ceased).

If more than one live vaccine is to be given they should either be given at the same time or an interval of one month left between doses. It is thought that a shorter interval than this may impair the body's immune response to each individual vaccine.

IMMUNISATION FOR SELECTED PATIENT GROUPS

1. **BCG** is given at birth to babies considered at increased risk of exposure to TB in early life; i.e. those with a close family history of TB or those whose parents or grandparents originate from countries with a high incidence of TB, or those babies living in areas with a high incidence of TB (an incidence of 40 per 100,000 or more is considered a high incidence – a list of countries with a high incidence of TB can be found at www.immunisation.nhs,uk/files/268967_bcgbaby.pdf)
2. **Hepatitis B** vaccine is given to babies of mothers identified to be surface antigen positive in pregnancy. Immunoglobulin should also be given if the mother is e-antigen positive as this denotes an increased risk of transmission. Hepatitis B vaccine should be given at birth, one month, two months and 12 months followed by serological testing. Completion of the immunisation course will prevent carrier status in 90–95% of infants.
3. **Pneumococcal** vaccine is indicated for unimmunised children in the following at risk groups:
   - Asplenia/splenic dysfunction e.g. homozygous sickle cell disease
   - Chronic respiratory disease e.g. Cystic Fibrosis
   - Infants with significant congenital heart disease
   - Immunocompromised (see live vaccines)
   - Chronic renal or liver failure or diabetes
   - Those with cochlear implants or CSF shunts
   - Previous pneumococcal meningitis or septicaemia.

   Dosage: aged 0–1 year, immunise according to routine immunisation schedule.

   Aged 1–5 years, 2 doses of Pneumococcal conjugate vaccine (7-valent) two months apart with one dose of polysaccharide vaccine (23-valent) after the second birthday.

   Aged 5 years and over, single dose of pneumococcal polysaccharide vaccine. Children with asplenia need boosting with polysaccharide vaccine every 5 years.
4. **Varicella zoster (VZ)** vaccine. Chicken pox is usually a mild, self limiting illness in children. However it may be severe or life threatening in the immunocompromised, pregnant women and neonates. VZ vaccine is indicated for:

- Health care workers working with high risk groups i.e. immunocompromised, pregnant women, neonates who have no antibody on serological testing
- Close contacts of immunocompromised individuals who have no antibody on testing.

Dosage: aged 1–13 require a single dose

Aged over 13 years, 2 doses separated by an interval of 4–8 weeks

Varicella vaccine is currently not recommended for routine use in the UK.

Varicella zoster immunoglobulin (VZIG) is recommended for individuals who fulfil all of the following 3 criteria:

- Significant exposure to chicken pox or herpes zoster (risk period is 1–2 days prior to the rash appearing until vesicles have crusted over)
- Immunocompromised or pregnant or a neonate
- Have no antibodies to VZ virus

Exposure to VZV in the first 20 weeks of pregnancy poses a risk of congenital Varicella syndrome (limb hypoplasia, cataracts, microcephaly)

Maternal chicken pox infection 7 days before to 7 days after delivery poses a risk of severe Varicella infection for the neonate as they will not have received protective maternal antibody transplacentally.

5. **Influenza** Vaccine is indicated for children over 6 months of age with any of the following risk factors:

- Chronic respiratory disease e.g., Cystic Fibrosis, chronic asthma which requires continuous or repeated courses of inhaled or oral steroids
- Significant congenital heart disease
- Chronic renal failure
- Diabetes
- Immunocompromised (see live vaccines), HIV, splenic dysfunction.

Influenza vaccine is inactivated and should be given intramuscularly.

Dosage: Age 6 months to 3 years, 0.25–0.5 ml.

Age 3–12 years, 0.5 ml. The dose should be repeated 4–6 weeks later if flu vaccine is being given for the first time.

Age 12 years and over, one single dose of 0.5 ml.

Flu vaccine is contraindicated in children who have had anaphylactic reaction to egg, but not those who are "egg allergic".

6. **Hepatitis A** Vaccine is indicated in the following circumstances:

- Travellers to endemic areas
- Haemophiliacs (given subcutaneously). There is a small risk of Hepatitis A from blood products
- Outbreaks. Vaccination helps control spread of the illness through communities. Close contacts of affected individuals should be given Human Normal Immunoglobulin (HNIG). Advice should be sought from a Consultant in Communicable Disease Control (CCDC) about the acute management of outbreaks.

A single dose of Hepatitis A vaccine gives immunity for up to 1 year. For long term immunity a booster dose after 6–12 months is required.

SOURCES

Immunisation Against Infectious Disease 1996 ("The Green Book") HMSO London – updated version available at www.dh.gov.uk/PublicationsAndStatistics/Publications/
Useful resource for parents and professionals: www.immunisation.nhs.uk

6

SOCIAL PAEDIATRICS

79

SUBSTANCE MISUSE IN CHILDREN AND YOUNG PEOPLE

DEFINITION

Numerous definitions, including 'maladaptive pattern of substance use manifested by recurrent and significant adverse consequences related to the repeated use of substances'.

EPIDEMIOLOGY AND AETIOLOGY

Reasons for involvement include peer pressure, experimentation and to boost self-esteem.

Reported rates of substance abuse (alcohol and drugs) in the UK are higher than elsewhere in Europe.

Recent evidence of drug use in pre-adolescent children (up to 5%).

Higher rates in young people who are vulnerable, including young people who are:

- 'looked after' by the local authority
- homeless
- local authority care leavers
- involved in offending, including those involved with the criminal justice system
- have parents who misuse drugs or alcohol
- disaffected from/excluded from school
- living in difficult family situations including those subject to abuse.

Reported drug misuse (2002) in England
Children aged 11–15 years
18% overall prevalence.

Prevalence increases sharply with age: 6% of 11 year olds; 36% of 15 year olds.

- 13% used cannabis (most frequent use)
- 1% used heroin
- 1% used cocaine
- 4% used a Class A drug*.

*Class A drugs – amphetamines, heroin, cocaine, ecstasy, magic mushrooms, LSD, unprescribed use of methadone.

Young people aged 16–24 years
30% use within the last year; 19% within the last month.

- 27% used cannabis
- 7% used ecstasy
- 5% used amfetamines
- 5% used cocaine
- 4% used poppers[†]
- 1% used crack
- 9% used a Class A drug.

Rates of use have stayed the same since 1996; however, there has been a significant increase in cocaine use (1–5%) and ecstasy use (4–7%). Use of amfetamines has dropped to 5% and LSD to 1%.

Solvent misuse
Glues, cleaning fluids, aerosols, petrol, Tipp-Ex, paint, varnish, nail polish, dyes, fire-extinguishers and room fresheners. Active ingredients are toluene, benzene, xylene and acetone.

Only a minority of young people abuse solvents. It is estimated that in the UK 0.5–1% of young people between 16 and 24 years of age will try inhaling solvents each year. The majority will experiment a few times and only a small minority will become chronic abusers.

- The total of all deaths from solvent abuse to 31 December 2003 was 2013.
- In children aged ≤14 years, there were 12 deaths in 2002 and 4 in 2003.
- In young people between 14 and 18 years of age there were 12 deaths in 2002 and 5 in 2003.

Although more boys than girls abuse solvents, the number of girls is increasing, currently accounting for 25% of cases. The highest rates occur in NE England, Scotland and Northern Ireland.

Gas fuel abuse accounts for the majority of deaths – 59% in 2002.

Prevalence of drinking alcohol in the last week (2000)
11–15 year olds ~24%.
Average of 10 units, usually beer, lager or cider.

PRESENTATION
Despite exposure to toxic substances, children and young people *do not* present in large numbers to health services:

Feeling out of it
Intoxication
Accidental/violent injury

[†]Poppers – a group of chemicals called alkyl nitrates.

Road traffic accidents
Sexually transmitted diseases
Teenage pregnancy
Respiratory diseases
Self-harm
Psychiatric disorders
Accidentally set fire to themselves (solvent abuse)
Associated with other risk-taking behaviours

Effects – short term
- Alter or amplify mood
- Alter perceptions
- May change personal and social inhibitions
- Impair reaction time
- Unusual stains or smells on body or clothing

Effects – long term
- Loss of interest in appearance, school work, hobbies
- Minor health problems, e.g. infections, coughs, accidents
- Loss or gain in appetite
- Lethargy, drowsiness and unsteady gait
- Deterioration in school work
- Furtive behaviour
- Leukaemia (benzene abuse)

ASSESSMENT
History
Past medical history
Prescribed medications
Allergies
Family medical history
Social history
Drug and alcohol usage history
Sharing needles
Sexual history
Criminal activity

Examination
Growth
Nutrition
Infestation (head lice, scabies)
Injuries?
Signs of drug or alcohol use, e.g. smell of alcohol, sniffing, venepuncture sites
Signs of liver disease (hepatitis B or C, alcohol)
Full examination
Assessment of mental status

Diagnostic tests

Urine drug toxicology.

Blood alcohol level.

Liver function tests.

Consider tests for sexually transmitted infections and blood-borne viruses
– Chlamydia, gonorrhoea, syphilis, HIV, hepatitis C.

> **ALERTS**
> - Homeless
> - Under 16 years of age
> - Intravenous drug use
> - Other risk-taking behaviour

WHO TO TALK TO

School nurse.

Social services.

GP.

Child and Adolescent Mental Health Services (CAMHS).

COMPASS (drug and alcohol support agency).

Other drug and alcohol support agencies.

Youth Offending Team (including preventative programme).

THERAPY

Drug and alcohol withdrawal programmes, e.g. COMPASS.

Treatment of individual conditions, e.g. head lice, depression.

FOLLOW-UP

Individual plan according to health needs.

KEY POINTS FOR PARENTS AND YOUNG PEOPLE

Young people and their parents will need advice and information on local
support services.

HEALTH PROMOTION

Recommended weekly alcohol intake.

Use of clean needles.

Use of barrier contraception.

SUPPORT ORGANISATIONS

Adfam (Families, drugs and alcohol) – www.adfam.org.uk
Charity working with families affected by drugs and alcohol.

BUPA fact sheet on substance misuse in young people – http://hcd2.
bupa.co.uk/fact_sheets/html/teen_drugs.html
DrugScope – www.drugscope.org.uk
National coordinating body for voluntary services and agencies working the drugs field.
National Drugs helpline 0800 776600 –
www.urban75.com/Drugs/helpline.html
Re-Solv (Society for the Prevention of Solvent and Volatile Substance Abuse)
Tel: 0808 8002345
www.re-solv.org (see also www.sniffing.org.uk, Re-solv's site for young people)
Charity dedicated to tackling solvent misuse.
COMPASS (Young People's Drug and Alcohol Service)
Huntingdon Street
Nottingham NG1 3JH
Tel: 0115 847 0445
Supports young people in Nottinghamshire and Yorkshire

SOURCES

Boreham R, Shaw A (eds) (2001) Smoking, drinking and drug use among young people in England 2000. National Centre for Social Research and National Foundation for Educational Research. London: TSO. Online. Available: www.archive.official-documents.co.uk/document/doh/sddyp/survey.htm

Goulden C, Sondhi A (2001) At the margins: drug use by vulnerable young people in the 1998/99 Youth Lifestyles Survey. London: Home Office Research, Development and Statistics Directorate. Online. Available: www.homeoffice.gov.uk/rds/pdfs/hors228.pdf

Home Office: Tackling Drugs, Changing Lives – www.drugs.gov.uk

McArdle P (2004) Substance abuse by children and young people. Archives of Disease in Childhood 89: 701–704

National Statistics (UK) – www.statistics.gov.uk

National Treatment Agency for Substance Misuse – www.nta.nhs.uk

St George's Hospital Medical School (2002) Annual report on mortalities from solvent and volatile substance abuse. London: St George's Hospital Medical School

7

80

SMOKING IN YOUNG PEOPLE

The UK Government has set a target to reduce the number of children aged 11–15 who smoke regularly (more than 1/week) from a baseline of 13% in 1996, to 11% by 2005, and 9% by 2010.

The Children's and Young People's (Protection from Tobacco) Act 1991 increased the penalties and provided for enforcement action against underage tobacco sales by local authorities.

EPIDEMIOLOGY AND AETIOLOGY

There are a variety of reasons why young people start to smoke:

- To fit in, be part of a group.
- To look cool (advertising, celebrities shown to smoke on TV).
- To experiment, just to try it out.
- Have a friend/friends who smoke.
- To look rebellious, be rebellious.
- To look older.

The proportion of regular smokers has been quite stable since 1998.

In 2002 10% of pupils aged 11–15 were regular smokers.

Prevalence of smoking is strongly related to age: 1% of 11 year olds; 23% of 15 year olds.

Since the early 1980s girls have been consistently more likely to smoke than boys. In 2002, 11% of girls were regular smokers compared with 9% of boys. However, boys smoked more cigarettes than girls – an average of 52/week for boys and 48/week for girls.

Associated with other risk-taking behaviour, e.g. alcohol and drug use, underage sex, etc.

PRESENTATION

Poorly controlled asthma.
Recurrent chest infections.
Conductive hearing loss.
Other risk-taking behaviours.

Stealing to pay for habit.
Chewing gum, mouth freshener use to hide smell.

ASSESSMENT
History
Need to ask all young people about smoking habits, regardless of the problem
they are presenting with, as unlikely to volunteer information.
Previous medical history (particularly asthma).
Family medical history.
Family members who smoke or are ex-smokers.
Age when started smoking.
Current smoking habits.
Concurrent drug use.

Examination
General appearance and demeanour.
Skin condition including injuries.
Signs of infection.
Full general examination.

THERAPY
Smoking cessation programmes, e.g. New Leaf.

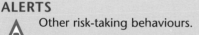

ALERTS

Other risk-taking behaviours.

WHO TO TALK TO
GP.
School nurse.
Smoking cessation counsellors.

HEALTH PROMOTION
Young people who feel that their parents would be upset with them if they
knew that they were smoking are *less* likely to start smoking.
The proportion of young people who remembered having lessons on
smoking has fluctuated over the years but has remained stable since
1999 at 65%.
Among older young people there was a positive correlation between
remembering lessons and whether they smoked (28% compared with
22%). However, it cannot be inferred that lessons lead to lower

smoking rates as previous rates have shown that perceived usefulness of lessons is also related to behaviour and pupils who are less likely to be in school (truanting or exclusion) are more likely to smoke.

SOURCES

Boreham R, McManus S (eds) (2003) Smoking, drinking and drug use among young people in England in 2002. London: TSO (*A survey carried out on behalf of the Department of Health by NatCen.*)

Boreham R, Shaw A (eds) (2001) Smoking, drinking and drug use among young people in England in 2000. National Centre for Social Research and National Foundation for Educational Research. London: TSO. Online. Available: www.archive.official-documents.co.uk/document/doh/sddyp/survey.htm

Department of Health – www.dh.gov.uk

Department of Health (1998) Smoking kills: a White Paper on tobacco. Cm 4177. London: TSO

National Statistics (UK) – www.statistics.gov.uk

81

TEENAGE PREGNANCY

DEFINITION
Pregnancy in a girl <18 years of age.

EPIDEMIOLOGY AND AETIOLOGY
The UK has the highest teenage pregnancy rate in Europe (Table 81.1).

PRESENTATION
May be asymptomatic/concealed pregnancy.
Request for pregnancy test.
Amenorrhoea.
Nausea and vomiting.
Breast tenderness.
Frequency of urine.
Abdominal swelling.

ASSESSMENT
History
Date of last menstrual period.
Contraceptive history.

Table 81.1 Conception data for England

Year	<18 years Number	<18 years % having TOP	<16 years Number	<16 years % having TOP
1998	41,089	42.4	7,885	52.9
1999	39,247	43.5	7,408	53.0
2000	38,690	44.8	7,617	54.5
2001	38,439	46.0	7,396	55.9

TOP, termination of pregnancy.

What are the symptoms?
Signs/symptoms of sexually transmitted infection (STI).
Age of partner (child protection issues).
Number of partners (risk of STI).
Partner/family support.
Previous medical history.
Family medical history.
Risk-taking behaviour.
What does she want to do about her pregnancy?
Who has she talked to about being pregnant?
Is her partner involved?

Examination
Height and weight.
Full examination.
Blood pressure.

Diagnostic tests
Urine pregnancy test for beta HCG.
USS to assess gestation if unsure of dates.

DIFFERENTIAL DIAGNOSIS

Polycystic ovarian syndrome.

ALERTS
- Young person <16 years
- Learning difficulties
- Chronic illness
- Lack of support
- Drug and alcohol use

WHO TO TALK TO

Encourage young person to involve mum/family member.
School nurse.
Local contraception and sexual health service.
SureStart plus.
Counselling service.
Social services.

WHEN TO REFER

If requesting termination of pregnancy (TOP).
Social services, if any suspicion of child protection issues.
SureStart plus if <16 years.

THERAPY

Continuing pregnancy.
Folic acid supplementation.
Avoidance of:

- smoking
- alcohol
- medications
- recreational drugs
- unpasteurised cheeses
- liver
- contact with cat litter.

Ensure food is fresh and well cooked.

Referral for termination of pregnancy
- Early medical TOP (if <9/52)
- Surgical TOP

HEALTH PROMOTION

STI prevention during pregnancy
Use of folic acid
Stopping smoking
Minimal alcohol
Healthy eating
Future contraception

SOURCES

Mellanby AR (1997) Preventing teenage pregnancy. Archives of Disease in
    Childhood 77: 459–462
National Statistics (UK) – www.statistics.gov.uk
Social Exclusion Unit – www.socialexclusion.gov.uk
SureStart – www.surestart.gov.uk
Teenage Pregnancy Unit, DfES – www.dfes.gov.uk/teenagepregnancy

7

82

TRANSITIONAL CARE

DEFINITION

Transition is 'the purposeful, planned movement of adolescents and young adults with chronic physical and medical conditions from child-centred to adult orientated health care systems' (Blum et al 1993).

'Young people' has become the preferred term for describing adolescents in today's health and social care arenas. There is much debate around the age parameters of adolescence. Although 13–18 years is generally acknowledged, for many young people, the period of adolescence starts much earlier; for others it continues well into their early twenties (RCPCH 2003).

DEVELOPING TRANSITIONAL CARE PATHWAYS

The importance of this process has recently been highlighted in the following documents:

- *National Service Framework for Children, Young People and Maternity Services* (DH 2004)
- *Bridging the Gap* (RCPCH 2003)
- *Adolescent Transition Care – Guidance for Nursing Staff* (RCN 2004).

AIMS OF TRANSITION

- To provide coordinated, uninterrupted healthcare that is:
  - patient centred
  - age and developmentally appropriate
  - culturally competent
  - comprehensive, flexible, responsive.
- To promote skills in communication, decision-making, assertiveness, self-care.
- To enhance a sense of control and interdependence in healthcare.
- To provide support for the parent(s)/guardian(s) of the young person during this process.

KEY ELEMENTS FOR AN EFFECTIVE TRANSITION POLICY

- A written transition policy
- A preparation period and education programme
- A coordinated transfer process with a named coordinator
- An interested and capable adult clinical service
- Administrative support
- Primary health care and social care support (Viner 1999, DH 2003).

Each speciality should identify a lead person for transitional care development in both child and adult services (DH 2003).

KEY ELEMENTS FOR TRANSITIONAL CARE

Transition should include the services of education, social care and the voluntary sector.

Service development must be undertaken in collaboration with the young people involved.

Transitional services must be multidisciplinary and include effective liaison with adult services and primary care.

WHEN SHOULD TRANSITION TAKE PLACE?

'Although it may be useful to set a target age, there is no 'right' time for transition. A flexible approach is called for that takes developmental readiness into account and links to other social transitions such as leaving school' (DH 2003).

Timing of transfer is dependent on:

- chronological age/maturity
- adherence
- dependence
- adolescent readiness
- parental readiness
- availability of adult specialist.

Flexibility is required in respect of the patient's health and ideally they should be in a period of disease remission during their ultimate transition to adult care.

PREPARATION FOR TRANSITION

Preparation should start in early adolescence with the aim of assessing understanding of disease and the rationale of therapy, source of symptoms, recognising deterioration and how to take appropriate action.

The young person should understand who to contact for health advice, when and how.

Young people should be encouraged to take control of their medication – parents should be encouraged to assist this process.

The concept of independent consultations should be introduced during the transitional phase. Parents should also be seen with the young person at some point in the consultation.

Consultations should take place in adolescent clinics and, where possible, with the same health professional at each visit.

Where possible, young people should see professionals of their preferred gender.

KEY POINTS FOR YOUNG PEOPLE AND THEIR FAMILIES

- *What Should A Really Good Hospital Look Like?* (version for children). Order number 3102
- *Standards for Children in Hospital* (version for parents). Order number 3103
- *What Should A Really Good Hospital Be Like?* (version for young people). Order number 31304

The above can be ordered from: Department of Health, PO Box 777, London SE1 6XH. Tel: NHS Response line 08701 555455, or email: doh@prolog.co.uk.

- *Careers*: www.connexions.gov.uk.
- *Consent*: www.dh.gov.uk (via A–Z listing: 'Consent: a guide for children and young people').
- *Generic health*: www.lifebytes.gov.uk, www.mindbodysoul.gov.uk, www.teenagehealthfreak.com.

SOURCES

American Academy of Pediatrics (2002) A consensus statement on health care transitions for young adults with special health care needs. Pediatrics 110: 1304–1306

Blum RW, Garell D, Hodgman CH et al (1993) Transition from child-centered to adult health-care systems for adolescents with chronic conditions: a position paper of the Society for Adolescent Medicine. Journal of Adolescent Health 14: 570–576

Department of Health (2003) Getting the right start: National Framework for Children, standards for hospital services. London: TSO

Department of Health (2004) National Service Framework for children, young people and maternity services – every child matters. London: TSO. Online. Available: www.dh.gov.uk

Forbes A, While A, Ullman R et al (2002) A multimethod review to identify components of practice which may promote the continuity in the transition from child to adult care for young people with chronic illness or disability. Online. Available: www.sdo.lshtm.ac.uk/continuityofcare.htm

McDonagh JE (2000) Child–adult interface: the adolescent challenge. Nephrology, Dialysis, Transplantation 15: 1761–1765

Royal College of Nursing (2004) Adolescent transition care – guidance for nursing staff. London: RCN. Online. Available: www.rcn.org.uk

Royal College of Paediatrics and Child Health (2003) Bridging the gap. London: RCPCH. Online. Available: www.rcpch.ac.uk

Viner RM (1999) Transition from paediatric to adult care. Bridging the gaps or passing the buck? Archives of Disease in Childhood 81: 271–275

SAFEGUARDING CHILDREN AND THE LAW

THE CHILDREN ACT 1989

Local authority social workers' actions are based on what the law requires and allows them to do. Children's social care, formerly known as social services have a statutory duty to safeguard and promote the well-being of children in their care. There is an expectation to inform the parents/carers of what is happening, unless to do so is inconsistent in safeguarding/promoting the child's welfare.

It is very useful for doctors to be aware of key sections of the Children Act 1989 so they can see how the framework of safeguarding children sits within the law. It also helps in understanding how best to communicate with social workers. Familiarity with parts of the Act will help understand the joint working process.

The document *Working Together to Safeguard Children* (DH 1999) is the government guidance for interagency cooperation under The Children Act 1989. The Department of Health was extensively involved in its compilation, along with the Home Office and Department for Education and Employment. The document should be complied with unless there are exceptional circumstances. Medical staff involved with caring for children should be aware of its contents.

Main principles

The necessary action to take in order to safeguard children involves obligations to ascertain wishes and feelings of family members.

It is better for children to be brought up within the family, where possible, if this is consistent with their welfare.

The welfare of the child is paramount when courts make decisions.

It is always preferable to have actions agreed with parents/carers on a voluntary basis. Court orders should only be used where the welfare of the child cannot be safeguarded without an order.

Parents have responsibilities for their children as opposed to rights. These responsibilities must be exercised in the best interests of the child.

THE CHILDREN ACT 1989 – SECTION 47

This section prescribes what social workers must do when they have reasonable cause to suspect that a child is suffering or likely to suffer significant (see below) harm, or a child in their area is brought into police protection. They have a statutory duty to:

- make enquiries to ascertain whether and to what degree there is a risk
- assess the needs of the child
- decide what action is necessary to safeguard and promote the child's welfare.

Thus, if a health professional makes a referral to social services because they have concerns about a child at risk, social services must consider their statutory responsibilities under this part of the Act.

Section 47 also empowers social workers to require other professionals to help them in these enquiries including by providing information, unless to do so would be unreasonable in the circumstances.

- *'Significant'*: The use of this word has a specific meaning and establishes a threshold of concern. In this context it means noteworthy or important. It is not actually defined in the Act, but left to the professional's judgement.
- *'Harm'*: Harm is defined as including ill treatment or the impairment of health or development and the seeing or hearing the ill treatment of others.

THE CHILDREN ACT 1989 – SECTION 17

A child is 'in need' if he is unlikely to achieve or maintain, or have the opportunity of maintaining, a reasonable standard of health or development without the provision for him of services by a local authority, or his health or development is likely to be significantly impaired or further impaired, without the provision for him of such services, or he is disabled.

Children's social care, (social services) has a duty to assess the child's needs and provide appropriate services. The *Framework for the Assessment of Children in Need and their Families* (DH 2000) provides the systematic approach that social workers are required to use to assess evidence about many aspects of a child's developmental progress, the parent's ability to respond to the child's needs and the wider family and environment. This framework can and should be used by doctors involved with children when that child may be 'in need', along with the 'Common Assessment Framework' which the government is currently developing.

Emergency Protection Order

This order lasts for 8 days (can be extended by 7 days). The local authority (or any other person) can apply to the court when there is belief that a child is suffering or likely to suffer significant harm unless that child is removed from where he/she is or kept in a particular place (e.g. a hospital). This order can also be applied for by a local authority if urgent access is unreasonably denied when making enquiries under Section 47. Whoever is granted the order (usually the local authority) acquires temporary parental responsibility.

Parental responsibility

This is defined as 'all the rights, duties, powers, responsibilities and authority which in law a parent of a child has in relation to their child and his property'. The emphasis has changed from rights to responsibilities – children are not the property of their parents. This responsibility diminishes with the increasing age and independence of the child.

Who has parental responsibility?

Where a child's parents are married at the time of the child's birth, each has parental responsibility.

Where a child's parents are not married at the time of the child's birth, the mother has parental responsibility. The father (in cases such as above) may acquire parental responsibility by:

- marrying the mother, or
- obtaining a court order, or
- having a formal agreement with the mother, or
- being present at the registration of the birth and being recorded as the father.

Others may acquire parental responsibility through the court by a residence order.

After adoption, the adopting parents have parental responsibility.

A local authority acquires parental responsibility with a care order (and shares it with the parents who have parental responsibility). The local authority must determine the extent to which parents exercise parental responsibility.

Thus parental responsibility may be held by more than one person at a time and can be exercised by one person independently.

Police protection

A police constable can remove a child or prevent the removal of a child for 72 hours if the officer believes that the child is suffering or is likely to suffer significant harm if action were not taken. The timescale means that a court order can be sought if thought necessary after further investigation. Police protection can be used, for example, if parents/carers want to remove a child from hospital, and by so doing would put the child's health or safely at significant risk.

HUMAN RIGHTS ACT 1998

Article 2 states that everyone has a right to life. Article 3 states that no one shall be subjected to inhuman or degrading treatment or torture. Child abuse and neglect are certainly degrading and can lead to loss of life.

All public authorities are expected to work to promote the safeguarding of children under these articles. While article 8 states that everyone has a right to *respect* for private and family life, it does not mean that there is a *right* to privacy, but respect for it. This is important when considering investigations required in safeguarding children – the safety of the child comes first.

THE CHILDREN ACT 2004

This Act provides overarching arrangements to promote the well-being of children, defined as:

- physical and mental health and emotional well-being
- protection from harm and neglect
- education, training and recreation
- the contribution made by them to society
- social and economic well-being.

It also places specific duties on a range of agencies to carry out their functions (including services to adults) having regard to the need to safeguard and promote the welfare of children.

A Children's Commissioner has been appointed. His function is to promote awareness of the views and interests of children and in particular to have regard to the United Nations Convention on the rights of the child.

Any reference to a child includes, in addition to a person under the age of 18, a person aged 18, 19 or 20 who:

- has been looked after by a local authority at any time after attaining the age of 16, or
- has a learning disability, and is receiving education or training.

Each children's services authority must ensure they safeguard and promote the welfare of children and young people. In order to improve the well-being of children, they must also take into account the importance of parents and carers. They must also promote cooperation between its partners – which include the police, Strategic Health Authorities, NHS Trusts and Primary Care Trusts.

This effectively means that all those who work in these services must communicate appropriately and effectively.

WHO TO TALK TO

Legal section of local social services for advice if needed.

7

SOURCES

Department of Health (1999) Working together to safeguard children. London: TSO

Department of Health (2000) The framework for the assessment of children in need and their families. London: TSO

The Children Act 1989. London: TSO. Online. Available: www.opsi.gov.uk/acts/acts1989/Ukpga_19890041_en_1.htm

The Children Act 2004. London: TSO. Online. Available: www.opsi.gov.uk/acts/acts2004/20040031.htm

The Human Rights Act 1998. London: TSO. Online. Available: www.opsi.gov.uk/acts/acts1998/19980042.htm

White W, Carr P, Lowe N (1995) The Children Act in practice. London: Butterworths

See also

Chapter 84 Social Services, Children's Social Care.

SOCIAL SERVICES/ CHILDREN'S SOCIAL CARE

DEFINITION

Children social care provide care and support to a wide variety of people, helping them to live better and fulfilling lives. Social care services also make a major contribution to tackling social inequality.

In 2004/5 the modernisation of social services became a national priority for the government.

Children's social care provide support for children, young people and families in whom there are concerns regarding child protection, i.e. children in need or children at risk for abuse, or a disabled child or children, vulnerable adults (mental health, learning difficulties, the elderly).

The Children Act 1989

This Act is the legislative authority for child welfare and protecting children from abuse. It states that the welfare of a child is paramount.

This Act places the statutory duty to enquire and act in relation to vulnerable children with one agency – the local social services authority.

Section 47 of the Children Act requires social services to carry out enquiries, or arrange for them to be carried out on their behalf, if a child in their area:

- is subject to an Emergency Protection Order
- is in police protection
- is in breach of a curfew notice
- whom they have reasonable cause to suspect is suffering, or likely to suffer, significant harm.

Section 17 (Children in Need) places a statutory duty on local authorities to safeguard and promote the welfare of children in need of services within their area.

A child is *in need* if:

- they are unlikely to achieve or maintain or have the opportunity of achieving or maintaining a reasonable standard of health or development without the provision of services by a local authority

- their health or development is likely to be significantly impaired or further impaired without the provision of such services
- they are disabled.

STATISTICS

At any time, up to 1.5 million of the most vulnerable people are relying on social services for care and support.

570,000 children and young people in England were referred to social services in the year ending 31 March 2002; 136,000 (24%) of referrals were re-referrals to the same department within 12 months of the previous referral.

PRESENTATION

The following should be presented to children's social care (social services department) (Fig. 84.1):

- Families with a disabled child or children.
- Children, young people and families where there are concerns about child abuse.

Any person or agency can refer to children's social care.
Anonymous referrals will be taken seriously.

ASSESSMENT

This should provide the basis for identifying the child's needs and strengths, and make decisions about services to be provided and priorities across all statutory and voluntary agencies working with children and families.

It requires a systematic and purposeful approach, using an assessment framework to gather and analyse relevant information within three domains:

- The child's developmental needs:
  - health
  - education
  - emotional and behavioural development
  - identity
  - family and social relationships
  - social presentation
  - self-care skills.
- Parenting capacity of caregiver to meet the child's needs:
  - basic care
  - ensuring safety
  - emotional warmth
  - stimulation
  - guidance and boundaries
  - stability.

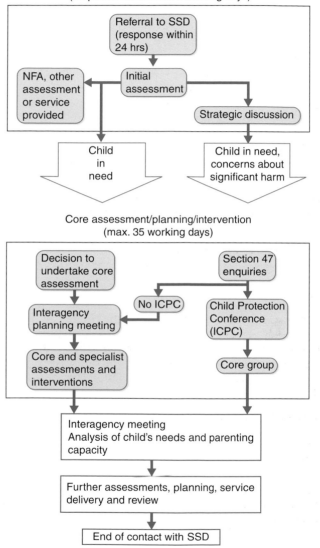

Fig. 84.1 Referral pathway. ICPC, initial child protection conference; NFA, no further assessment; SSD, social services department, children's social care.

- Family and environmental factors:
  - family history and functioning
  - wider family
  - housing
  - employment
  - income
  - family's social integration
  - community resources.

Children's social care must decide whether there is enough evidence to do a Section 47 (Children Act) enquiry. Approximately 50% of enquiries proceed to an initial child protection conference (ICPC) and 80% of these lead to registrations on the child protection register (data from year ending 31 March 2002).

In England, on 31 March 2002, 25,700 children and young people were on the child protection register.

ALERTS

- Disabled children
- Homeless
- Under 16 years of age
- Drug and alcohol misuse
- Other risk-taking behaviour
- Criminal activity
- Presence of a Schedule 1 offender (person convicted of a crime against a child)

WHO CHILDREN'S SOCIAL CARE TALK TO

Anyone involved with the family and children:

- Family members
- Friends
- GP
- Health visitor, midwife, nurses
- Paediatricians
- Other health professionals, e.g. speech and language therapists
- Education – teachers, Education Welfare Officer
- Voluntary services.

FOLLOW-UP

Individual plan according to the family's/child's needs.

KEY POINTS FOR PARENTS

Social services departments are there to support them and their children.

Only in very extreme circumstances, if a family is unable to work with social services *and* there is a significant risk that a child may come to serious harm, then a child/children will be removed against the wishes of a parent.

SUPPORT ORGANISATIONS

Respite care.
Babysitting.
Outreach services.
Parenting classes.
Local child protection procedures for local contacts etc. (should be available in any setting where children are seen).

SOURCES

Department of Health – www.dh.gov.uk
Referrals, assessments, and children and young people on child protection registers in England 2001–2002 – www.statistics.gov.uk
The Children Act 1989. London: TSO. Online. Available: www.opsi.gov.uk/acts/acts1989/Ukpga_19890041_en_1.htm

See also

Chapter 83, Safeguarding children and the law.

85

CHILD PROTECTION

DEFINITION

Child abuse is criminal conduct of a particular reprehensible character: children are highly vulnerable members of society. Child abuse is also a form of criminal conduct peculiarly hard to combat, because its existence is difficult to discover. Babies and young children are unable to complain, older children too frightened. If the source of abuse is a parent, the child is at risk from his primary and natural protector within the privacy of his home. This both increases the risk of abuse and means that investigation necessitates intrusion into highly sensitive areas of family life, with the added complication that the parent who is responsible for the abuse will give a false account of the child's history.

House of Lords (2005).

Appropriate recognition and management of situations when abuse of a child is suspected can be very anxiety provoking. Part of the reason is because many basic premises learned as a doctor seem to be different. Faith in parents may be misplaced and it is difficult to come to terms with the elements of deception that can occur. Other problems are:

- difficulty in diagnosis
- multiagency involvement
- multiprofessional involvement
- extensive chronology and time span
- multiple presentations at different venues
- documentation issues
- confidentiality
- only one aspect presenting to individual professionals.

You must be familiar with your local Area Child Protection Committee (ACPC) procedures (ACPCs will be replaced by Local Safeguarding Children Boards [LSCBs] to be established by April 2006).

Children of any colour, background, race or religion may suffer abuse, and those with special needs may be particularly vulnerable.

The House of Lords has recently emphasised that doctors with child patients have a duty to act 'single-mindedly in the interests of the child' and not the parents.

Definitions (as in *Working Together to Safeguard Children* [DH 1999])

- *Physical abuse*: May involve, hitting, shaking, throwing, poisoning, burning or scalding, drowning or suffocating, or otherwise causing physical harm to a child or deliberately causing ill health to a child who they are looking after.
- *Sexual abuse*: Involves forcing or enticing a child or young person to take part in sexual activities, whether or not the child is aware of what is happening. The activities may involve physical contact, including penetrative or non-penetrative acts. They may include non-contact activities, such as involving children in looking at, or in the production of, pornographic material or watching sexual activities, or encouraging children to behave in sexually inappropriate ways.
- *Neglect*: The persistent failure to meet a child's basic physical and/or psychological needs, likely to result in the serious impairment of the child's health or development. It may involve a parent or carer failing to provide adequate food, shelter or clothing, failing to protect a child from physical harm or danger, or the failure to ensure access to appropriate medical care or treatment. It may also include neglect of a child's emotional needs.
- *Emotional abuse*: The persistent emotional ill-treatment of a child such as to cause severe or persistent adverse effects on the child's emotional development. It may involve conveying to children that they are worthless or unloved, inadequate, or valued only insofar as they meet the needs of another person. It may involve causing children frequently to feel frightened or in danger, or the exploitation or corruption of children. Some level of emotional abuse is involved in all types of ill-treatment of a child, though it may occur on its own.

Types of abuse can overlap in the same child and different types can happen to the same child at different times, e.g. physical and sexual abuse can occur together.

Remember – according to the Children Act 1989, any person under 18 year of age is considered a child.

EPIDEMIOLOGY AND AETIOLOGY

Year ending 31st March 2004 (England)

Referrals to children's social care formerly known as social services social services departments = 572,700.

Children on child protection registers (CPRs) = 26,300. This represents 24 children per 10,000 of the population aged under 18.

Category
- Neglect – 41%
- Physical abuse – 19%
- Emotional abuse – 18%

- Sexual abuse – 9%
- Mixed categories – 14%

Length of time on the register
7% of children removed from the register had been on it for over 2 years. The registration figures are the 'tip of the iceberg' as children's names are only placed on the CPR when a protection plan is needed, i.e. children who are abused but assessed to be 'safe' and not in need of a protection plan do not have their names put on the register.

Risk factors
Child abuse occurs throughout society, but certain groups tend to feature more often:

- *Child factors*: Preterm babies, babies under 1 year old.
- *Adult factors*:
  - parents with learning difficulties
  - history of domestic violence
  - single parent families
  - Schedule 1 offender in the household (someone who has been convicted of an offence against a child – Schedule 1 of the Children and Young Persons Act 1933 details a list of serious offences against a child up to the age of 18 years; the offences range from murder, assault and neglect to sexual abuse and abduction). The term "risk of harm to children" is now replacing schedule 1 offender.
  - mental health problems
  - drug and alcohol misuse
  - teenage mothers.

PRESENTATION
The possibility of a child protection issue may arise because of suspicious symptoms and signs. Child abuse can present as a disclosure from the child/young person or as allegations by a parent/carer, social worker or police officer.

Physical abuse
Any injury in a non-mobile child should arouse suspicion – the presence of even a minor injury in a baby is extremely significant, for example:

- burns
- scalds
- bruises – the following are especially worrying:
  - facial bruises
  - bruises around the mouth, torn frenulum
  - grasp marks or finger-tip bruising on the chest
  - marks on unusual sites or areas normally hidden from view, e.g. behind the ears, the scalp, back, buttocks, neck, genitalia

- bites
- fractures
- shaken baby syndrome
- retinal haemorrhage, subdural
- haemorrhage
- abdominal injury.

Remember – fabricated/induced illness may present as part of physical abuse. This is an extremely difficult situation and usually requires the collective gathering of information from several sources over a considerable time span (see below).

Sexual abuse
Remember – in cases of sexual abuse there are often no specific abnormal physical findings.
Disclosure must always be taken seriously.
The following are strongly suggestive of sexual abuse:

- sexually transmitted diseases
- pregnancy
- bruising/tears in the perineal area
- inappropriate sexualised play and/or language
- abuse of another child.

Sexual abuse should be considered as part of the differential diagnosis in the following circumstances:

- recurrent UTI
- enuresis
- recurrent abdominal pain
- soiling
- behaviour problems
- sleeping disturbances
- self-harm
- rectal/vaginal bleeding
- bruising on thighs
- anal trauma
- genital warts.

Neglect
Non-organic failure to thrive.
Not receiving enough food.
Exposed through lack of supervision to injuries, including ingestion of drugs.
Exposed to an inadequate, dirty and/or cold environment.
'Home alone'.
'Deprivation hands and feet' – deep pink/bluish tinge to the hands and feet which also have a puffy appearance. This may be confused with cardiac conditions.

Parents/carers failing or refusing to seek medical advice or treatment.
Repeated attendances for minor injuries to different professionals, e.g. Emergency Department, GP surgery, health visitor.
Lack of stimulation.
Inadequate environment to enable child to develop physically and emotionally.

Emotional abuse
Abnormally passive, lethargic behaviour.
Attention seeking.
Soiling, faecal smearing.
Excessive drinking.
Persistent eating of inedible substances.
Self-mutilation.
Severely delayed social development.
Speech and language delay due to actions/inactions of parent/carer.
Weight and height disproportionately low that cannot be explained by medical reasons.

ASSESSMENT

In all cases, note:

- name of adult accompanying the child
- relationship of adult to child
- primary carer's name
- who has parental responsibility (see Chapter 83)
- if the child/family already has a social worker
- if the child is subject to a court order.

Check:

- that the child has a GP
- who the health visitor is
- name of school (if appropriate).

Consider:

- if the child's or carer's first language is English (if not, an interpreter is needed)
- if the child is disabled, are other communication skills required?

History
A careful history should be taken, but special considerations apply in some cases, e.g. sexual abuse, possible fabricated or induced illness (see below).
If the child is old enough, an opportunity should be offered to interview the child without the parent/carer present, but with the parent's/carer's consent whenever possible. If consent is withheld, the reason should be documented and advice sought. However, if it is in the

child's best interests to be talked to/seen alone, then the doctor should do so with or without consent and record/justify why this has been done. If the person with parental responsibility is not available to give consent to interview or examine, the same principles apply.
Has the child been seen elsewhere, e.g. local Emergency Department or a hospital outside the area?

Physical abuse
Is the history compatible with:

- the injury?
- age of child?
- developmental capabilities?

Is the site of injury unusual? – e.g. soles of feet.
Is there a recognisable pattern to the bruising? – e.g. finger-tip bruising on the chest wall (consider 'shaken baby' syndrome).
Is the history given to different professionals consistent?
How detailed is the history?
Has there been any delay in seeking advice?

Sexual abuse
If a child discloses sexual abuse to you – record in the child's own words, reassure the child but do not make promises of secrecy.
Take just enough history to confirm sexual abuse has taken place – remember this includes activities such as being made to look at inappropriate activities or images.
Do not question the child in detail – this will be done by a social worker and a police officer who are specially trained in this field.

Neglect
Failure to give adequate healthcare, e.g. repeated non-attendance for hospital/GP appointments.
Repeated attendances for minor injuries, especially to different sources of advice.
Refusal to seek or cooperate with medical advice, e.g. not giving treatment for diabetes or failing to have a hearing difficulty treated.
Use the assessment framework to help build up a picture.

Examination
In all cases:

- The consent of the parent/carer should be obtained where possible.
- The child's growth should be plotted on a centile chart.
- Carry out a general developmental assessment.
- Note the child's overall appearance, e.g. state of hair, skin, if appropriately dressed.
- Observe interaction with parent/carer.

Physical abuse

Use of photographs – requires consent and usually is best done by a medical photographer – discuss with a senior colleague.

Record all marks on a body map:

- pattern of bruising, e.g. hand marks or finger-tip bruising, bites
- marks made by implements, e.g. strap or buckle marks.

Remember to look in places usually hidden (e.g. scalp) and areas concealed by clothing (e.g. buttocks, trunk).

Site of injury is important:

- buttocks, lower back and outer thighs are often related to punishment
- injury to head and neck is suggestive of abuse, e.g. slap marks to face
- bruises to trunk and abdomen are suggestive of abuse; bruises to external ear are unlikely to be caused by accidents; (in general, bruises distal to elbow and knee are more likely to be accidental)
- distribution of scald
- presence of 'frozen watchfulness'
- retinal examination (by ophthalmologist) when shaking is suspected.

Sexual abuse

Only examine the genitalia if it is necessary to exclude trauma requiring emergency treatment or to reassure the child.

Make sure that you are aware of the arrangements that are in place in your area for specific examinations for suspected sexual abuse. This usually takes place after referral to social services, by specially trained paediatricians/police surgeons.

Neglect

Particular attention to growth, development and appearance.

Hygiene.

Deprivation hands and feet – deep pink/bluish, slightly oedematous hands and feet.

Emotional abuse

This type of abuse virtually always occurs in conjunction with the other three types, but can be the most difficult to diagnose should it occur alone.

Observe appropriateness of reaction to others, language development and self-esteem (see 'Presentation', above).

Diagnostic tests

Physical abuse

In many circumstances, the diagnosis depends on the history and clinical presentation. The following may be required and initiated after discussion with a senior colleague:

- Hb, FBC, platelet count, clotting studies – particularly if there is extensive or unusual bruising.

- X-ray of the affected part.
- Skeletal survey – consider in all babies and children under 2 years old (discuss with senior colleagues, consult local guidelines).
- CT scan of head.

Sexual abuse
To be initiated by a senior colleague with special expertise in this field.
Photographs – usually using a colposcope.
Relevant vaginal, anal and perineal swabs for infection and for forensic purposes.

Neglect
Appropriate investigations for failure to thrive may be required (see Chapter 30).

DIFFERENTIAL DIAGNOSIS
Birthmarks, e.g. Mongolian blue spot.
Bleeding, clotting disorders.
Skin disorders, especially infections.
Bone disorders.
Causes of failure to thrive (see Chapter 30).
Gynaecological disorders.

OTHER ACTIONS
Information gathering is of prime importance in child protection; a solitary consultation rarely reveals the whole picture.
Check the child protection register – but lack of information should not prevent a referral to social services.
Contact the child's GP, health visitor and midwife.
If a child has been seen in hospital or the Emergency Department, find out about the circumstances.
Strategy meetings may be called by health professionals to pool information and discuss further action. Participants should be those professionals who know the child and family and may also include a social worker.
Sometimes it is clear what has to be done. If not, it is most important to ask advice. Senior experienced nurses can be very helpful, as well as local named and designated doctors in child protection.

ALERTS

You must be familiar with your Local Safeguarding Children's Boards (LSCB's) procedures.
Other helpful advice is provided by the booklet *What To Do If You're Worried A Child Is Being Abused* (DH et al 2003). Regular updating in child protection is also essential.

WHO TO TALK TO

You should discuss cases of concern with the appropriate responsible paediatrician.

There is also a named doctor/nurse for child protection in each Trust and a designated doctor/nurse in each area who will be available to advise.

It may also be helpful to talk to the appropriate local social worker.

You must be aware of the LSCB's child protection procedures.

Communication with parents/carers

While professionals should seek, in general, to discuss any concerns with the family, and where possible, seek their agreement to making referrals to children's social services, this should only be done where such discussion and agreement seeking will not place a child at increased risk of significant harm.

Department of Health (1999).

Sexual abuse is one instance where it may not be appropriate to share information with parents/carers before referral. Pressure may be put on the child to retract any allegations. Also, the child may be put at risk of being physically abused.

Where fabricated/induced illness (see below) is suspected, the timing of discussing concerns with the parents/carers is crucial and can only be undertaken when this will not put the child at risk. Senior professionals must always be involved with this decision.

Documentation in the notes must clearly state what has been said and to whom. If concerns are not shared with parents/carers, the reasons should be recorded and shared with relevant professionals.

WHEN TO REFER

Any child who is at risk from significant harm, or has suffered significant harm, must be referred to children's social care. A verbal referral must be followed up in writing within 48 hours and copies kept in the medical records and sent to the GP and/or health visitor.

Be clear in your referral about your concerns and where available use the locally approved form. This should have prompts for the information required by children's social care.

If the child is in hospital, the named doctor/nurse should be informed.

Health staff do not have statutory duties of investigation.

Physical abuse

A child with serious injuries and/or requiring hospital investigations must be admitted to hospital, with the relevant information shared with hospital staff. The referring doctor must also make the referral to social services. This action should be clear to the receiving doctor – the referring doctor and the receiving doctor must be clear with each other who is referring to social services.

Remember the vulnerability of babies and very young children.

Do not forget about the safety of siblings.

If abuse is strongly suspected, but further advice is required, follow the local arrangements to obtain a second opinion.

Sexual abuse
Any child who tells you that he/she has been touched inappropriately, or abused as under the definition of sexual abuse (see above), must be referred to social services.

Do not make promises of secrecy, but it may not be appropriate to tell the parents/carers at this stage. Each situation needs to be assessed.

Sometimes an adult makes allegations about another adult sexually abusing a child. This must also be referred.

Neglect and emotional abuse
It is often difficult to decide when thresholds are reached for referral to social services in these circumstances. Interprofessional/interagency meetings for pooling of information and compiling a chronology are helpful and can be convened by health staff.

Note-keeping
All notes must be clearly kept, contemporaneous where possible, signed and dated.

There must be good communication between professionals involved, e.g. GPs, hospital and community, as well as social workers and police.

Fabrication or induction of illness in a child by a parent/carer
This is considered to be rare, but accurate statistics are difficult to obtain due to almost certain under-reporting. However, up to 10% of those children affected by parents/carers fabricating or inducing illness die and about 50% experience long-term morbidity.

There are three main ways a carer may fabricate or induce illness in a child; they are not mutually exclusive.

- Fabrication of signs and symptoms – may include the past medical history.
- Fabrication of signs and symptoms and falsification of hospital charts, records and specimens of bodily fluids. May include falsification of letters and documents.
- Induction of illness by a variety of means.

The following are examples of behaviours of parents/carers:

- Administering medication or other substances to deliberately induce symptoms.
- Suffocation to induce apnoea attacks.
- Interfering with treatments (over- or underdosing) or medical equipment.
- Claiming that the child has symptoms which cannot be checked unless observed directly, e.g. fits, vomiting.

7

- Exaggerating symptoms.
- Interfering with test results, e.g. adding blood to urine or stool specimens.

The above situations lead to repeated unnecessary investigations and treatments, including operations, by medical staff. The child may spend extended amounts of time in hospital undergoing painful procedures. The parents tend to be very involved in the care of the child.

Children in this group usually have extensive medical histories and have been seen in several different hospitals and geographical areas. It may be a considerable time before fabrication or induction of illness is considered.

Such concerns may arise when:

- reported symptoms and signs are not explained by any medical condition which the child may have
- examination and investigation results do not explain reported symptoms and signs
- inexplicable poor response to medication
- new symptoms arise when old ones resolve
- when the carer is absent, reported signs or symptoms do not occur
- the child's normal daily activities are restricted more than would be expected for the condition which the child is known to have.

If fabrication or induced illness is suspected, it is most important to consult with colleagues – the consultant paediatrician responsible, GP, health visitor, nursing staff and relevant other agencies such as children's social care, education and the relevant legal team. The named and designated doctor and nurse for child protection should also be informed and consulted.

A full review of all the signs, symptoms, investigations, treatments and outcomes is necessary – this is best done by a chronology.

Referral to children's social care should be made. This is only discussed with parents/carers when such discussion will not put the child at increased risk of significant harm.

Detailed action depends on the individual situation. The management of such cases is complex and needs to be dealt with by senior staff, in conjunction with social services and the police.

THERAPY

General

Child abuse betrays the core relationships that children need to develop. Trust, a sense of identity and attachment are all affected. Abused children may have low self-esteem, leading to an inability to manage strong emotions. This can lead to aggressive, impulsive behaviour.

Abusive parenting causes *disorganised attachment*. The child responds to the parent in an abnormal pattern such as freezing or staring into space. Such children find it difficult to form close relationships later on, with implications for foster parenting or peer relationships.

Inconsistent messages to children from carers lead to *ambivalent attachment* where a child wants the comfort of the carer but is unable to accept it. Unresponsiveness in the carer to a child's needs leads to *avoidance attachment*. In this situation the child is not affected by the parent's presence or otherwise. This pattern can lead to depression, self-harming, bulimia or substance abuse.

Sexual abuse can affect the ability to form normal adult relationships.

Each circumstance needs assessing to see what is required. Help from a psychiatrist/psychologist may be needed for the child/family. Alternatively, input from a health visitor, social worker or organisations such as SureStart may be more appropriate.

Physical abuse

Obviously, any resulting physical trauma should be managed appropriately. This can encompass a wide range of situations from treatment of burns to management of head injuries. Specialist care may be required.

Sexual abuse

Consider the following:

- screening/treatment of sexually transmitted disease
- repair of trauma to the genital tract
- pregnancy testing
- termination of pregnancy
- antenatal care
- emergency contraception.

Neglect and emotional abuse

Education with regard to:

- home safety
- appropriate responses to the child's physical needs, e.g. feeding, clothing
- appropriate responses to the child's emotional needs, e.g. playing, cuddling, boundary setting
- appropriate responses to the child's changing needs as development progresses.

FOLLOW-UP

Attendance at child protection case conferences (both initial and review conferences) is an integral part of work in this field and the medical input is essential in many cases. In all circumstances where a medical practitioner has been involved, a written report should be provided when requested by the organiser of the conference. The doctor may be part of the child protection plan agreed at a child protection case conference and is frequently involved in follow-up where a child is 'in need' (see below).

Child in need

Safeguarding issues should not be perceived separately from the many needs of children and their families. There is a range of services available and children's social care have special funding to help the 'child in need' (see Chapter 83).

The aim should be to provide support. The assessment framework (see above) should be used in conjunction with social services to develop an overall picture of the circumstances.

Serious case reviews

The LSCB instigates a case review when a child dies or is seriously injured and abuse or neglect is known or suspected to be a factor.

The purpose of the review is to learn any lessons about the way local professionals/agencies work together, to formulate an appropriate plan so the lessons are acted upon and to improve interagency working.

Any person involved in the care of the child or family may be interviewed and their notes scrutinised. This is carried out by a senior member of the appropriate profession/agency. The designated or named doctor/nurse will conduct the health aspect of the review. This can be a stressful process for those being interviewed, and emphasises the need for careful management and good practice.

Confidentiality

Doctors are not used to sharing information with non-medical colleagues. However, the General Medical Council guidance is clear:

If you believe a patient to be a victim of neglect or physical, sexual or emotional abuse and that the patient cannot give or withhold consent to disclosure, you must give information promptly to an appropriate responsible person or statutory agency, where you believe that the disclosure is in the patient's best interests. If, for any reason, you believe that disclosure of information is not in the best interests of an abused or neglected patient, you should discuss the issues with an experienced colleague. If you decide not to disclose information, you must be prepared to justify your decision.

Disclosures may also be necessary in the public interest (see GMC 2004, p. 12).

SOURCES

Department of Health (1999) Working together to safeguard children. London: TSO

Department of Health (2000) Framework for the assessment of children in need and their families. London: TSO

Department of Health (2002) Safeguarding children in whom illness is fabricated or induced. London: TSO

Department of Health, Home Office, Department for Education and Skills (2003) What to do if you're worried a child is being abused. London: Department of Health Publications

General Medical Council (2004) Confidentiality: protecting and providing information. London: GMC

Hobbs CJ, Hanks HGI, Wynne JM (1999) Child abuse and neglect. Edinburgh: Churchill Livingstone

House of Lords April (2005) JD (FD) (Appellant) v. East Berkshire Community Health NHS Trust and others (Respondents) and two others (FC).

Lord Laming (2003) The Victoria Climbie Inquiry. London: TSO

Polnay J (2001) Child protection in primary care. Oxford: Radcliffe Medical Press

Royal College of Paediatrics and Child Health and The Association of Forensic Physicians (2004) Guidance on paediatric forensic examinations in relation to possible child sexual abuse. London: RCPCH

Royal College of Physicians of London (1997) Physical signs of sexual abuse in children, 2nd edn. London: RCP

The Children Act 1989. London: TSO. Online. Available: www.opsi.gov.uk/acts/acts1989/Ukpga_19890041_en_1.htm

See also

Chapter 30, Poor weight gain – weight and growth faltering in young children; Chapter 83, Safeguarding children and the law, Chapter 84, Social services.

7

86

CHILDREN LOOKED AFTER

DEFINITION

- *Accommodated* – looked after by the local authority as a voluntary agreement with those who have parental responsibility.
- *In care* – as a consequence of a court order where the local authority is granted parental responsibility (Children Act 1989)

EPIDEMIOLOGY AND AETIOLOGY

In England, on 31 March 2002, 59,700 children were looked after:

- 38,400 were on care orders
- 66% were in foster placements
- 62% were looked after because of abuse or neglect

(data includes 2200 unaccompanied asylum seekers, half of whom were under 16).

PRESENTATION

Children entering the looked-after system are much more likely than others to have incomplete child health surveillance, unidentified health, mental health (common) and health promotion needs.

ASSESSMENT

Initial assessment by a doctor on entering care, leading to a healthcare plan. These are reviewed by a nurse or doctor every 6 months for children under the age of 5 and yearly in older children.

Assessments include physical and mental health and health promotion.

Assessments should be sensitive to the child's needs, wishes and fears and flexible enough to accommodate these. Children who have experienced abuse or neglect may have a high degree of fear and mistrust of adults. Children need to be prepared and informed about what is involved (DH 2002).

History

Information will need to be collected from community, hospital and computerised records of past medical history and family history.

Examination

Assessment should cover:

- immunisation
- child health screening, including dental
- assessment of current and/or unrecognised health and mental health concerns
- review and advice on known existing health problems
- identification of outstanding appointments
- identification of mental health, behavioural and emotional problems
- recognition of developmental or learning concerns
- discussion of age-appropriate lifestyle issues – diet, exercise, smoking, alcohol, use of drugs, sexual health and need for contraception advice and protection from STIs
- planning of appropriate action and ensuring recommendations are carried through
- planning of follow-up.

ALERTS

High risk of teenage pregnancy, poor educational outcomes, future unemployment, homelessness, offending behaviours and mental health problems in teenagers leaving care. Well-coordinated services and integration of care are necessary to improve these outcomes.

The same principles of competency apply to self-consent and confidentiality as to any other young person. In other circumstances it is essential to ascertain whether consent is required from parents or if the local authority social worker has this authority.

Medical records must follow the child in order to prevent important information getting lost. Authorities are required to fast track the medical records of children looked after.

7

WHO TO TALK TO

Children's social care, and allocated case worker.

Serious mental health problems are common – important to have close contact with CAMHS.

Education services – children may have missed school, moved school frequently, be excluded or have problems with truancy. Learning difficulties are also more common.

WHEN TO REFER

Refer to dedicated services wherever available.
Need to check attendance, recommendations and compliance.

FOLLOW-UP

6-monthly under 5 years of age, yearly thereafter.

HEALTH PROMOTION

Health promotion is an essential part of the programme and should include standards for the environment in which the child or young person is living (Chambers et al 2002).

ADDITIONAL POINTS

The designated doctor and nurse for children looked after are responsible for overseeing the update, quality and implementation of healthcare plans.

SOURCES

Chambers H, Howell S, Madge N, Olie H (2002) Healthy care – building an evidence base for promoting the health and wellbeing of looked after children and young people. London: National Children's Bureau

Department of Health (2002) Promoting the health of looked after children. London: TSO

The Children Act 1989. London: TSO. Online. Available: www.opsi.gov.uk/acts/acts1989/Ukpga_19890041_en_1.htm

See also

Chapter 83, Safeguarding children and the law.

YOUNG CARERS

DEFINITION

A child or young person under the age of 18 who provides care, assistance or support to another family member.

EPIDEMIOLOGY AND AETIOLOGY

3 million children under the age of 16 in the UK (23% of children) live in households where one family member is hampered in daily activities by a chronic physical or mental disability or illness. Of these, 51,000 will be young carers.

PRESENTATION

Children who are young carers frequently do not present either because of fear that authorities might take them into care if they are identified as not coping ('silence and secrets') or because adult services are not proactive in addressing the impact of adult illnesses upon children in the household.

ASSESSMENT

Problems that need to be addressed include:

- limited social and leisure activities
- absence from school
- lack of understanding by peers
- emotional problems, fears about the future
- health problems, e.g. injuries from lifting an adult, fatigue
- inappropriate responsibility
- lack of medical information about the adult's condition.

WHO TO TALK TO

Multidisciplinary discussion, involving the primary healthcare team, adult specialists, community paediatrics, social services and education, is often needed.

Needs sensitive handling in view of the frequent fear of professionals and confidentiality issues.

WHEN TO REFER

Many towns now have dedicated young carer support workers.
Carers UK is a national organisation highlighting the needs of carers of all ages.

THERAPY

Needs of young carers include:

- recognition and respect
- information about care, medical conditions, practical tasks, welfare benefits and services
- support and services
- time off
- choice to care as well as receiving external services
- someone to talk to.

FOLLOW-UP

Offer of regular follow-up to the child as well as the adult.

KEY POINTS FOR PARENTS

Adults usually feel uncomfortable about the responsibility given to children and the inappropriateness of some tasks such as intimate care. They need to be informed by their adult health professionals that there are services to prevent the impact on children and that referrals will be made.

SUPPORT ORGANISATIONS

Carers UK – www.carersuk.org.

88

REFUGEES AND ASYLUM SEEKERS

DEFINITION (UK)

An 'asylum seeker' is someone who has applied for refugee status.
A 'refugee' is a person who:

...owing to a well founded fear of being persecuted for reasons of race, religion, nationality, membership of a particular social group or political opinion is outside the country of his nationality and is unable, or owing to such fear, is unwilling to avail himself of the protection of that country; or who, not having a nationality and being outside the country of his former habitual residence, as a result of such events, is unable to or, owing to such fear, is unwilling to return to it.

UN Convention (1951).

EPIDEMIOLOGY AND AETIOLOGY

In 2002 there were 84,130 applications for asylum in the UK; of these, 25% were under the age of 20.
There were 6200 unaccompanied children age 17 or under. The main countries of origin were Iraq, Zimbabwe, Afghanistan, Somalia and China.

PRESENTATION

May present for routine child health surveillance or with problems (especially mental health), resulting from previous experiences as well as difficulties in adjustment to life in a new country.

ASSESSMENT

Important information relating to past medical history may not be available, including basic information such as birth weight, gestation or date of birth.
Interpreters may be required.
They are likely to be unfamiliar with UK healthcare and that a consultation is confidential. Reassurance is needed.
Advice must be given with an understanding of the family's culture.

It is important to ensure that they are registered with a general practitioner and a dentist.

A holistic approach is required, assessing the physical and mental well-being of the family as a whole.

History

Medical history and family history, where available.

Whereabouts of family members; have parents died?

Previous education.

Experiences – before, during and after arrival in the UK.

Emotional and behavioural problems – fears, sleep problems, withdrawn, poor appetite, lethargy, somatic symptoms, bullying, post-traumatic stress disorder.

Examination

Check growth and nutrition.

Assess development.

Are there any old injuries?

Female genital mutilation still seen in girls from some African countries.

Diagnostic tests

Consider tests for tropical and infectious diseases – malaria, hepatitis B, tuberculosis.

Possibility of HIV/AIDS, especially if from a country with a high prevalence.

Neonatal biochemical screening may not have been carried out in the country of origin.

WHO TO TALK TO

In some areas where there are high numbers of refugees and asylum seekers, specialised teams may have been set up.

Specialist advice may be needed on infectious disease screening, management and immunisation.

Specialist clinics are available for children who have been victims of torture.

Families may need advice on welfare benefits.

THERAPY

Remember to offer routine immunisation – advice on older children or those with uncertain immunisation histories may be needed from the district immunisation coordinator.

Referral may be needed to specialised counselling or CAMHS services, with these decisions being influenced by individual histories and knowledge of cultural and religious beliefs.

FOLLOW-UP

Individual plans are needed, but ongoing surveillance of growth, nutrition, development, physical and mental health may be required.

KEY POINTS FOR PARENTS

Parents will need advice and information on the structure of and access to health services for children.

HEALTH PROMOTION

Important topics are nutrition, hygiene, sexual health – advice must take account of the family's culture and religious beliefs.

ADDITIONAL POINTS

Doctors are advised to be cautious when requested to assess the age of children where there is no documentation of date of birth. Assessments may be misleading, inaccurate and unhelpful.

SOURCES

King's Fund and Royal College of Paediatrics and Child Health (1999) The health of refugee children. London: King's Fund/RCPCH

PROBLEMS IN DEPRIVED AREAS

DEFINITION

'Deprivation' is a *relative* lack of material and/or psychological support, usually a consequence of poverty.

Various indices have been used to illustrate the scale of deprivation in a particular area. The Jarman index (Jarman 1983) is the most often used; others include the Townsend index (Townsend et al 1988) and the social index.

EPIDEMIOLOGY AND AETIOLOGY

There are 11.7 million dependent children in England and Wales and a disproportionate number of British children are born into low-income households: 2.6 million children have lone parent households and 2.7 million children are in low-income households.

PRESENTATION

Deprivation affects child health in many ways:

Recurrent infections
Conductive hearing loss
Enuresis
Iron deficiency anaemia
Faltering growth
Obesity
Dental caries
Recurrent admissions to hospital
Recurrent accidents
Teenage pregnancy
Child abuse and neglect
School truancy
Poor educational attainment
Conduct disorders
Low self-esteem
Low expectations

Repeated house moves, homelessness
Self-harm
Juvenile crime

ASSESSMENT
History
- Family history:
  - learning difficulties
  - non-chromosomal anomalies (associated with increasing deprivation).
- Environment:
  - current housing
  - homelessness
  - neighbourhood
  - heating
  - bathrooms
  - kitchen.
- Income:
  - employment
  - benefits.
- Family structure:
  - number of people in the household
  - marital status
  - clarification of parental responsibility.
- Culture:
  - language spoken at home
  - inherited diseases
  - consanguinity
  - other factors, e.g. high proportion of TB in South-East Asian families.
- Stimulation:
  - history of mental health problems in parents.
- Nurture and affection:
  Deprivation has a negative and direct effect on parental behaviour, e.g.
  - child abuse
  - behaviour and conduct disorders
  - truancy, school failure
  - juvenile crime rates
  (correlate with maternal deprivation).
- Diet:
  - faltering growth
  - obesity
  - iron deficiency anaemia.
- Access to services:
  - lack of telephone
  - personal transport

7

- poor public transport
- poor literacy skills.
- Life events:
  - death of a parent or sibling
  - divorce
  - ill health
  - debt
  - homelessness.
- Temperament.

Examination

Height (cm) and centile
Weight (kg) and centile
BMI
General appearance and demeanour
Skin condition including injuries
Clinical signs of anaemia
Signs of infection
Condition of teeth and gums
Signs of self-harm
Hearing impairment
Behaviour

Diagnostic tests

Dependent on clinical findings, e.g. FBC and ferritin.

DIFFERENTIAL DIAGNOSIS

Child abuse.
Immunodeficiency.
Malabsorption.

Therapy

Treatment of individual conditions, e.g. anaemia.
Involvement of SureStart programme.
Referral to other services as appropriate, e.g. speech and language therapy, community paediatrician, Child and Adolescent Mental Health Services (CAMHS).
Liaison with social services.

ALERTS

- Recurrent non-attendance at appointments
- Recurrent accidents
- Non-biological faltering growth
- Lack of immunisations
- Physical abuse

WHO TO TALK TO

GP.
Health visitor.
School nurse.
Social services.
School (with parental consent).

HEALTH PROMOTION

There is good evidence that targeting areas of deprivation may improve outcomes. Mothers receiving antenatal intervention had babies who had a higher mean birth weight, fewer VLBW babies, fewer obstetric admissions to hospital, higher rate of spontaneous onset of labour, less likely to require epidural anaesthesia and mothers and babies who were significantly healthier.

ADDITIONAL POINTS

SureStart programme
- Government policy to prevent social exclusion.
- Targeted at preschool children and their families in areas of deprivation.

The initiative was a result of a review of services for young children which examined the problems of multiple disadvantages for young children, variation in the quality of services provided for children and families, and the need for a community-based programme of early intervention as the early years of a child's development are crucial for long-term good health.

The aim is to work with parents and preschool children to promote physical, intellectual, social and emotional development of children, particularly those who are disadvantaged.

In each SureStart area, locally based programmes are encouraged to build on existing services and to ensure a range of core services, including:

- outreach services and home visiting
- support for parents and families
- good quality play, learning and childcare
- primary and community-based healthcare and advice about child and family health, and child development
- support for those with special needs.

Extra services are also provided, but vary according to the needs of the local population:

- skills training for parents
- personal development courses
- practical advice and support, e.g. debt counselling
- language/literacy training.

The objectives are:

- to improve social and emotional development
- to improve health
- to improve the ability to learn
- to strengthen families and communities
- to increase productivity.

SOURCES

Blaxter M (1981) The health of children. A review of research on the place of health in cycles of disadvantage. SSRC/DHSS Studies in deprivation and disadvantage, Vol. 3. London: Heinemann

Department for Work and Pensions (2003) Households below average income. Online. Available: www.dwp.gov.uk/asd/hbai/hbai2003/contents.asp

Department of Health (2003) Health inequalities. Online. Available: www.dh.gov.uk/PolicyAndGuidance/HealthAndSocialCareTopics/HealthInequalities/fs/en

Jarman B (1983) Identification of underprivileged areas. BMJ 286: 1705–1709

National Statistics (UK) – www.statistics.gov.uk

Oakley A, Rajan L, Grant A (1990) Social support and pregnancy outcome. British Journal of Obstetrics and Gynaecology 97: 155–162

Reading R (1997) Poverty and the health of adolescents. Archives of Disease in Childhood 76: 463–467

Roberts H, Hall DMB (2000) What is SureStart? Archives of Disease in Childhood 82: 435–437

Spencer N (2000) Poverty and child health, 2nd edn. Oxford: Radcliffe Medical Press

SureStart – www.surestart.gov.uk

Teranishi H, Nakagawa H, Marmot M (2000) Social class difference in catch up growth in a national British cohort. Archives of Disease in Childhood 84: 218–221

Townsend P, Phillimore P, Beattie A (1988) Health and deprivation: inequality and the North. London: Croom Helm

90

FINANCIAL HELP

DEFINITION

Financial help is needed for all children in order to provide the necessities of life.

EPIDEMIOLOGY AND AETIOLOGY

For about a third of all children the state provides additional benefits to supplement the income of parents and to alleviate the adverse effects of poverty.

Additionally, children with disabilities can claim targeted benefits: 400,000 children with disabilities; 100,000 children with severe disabilities.

PRESENTATION

All children of parents on low income.
All children suffering ill health because of disability.

ASSESSMENT

Medical reports are usually required for those claiming benefits because of a disability. The quality and content of the reports can greatly influence the level of benefit paid.

Key benefits include the following:

- Disability living allowance (DLA) (separate components for care and mobility).
- Invalid care allowance paid to an adult of working age who looks after someone in receipt of DLA.
- Income support is a means-tested benefit for those on low income who work 16 hours a week or less or who do not have to be available for work.
- Working families' tax credit is a means-tested benefit for families who have children and where the claimant works for 16 hours or more.
- Social fund for payment for specific items.
- Community care grants to help families under stress.

7

- Housing benefit.
- Council tax benefit.
- Payments for fares to hospital.

ALERTS

All health professionals should be aware of the relationship between poverty and ill health and the additional costs of looking after children with disabilities. They should be encouraging parents to apply and to regard this as an integral part of the consultation.

WHO TO TALK TO

Welfare rights workers.
Citizens Advice Bureau.
Social workers.
Government Department of Work and Pensions.

WHEN TO REFER

The benefit system is complicated and there is a complex relationship between the payment of many of the benefits.

There should be a very low threshold of advising parents to get expert help

ADDITIONAL POINTS

Numerous local and national charitable bodies frequently provide help. There is usually a local directory of these.

SUPPORT ORGANISATIONS

Family Fund
Unit 4, Alpha Court
Monks Cross Drive
Huntington
York YO32 9WN
Tel: 08451 30 4542
www.familyfund.org.uk
Provides help to families caring for a child with a severe disability

SOURCES

Child Poverty Action Group – www.cpag.org.uk
Citizens Advice – www.nacab.org.uk
Department for Work and Pensions – www.dss.gov.uk

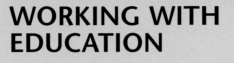

SECTION

8

WORKING WITH EDUCATION

91

WHO'S WHO IN EDUCATION

DEFINITION

The aim of education is to give children an excellent start in life, enable young people to equip themselves with life and work skills and encourage adults to achieve their full potential.

ORGANISATION (figs 91.1, 91.2)

Nationally

The Department for Education and Skills (DfES) is responsible for administering education in England and Wales, and is governed by legislation. Different legislation exists for Scotland and Northern Ireland. The Secretary for Education heads this department.

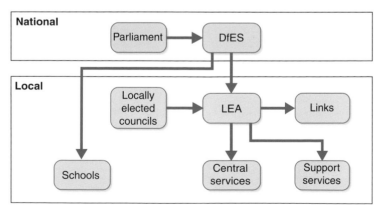

fig. 91.1 Relationship of structure of education at national and local government level. DfES, Department for Education and Skills; LEA, local education authority.

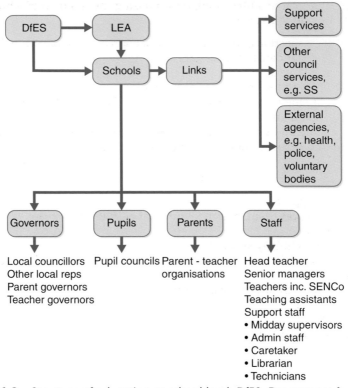

fig. 91.2 Structure of education at school level. DfES, Department for Education and Skills; LEA, local education authority; SENCo, special needs coordinator (responsible for school policy, monitoring and review of individual children with special educational needs, liaison with parents, health services, social services (SS) and LEA specialist support services).

The DfES:

- ensures that the legislation is carried out at a local level
- issues policies and guidance
    - oversees a variety of bodies
    - commissions research.

Locally

Education is administered by elected councils with a department, the local education authority (LEA), which employs officers to carry out the functions.

STANDARDS

All schools have to teach the national curriculum set out by the DfES. This includes programmes of study and attainment targets. Pupils are tested at key points of their education by standard assessment tasks (SATs).

The DfES has placed a high emphasis on raising the standard of schools in England and Wales by:

- OFSTED inspections, independent inspections of schools through the Office for Standards in Education
- setting of targets
- publication of test results 'league tables'
- the requirement that LEAs support schools that are failing to achieve desired standards
- the naming and shaming of failing schools and ultimately closing those that persist in not meeting the standards.

SUPPORT ORGANISATIONS

Behaviour support
Inclusion support (help, maintain children with disabilities in
    mainstream)
Education psychology service
Connexions (advises on careers and further education for 14–19 year
    olds)
Social services (children's social care)
School nursing
Primary care
Community paediatrics

SOURCES

Department for Education and Skills – www.dfes.gov.uk

8

SPECIAL MEDICAL NEEDS IN EDUCATION

DEFINITION

Most children will have, at some time, a health problem that interferes with their education. This may be just a short absence from school or the need to have short-term medication while at school.

Children with chronic illnesses may need to have special arrangements made for them so that they can receive treatment during school time. Some complex problems will require special provision to allow the child to access the curriculum. This may include education other than in a mainstream school or additional support in school.

EPIDEMIOLOGY AND AETIOLOGY

Around 5% of children have a longstanding illness which limits their functional capacity.

100,000 children each year require education outside of school because of illness or injury.

IMPACT OF MEDICAL PROBLEMS ON EDUCATION

There are a number of reasons why medical needs may interfere with education. These include:

- school absence
- poor health in school
- physical access
- sensory difficulties
- treatment required in school day
- self-care in school day
- effects of medication on learning
- social and emotional impact.

ASSESSMENT

Any child who may have medical needs that need to be addressed in school should have an assessment by the school doctor or community paediatrician; alternatively, these professionals should be able to gather information from health professionals already involved.

For children with significant problems, an individual healthcare plan should be drawn up, in liaison with the parents and the school.

WHO TO TALK TO

Hospital staff, specialist nurses (e.g. for diabetes, epilepsy, oncology).
School nurse/doctor.
Health commissioners (re: funding for support in school).
Parents, carers.

THERAPY

Medication or special procedures related to feeding, toileting, tracheostomy care, etc. may be required.

May need therapy in school, e.g. physiotherapy for cystic fibrosis.

Although health professionals may be involved in planning the care and providing training, therapy is usually carried out by learning support assistants or care assistants employed by the school.

FOLLOW-UP

Most children with ongoing medical needs will be under regular review by the relevant medical specialists.

Paediatricians who have responsibility for liaison with the school will need to review the child's needs, but should avoid unnecessarily adding to the number of medical appointments the child has to attend.

The individual healthcare plan should be reviewed at least annually, and updated if necessary.

KEY POINTS FOR PARENTS

Parents should be involved at all stages of discussing the special provision for their child.

They will have a central role in advising what the child's healthcare plan should include, and may be involved in training the staff who will implement it.

Parents need to understand what school staff are willing and able to do.

ADDITIONAL POINTS

- *Difficulties with funding*: It is not always clear whether health or education is responsible.
- *Medication in schools*: Some school staff will not administer medication.
- *Transport*: For a child with complex care needs, the transport and escort staff will also need to be trained.

SOURCES

Department for Education and Skills (2000) Supporting pupils with medical needs. London: DfES

Department for Education and Skills (2001) Access to education for children and young people with medical needs. London: DfES

See also

Chapter 93, Special educational needs; Chapter 95, Education legislation.

SPECIAL EDUCATIONAL NEEDS

DEFINITION

A child is said to have special educational needs (SEN) if they have a learning difficulty that calls for special educational provision to be made. The term 'learning difficulty' is used where a child:

- has a significantly greater difficulty in learning than the majority of children of his age, *or*
- has a disability that prevents or hinders him from making use of educational facilities generally provided for children of his age in schools within the area of the local education authority, *or*
- is under 5 years of age and would be likely to fall into the above categories if special educational provision were not made.

EPIDEMIOLOGY AND AETIOLOGY

A child may have SEN as result of a variety of problems, singly or in combination.

The Department for Education and Skills (DfES) describes four areas of need, with subdivisions (as used by OFSTED) described below:

- Cognition and learning needs:
  - specific learning difficulty (SpLD)
  - moderate learning difficulty (MLD)
  - severe learning difficulty (SLD)
  - profound and multiple learning difficulty (PMLD).
- Behaviour, emotional and social development:
  - behaviour, emotional and social difficulty (BESD).
- Communication and interaction needs:
  - speech, language and communication needs (SLCN)
  - autistic spectrum disorder (ASD).
- Sensory and/or physical needs:
  - visual impairment (VI)
  - hearing impairment (HI)
  - multisensory impairment (MSI)
  - physical disability (PH).

8

In addition, there will be children who have medical problems that interfere with their learning.

20% of children will have some sort of SEN during their school career.

3% of children have a statement of SEN – this varies enormously from area to area, ranging from 1% to almost 5%.

The majority of children with SEN will have them met in mainstream schools.

Just over 1% of children attend special schools in the UK.

PRESENTATION

Children with significant disability are likely to be known to health services early in life and SEN predicted well before starting their formal education.

Where problems are less severe, these may be picked up only when the child starts to struggle at school.

Sometimes presentation is more subtle, e.g. a child who is reluctant to attend school, or is badly behaved there, may be so because they are having difficulties learning.

ASSESSMENT

The process for assessment of SEN is described in the *Special Educational Needs Code of Practice* (DfES 2001).

All children not making expected progress should have assessment by school staff of their strengths and difficulties (School Action). They will decide how they can address this and set up an individual education plan (IEP) for the child.

Once it is established that there is a significant learning problem further consultation will be necessary (School Action Plus).

May include education professionals (specialist teachers, educational psychologists) and health professionals (school nurse, paediatrician, speech and language therapist, clinical psychologist) who should further investigate the nature of the difficulty, i.e. is it a general learning problem or specific?

The medical role at this stage is to identify any treatable problems that may be contributing (illness, vision or hearing problems), look for any underlying explanation for the problem by reviewing the medical history, examining and investigating as necessary.

Assessment should always be multidisciplinary and may be facilitated by meetings of all involved. For children with severe or complex difficulties a statutory assessment of SEN may be initiated (see Chapter 95).

School placements

Children with SEN will normally have them met in a mainstream school, with appropriate support. Other placements will occur where this is not possible or when such provision would be incompatible with the education of other students. Alternatives include special units within a mainstream school, pupil referral units (behaviour problems) and special schools. Home tuition may be provided for children who have been excluded, have school refusal or medical problems.

WHO TO TALK TO

Assessment must be multidisciplinary and include a broad range of health and educational professionals.

FOLLOW-UP

Once identified as having SEN, a review of the child's IEP should take place at least twice a year. The school can invite contributions from other agencies.

Children with a statement of SEN will have an annual review of the statement. Annual review in Year 9 and subsequently also includes drawing up and then review of a transition plan to help prepare for Post 16 provision and school leaving. The Connexions service is involved at this stage. Involved heath professionals should contribute.

KEY POINTS FOR PARENTS

LEAs vary in their approach to provision for SEN. Many children are adequately provided for without the need for a statement of SEN.

Parent partnership services must be set up in each LEA to provide parents with advice and information on SEN.

HEALTH PROMOTION

Children with SEN may also be at risk of health problems, e.g. those with specific syndromes.

Problems with vision, hearing, sleep, nutrition, toileting, etc. are all more common in children with SEN.

Many children with learning problems suffer from lack of confidence and poor self-esteem, possibly leading to mental health problems.

ADDITIONAL POINTS

Parents of children with SEN may well have had special needs themselves. Care needs to be taken to help them understand their child's difficulties and the support they require.

SUPPORT ORGANISATIONS

Connexions (career guidance for 14–19 year olds) – www.connexions. gov.uk

SOURCES

Department for Education and Skills (2001) Special educational needs: code of
   practice. London: DfES. Online. Available:
   www.teachernet.gov.uk/_doc/3724/SENCodeOfPractice.pdf

See also

Chapter 92, Special medical needs in education; Chapter 94, Checklist for
   advice to local education authorities; Chapter 95, Education legislation.

CHECKLIST FOR ADVICE TO LOCAL EDUCATION AUTHORITIES

PRINCIPLES

Report must be returned within 6 weeks of request, unless child is unknown to the service.

There is usually advance notification that the need for an assessment is being considered.

Must be written in easily understood language.

Should provide information on how the child's health is likely to affect his/her education.

Should be agreed in consultation with parents. There may be information that they are sensitive about. Parents should never acquire important new information about their child for the first time in a report for the LEA.

School paediatrician is responsible for requesting and collating any necessary specialist or paramedical reports, e.g. from speech therapy, physiotherapy, child psychiatry.

It is essential to include strengths as well as weaknesses – children need to feel good about their achievements.

There may also be special medical needs that should be met in school and which do not cause learning difficulties.

EPIDEMIOLOGY AND AETIOLOGY

20% of children will have a special educational need at some point; a much smaller number will have a formal statement.

CONTENT OF THE MEDICAL REPORT

The following areas need to be considered although some may not be relevant for a particular child:

- Brief description of medical problems/conditions – in many cases there is no medical diagnosis.
- Medical history, including development.
- Problem list using functional approach, e.g. mobility, hand function, communication.

- Growth.
- Emotional and behavioural difficulties.
- Relevant information on family and social problems on a need-to-know basis.
- Include positive attributes, i.e. what the child can do.
- Self-help skills – toileting, feeding, dressing, washing.
- Should any restrictions be placed on the child's activities?
- Include significant negatives, e.g. normality of vision or hearing.
- With sensory impairments, give technical data (e.g. visual acuity, auditory thresholds) as well as a functional explanation of abilities (e.g. can the child see the outline of a person, read a facial expression, hear a car coming).
- Might the child's abilities fluctuate in the short term or deteriorate in the long term?

Summary of recommended medical facilities and resources
Medical and nursing supervision.
Physical environment, e.g. access, lighting, acoustics.
Emotional climate and social regimen.
Provision of aids, e.g. mobility, auditory, visual.
Medication needed in school – routine and in emergency situations, administration, side effects.
Diet and help with feeding.
Health resources, e.g. speech therapy, occupational therapy, orthoptics.
Help with daily living, e.g. feeding, dressing, washing, toileting, guarding against common dangers.
Medical follow-up.
Transport to school.

FOLLOW-UP
Medical advice will need updating when individual education plans are reviewed or when clinical needs change.

KEY POINTS FOR PARENTS
Information on organisations or support services from voluntary groups can be very helpful to parents.

SOURCES
Department for Education and Skills (2001) Special educational needs: code of practice. London: DfES. Online. Available: www.teachernet.gov.uk/_doc/3724/SENCodeOfPractice.pdf

EDUCATION LEGISLATION

EDUCATION ACT 1996

Extensive piece of legislation covering statutory systems, funding, curriculum, attendances and admissions. Part 4 addresses special educational needs (SEN).

A child is said to have SEN if they have a learning difficulty which calls for special educational provision to be made.

The term 'learning difficulty' is used where a child:

- has a significantly greater difficulty in learning than the majority of children of his age, *or*
- has a disability that prevents or hinders him from making use of educational facilities generally provided for children of his age in schools within the area of the local education authority, *or*
- is under 5 years of age and would be likely to fall into the above categories if special educational provision were not made.

Special educational provision means provision that is different from that made generally for other children of the same age in schools maintained by the local education authority (other than special schools) or grant-maintained schools in their area or, in a child under 2, educational provision of any kind.

Principles introduced in the 1996 Education Act have been built on and amended in the subsequent Special Educational Needs and Disability Act 2001 and the Code of Practice 2001, described below.

SPECIAL EDUCATIONAL NEEDS AND DISABILITY (SEND) ACT 2001

Key points include:

- strengthened rights for pupils with SEN to mainstream educational provision
- new duties on LEAs to:
  - advertise parent partnership services

- make arrangements for resolving disagreement between schools, parents and the LEA
- inform parents when any SEN provision is made for their child
- time limits for completing assessment of SEN and issuing a statement of SEN where appropriate
- specific procedures for reviewing statements
- extension of parents' rights to appeal against LEA decisions on assessment and statements of SEN, independent Special Educational Needs Tribunal to hear those appeals and time limits to implement tribunal decisions
- duty on schools to draw up, publish and report on their SEN policy.

Part 2 of the SEND Act came into force in 2002 and amends the Disability Discrimination Act by introducing new legislation to prevent discrimination against disabled people in their access to education, including in schools.
The key duties are:

- not to treat disabled pupils less favourably
- to make reasonable adjustments to avoid putting disabled pupils at a disadvantage.

THE SPECIAL EDUCATIONAL NEEDS (SEN) CODE OF PRACTICE 2001

The fundamental principles are that:

- a child with SEN will have their needs met
- the child will normally be educated in a mainstream school
- the views of the child should be taken into account
- parents have a vital role in supporting their child's education
- children with SEN should be offered full access to a broad, balanced and relevant curriculum
- those involved with SEN should work in partnership with other agencies.

The code recommends a staged approach to making provision:

- *Identification*: Teacher identifies child as making inadequate progress.
- *School Action*: School informs parents. Information gathered, special provision organised, and individual education plan (IEP) drawn up.
- *School Action Plus*: Outside specialists consulted as to how child's needs could be met in school.
- *Statutory assessment*: LEA considers need for statutory multidisciplinary assessment.
- *Making a statement*: LEA uses multidisciplinary assessment to make a statement, and then reviews and monitors provision.

ASSESSMENT

Statutory assessment of special educational needs

The parents or the school can request an assessment.

Other agencies (health or social services) can alert the LEA that a child may need an assessment. The education authority will gather evidence and decide whether they should proceed.

Statutory assessment must include:

- parental advice
- educational advice
- medical advice
- psychological advice
- social services advice.

Once complete, the LEA decides whether to issue a statement of SEN.

The whole process from considering an assessment to finalising a statement should take 6 months. There are time limits for each stage.

See also

Chapter 93, Special educational needs.

8

REFERENCE CHARTS AND TABLES

ESSENTIAL CORE DATA SET

On a national basis in the UK, information about children's health and development is not currently collected in a standard way. Different agencies are involved, collecting differing pieces of information in differing formats.

The Child Health Informatics Consortium has tried to address this problem with the formation of the Essential Core Data Set, a set of 37 individual pieces of information to be collected for every child.

The Core Data Set will enable us to compare individuals against standards reflecting best practice. This will support the initiatives of clinical governance, reduction of inequalities in health, and ensure the best possible future for our children in the 21st century.

The Essential Core Data Set will eventually form the basis of a child health electronic health record.

Data will be collected from birth to 16 years of age. Some examples of items to be collected are:

- at birth, NHS numbers of mother and child, birth weight, gestational age, neonatal screening test results, etc.
- developmental reviews completed, breast feeding status, immunisations completed at key ages
- status with regard to child protection registration and disability status
- hospital outpatient attendances and Emergency Department attendances.

SOURCES

Child Health Informatics Consortium (2000) Monitoring the health of the nation's children. Online. Available: www.chiconsortium.org.uk

9

DEVELOPMENT

0–5 YEARS

The boxes corresponding to the child's chronological age are filled in (horizontal axis) against the age-related developmental items on the left. One box must be filled in for each item achieved.

90% of children will complete items above the black line. Those 10% scoring below the line should be referred or reassessed within 1 month. Allowances must be made for prematurity when filling out these charts.

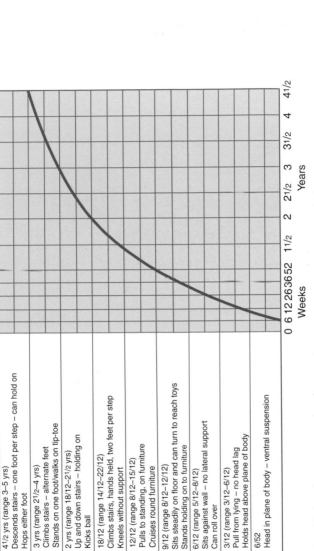

4½ yrs (range 3–5 yrs)
Descends stairs – one foot per step – can hold on
Hops either foot

3 yrs (range 2½–4 yrs)
Climbs stairs – alternate feet
Stands on one foot/walks on tip-toe

2 yrs (range 18/12–2½ yrs)
Up and down stairs – holding on
Kicks ball

18/12 (range 14/12–22/12)
Climbs stairs, hands held, two feet per step
Kneels without support

12/12 (range 8/12–15/12)
Pulls to standing, on furniture
Cruises round furniture

9/12 (range 8/12–12/12)
Sits steadily on floor and can turn to reach toys
Stands holding on to furniture

6/12 (range 5/12–8/12)
Sits against wall – no lateral support
Can roll over

3/12 (range 3/12–6/12)
Pull from lying – no head lag
Holds head above plane of body

6/52
Head in plane of body – ventral suspension

0 6 12 26 36 52   1½   2   2½   3   3½   4   4½
Weeks   Years

Fig. 97.1   Gross motor development.

9

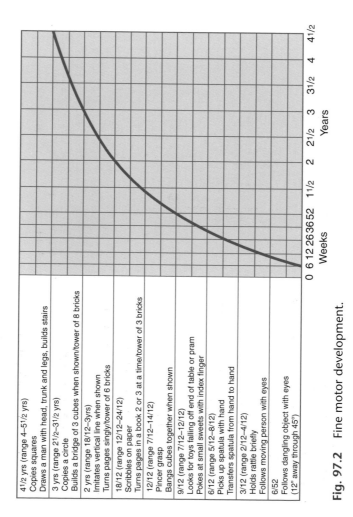

Fig. 97.2 Fine motor development.

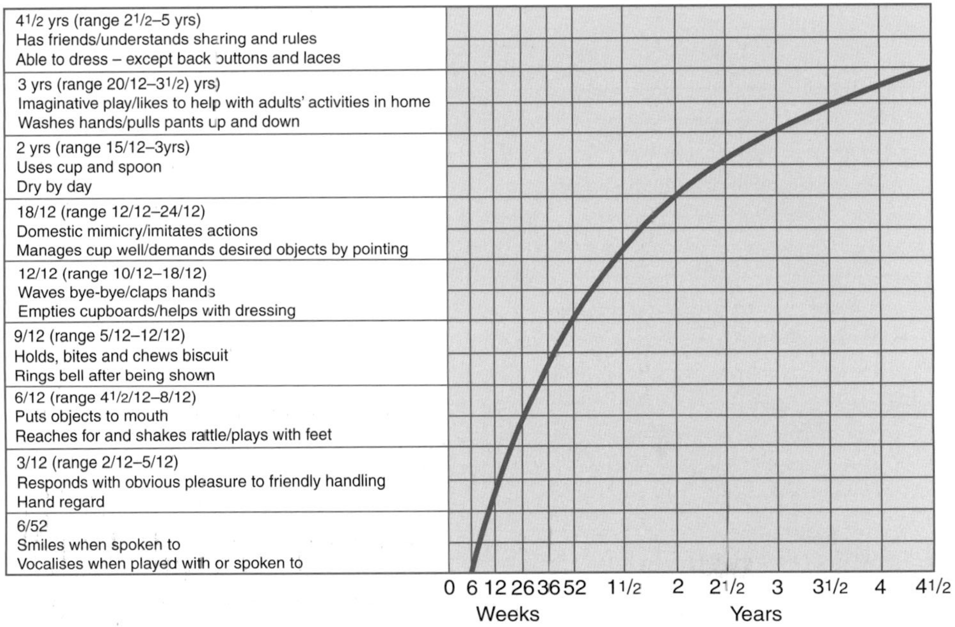

41/2 yrs (range 21/2–5 yrs)
Has friends/understands sharing and rules
Able to dress – except back buttons and laces

3 yrs (range 20/12–31/2) yrs)
Imaginative play/likes to help with adults' activities in home
Washes hands/pulls pants up and down

2 yrs (range 15/12–3yrs)
Uses cup and spoon
Dry by day

18/12 (range 12/12–24/12)
Domestic mimicry/imitates actions
Manages cup well/demands desired objects by pointing

12/12 (range 10/12–18/12)
Waves bye-bye/claps hands
Empties cupboards/helps with dressing

9/12 (range 5/12–12/12)
Holds, bites and chews biscuit
Rings bell after being shown

6/12 (range 41/2–8/12)
Puts objects to mouth
Reaches for and shakes rattle/plays with feet

3/12 (range 2/12–5/12)
Responds with obvious pleasure to friendly handling
Hand regard

6/52
Smiles when spoken to
Vocalises when played with or spoken to

0 6 12 26 36 52   11/2   2   21/2   3   31/2   4   41/2
Weeks   Years

Fig. 97.3 Social development.

9

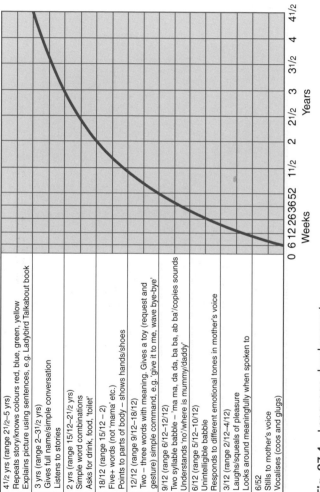

4½ yrs (range 2½–5 yrs)
Repeats story/knows colours red, blue, green, yellow
Explains picture using sentences, e.g. Ladybird Talkabout book

3 yrs (range 2–3½ yrs)
Gives full name/simple conversation
Listens to stories

2 yrs (range 15/12–2½ yrs)
Simple word combinations
Asks for drink, food, 'toilet'

18/12 (range 15/12 – 2)
Five+ words (not 'mama' etc.)
Points to parts of body – shows hands/shoes

12/12 (range 9/12–18/12)
Two – three words with meaning. Gives a toy (request and
gesture) simple command, e.g. 'give it to me, wave bye-bye'

9/12 (range 6/12–12/12)
Two syllable babble – 'ma ma, da da, ba ba, ab ba'/copies sounds
Understands 'no'/where is mummy/daddy'

6/12 (range 5/12–10/12)
Unintelligible babble
Responds to different emotional tones in mother's voice

3/12 (range 2/12–4/12)
Laughs/squeals of pleasure
Looks around meaningfully when spoken to

6/52
Stills to mother's voice
Vocalises (coos and glugs)

0 6 12 263652   1½   2   2½   3   3½   4   4½
Weeks   Years

Fig. 97.4 Language development.

98

GROWTH CHARTS AND MISCELLANEOUS CHARTS

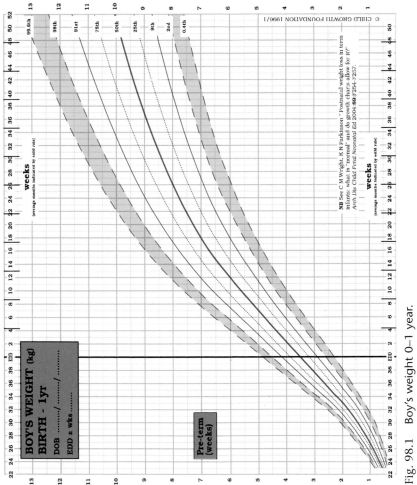

Fig. 98.1 Boy's weight 0–1 year.

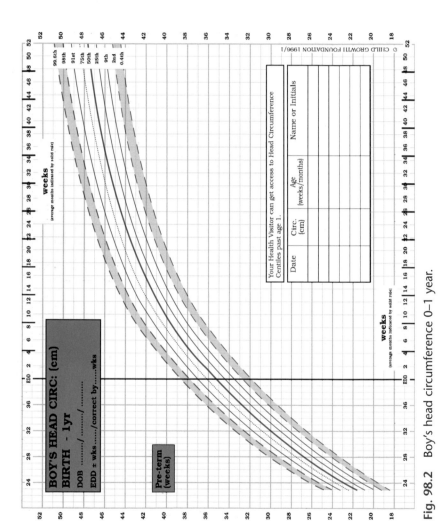

Fig. 98.2 Boy's head circumference 0–1 year.

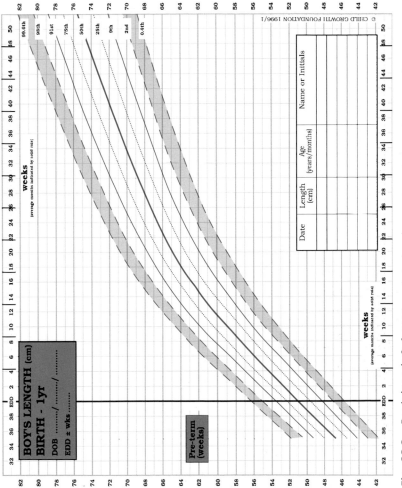

Fig. 98.3 Boy's length 0–1 year.

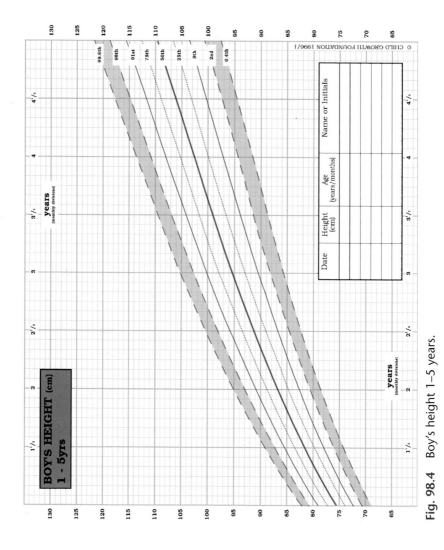

Fig. 98.4 Boy's height 1–5 years.

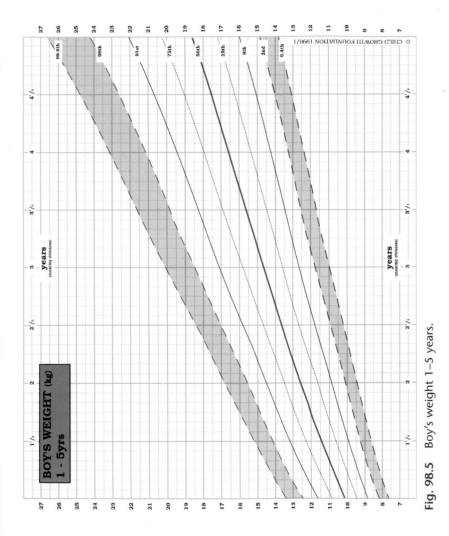

Fig. 98.5 Boy's weight 1–5 years.

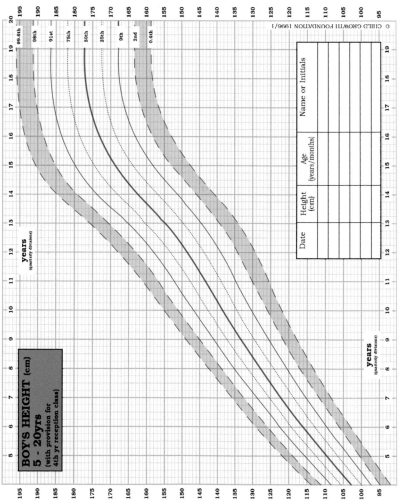

Fig. 98.6 Boy's height 5–20 years.

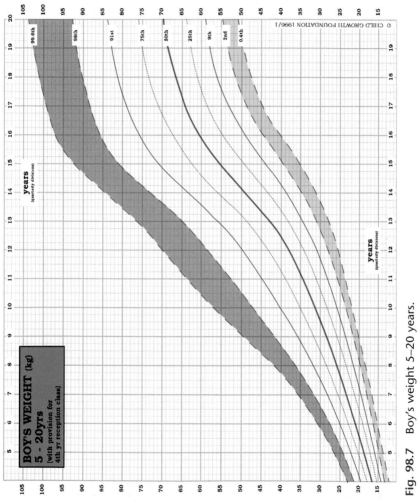

Fig. 98.7 Boy's weight 5–20 years.

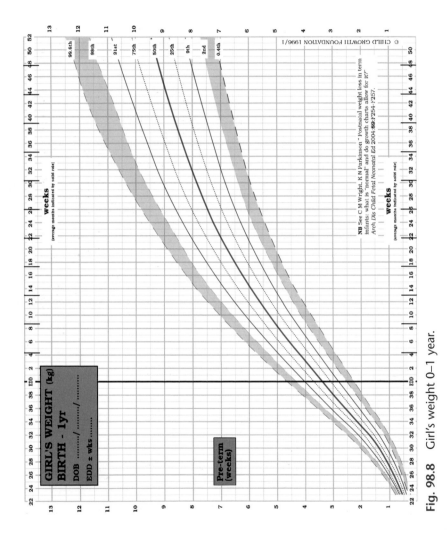

Fig. 98.8 Girl's weight 0–1 year.

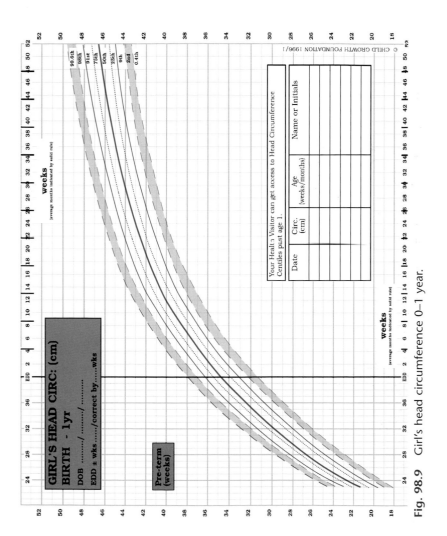

Fig. 98.9 Girl's head circumference 0–1 year.

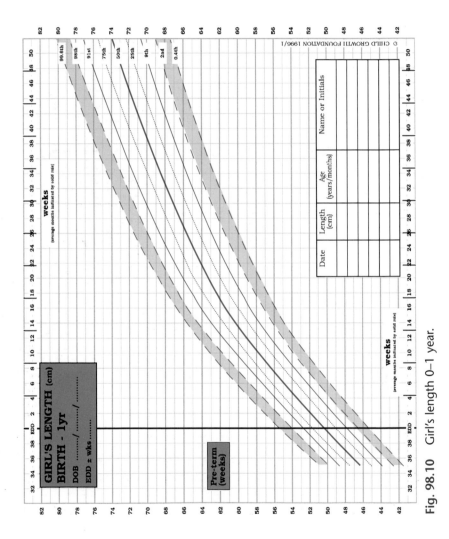

Fig. 98.10 Girl's length 0–1 year.

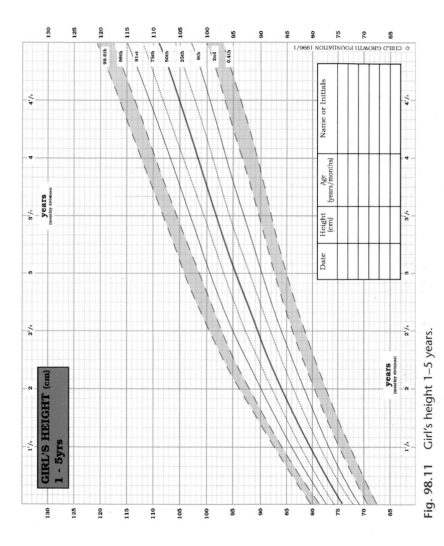

Fig. 98.11 Girl's height 1–5 years.

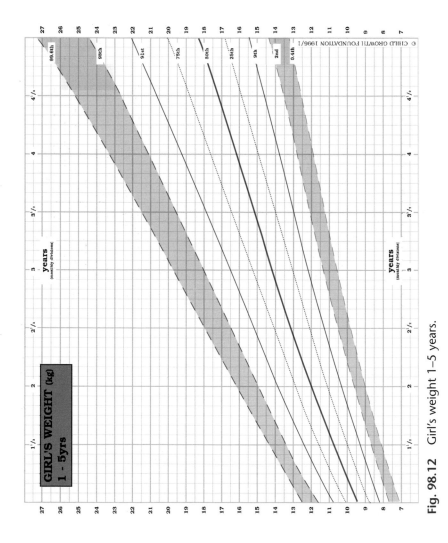

Fig. 98.12 Girl's weight 1–5 years.

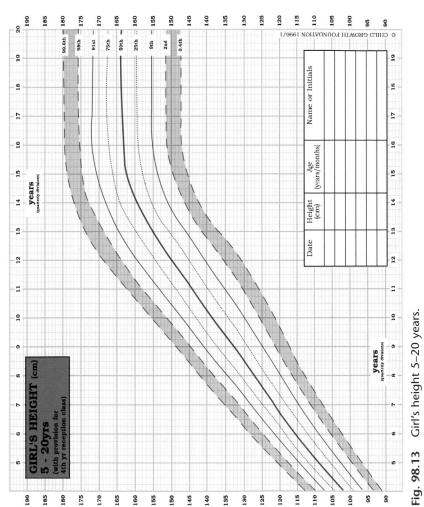

Fig. 98.13 Girl's height 5–20 years.

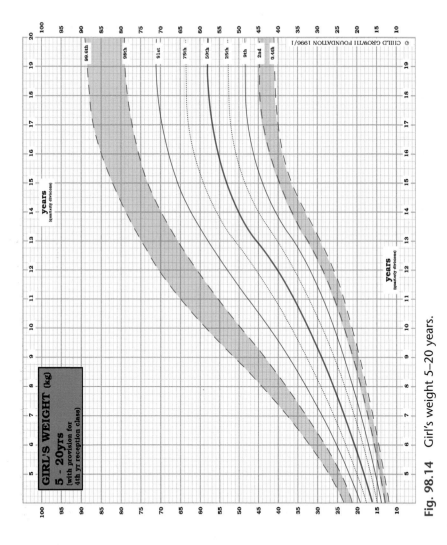

Fig. 98.14   Girl's weight 5–20 years.

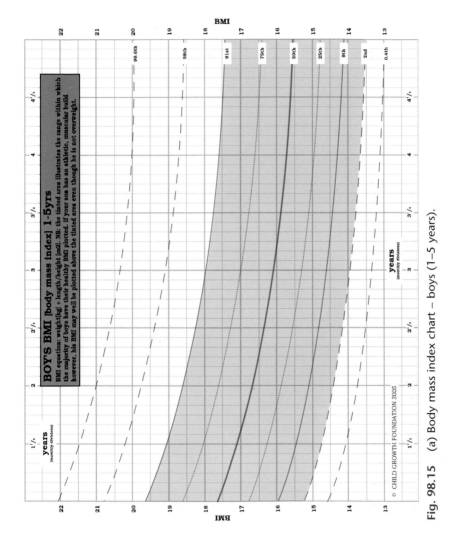

BOY'S BMI [body mass index] 1-5yrs

BMI equation: weight[kg] ÷ length/height [m2]. NB: the tinted area illustrates the range within which the majority of boys have their healthy BMI plotted. If your son has an athletic, muscular build however, his BMI may well be plotted above the tinted area even though he is not overweight.

© CHILD GROWTH FOUNDATION 2005

Fig. 98.15 (a) Body mass index chart – boys (1–5 years).

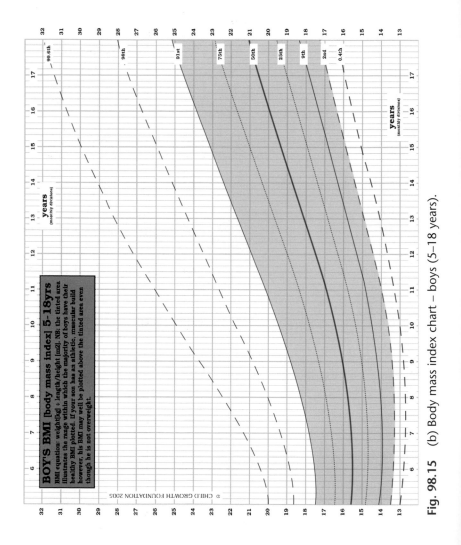

BOY'S BMI (body mass index) 5-18yrs

BMI equation: weight(kg) ÷ length/height (m2). NB: the tinted area illustrates the range within which the majority of boys have their healthy BMI plotted. If your son has an athletic, muscular build however, his BMI may well be plotted above the tinted area even though he is not overweight.

© CHILD GROWTH FOUNDATION 2005

Fig. 98.15 (b) Body mass index chart – boys (5–18 years).

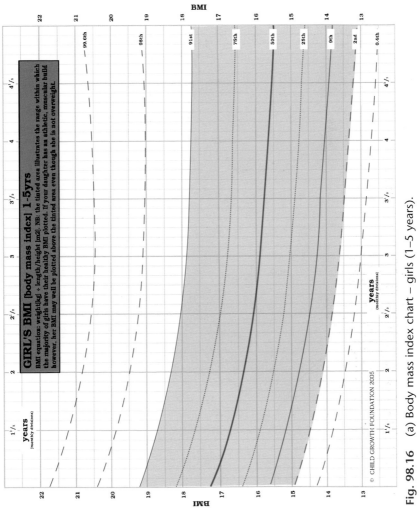

GIRL'S BMI [body mass index] 1-5yrs

BMI equation: weight[kg] ÷ length/height [m2]. NB: the tinted area illustrates the range within which the majority of girls have their healthy BMI plotted. If your daughter has an athletic, muscular build however, her BMI may well be plotted above the tinted area even though she is not overweight.

© CHILD GROWTH FOUNDATION 2005

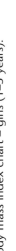

Fig. 98.16 (a) Body mass index chart – girls (1–5 years).

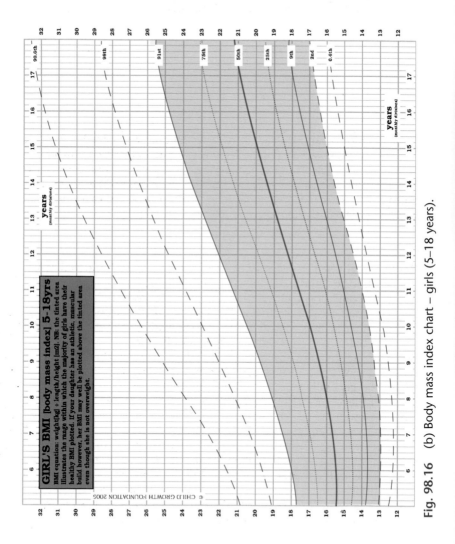

GIRL'S BMI [body mass index] 5-18yrs

BMI equation: weight[kg] ÷ length/height [m2]. NB: the tinted area illustrates the range within which the majority of girls have their healthy BMI plotted. If your daughter has an athletic, muscular build however, her BMI may well be plotted above the tinted area even though she is not overweight.

© CHILD GROWTH FOUNDATION 2005

Fig. 98.16 (b) Body mass index chart – girls (5–18 years).

99

LABORATORY NORMAL VALUES

BACKGROUND

In general, biological variables – such as laboratory normal values or reference ranges – are normally distributed and an arbitrary cut-off can be chosen, e.g. defining abnormal values as above and below two standard deviations (2 SD) from the mean, or those in the top and bottom 2%. This is a statistical view of the normality of values in a given population of values.

CAUTIONS

- Doctors might be interested in making a diagnosis and undertaking intervention to improve quality of life or prognosis at a value within this statistically normal range, e.g. by using statins to reduce adverse lipids in adults at risk of atheroma-related coronary artery disease.
- On the other hand, there are some diseases which may be diagnosed or suggested by abnormal laboratory values but only when far in excess of the statistically normal range. Becker and Duchenne muscular dystrophies are relatively common dystrophinopathies which can generally be excluded by a normal plasma creatine kinase (CK, CPK) level (60–300 IU/l). However they can also be excluded by a high CK well outside the normal range, being suggested at CK values above, often way above, 5000 IU/l.
- Some values are particularly susceptible to artefact. Plasma values for potassium, lactate, CK and platelet concentrations can be affected by trauma, haemolysis and difficulty getting the blood to flow freely.
- In addition, samples taken into the wrong bottle may be useless, e.g. blood for glucose and lactate should be taken into fluoride oxalate (beware different laboratories use different colour codes on the bottles).
- Some estimations need to be done immediately, e.g. plasma ammonia levels rise with time in the bottle and should be measured within 30–60 minutes of venepuncture. The laboratory will need warning for this and other complex tests, e.g. white cell enzymes.

- For some tests different laboratories have different normal ranges of values or reference ranges, or even express the results in different units, e.g. for antiepileptic drug (AED) concentrations. If in doubt, check with your own laboratory.
- Very rarely labelling or processing errors can arise. The occurrence of one abnormality that does not fit with the other clinical and laboratory evidence should be regarded with caution and perhaps repeated or ignored.
- The clinical significance of an abnormal value may depend on the child's clinical state, e.g. the target ranges quoted for AEDs were generally induced from small adult studies, and individual children may not conform to them. One child may be toxic at a modest plasma phenytoin level whereas another will be well and need a high level above the 'target range' to get benefit. The unnecessary reduction of AEDs due to their unnecessary measurement and inexperienced interpretation can precipitate status epilepticus.
- Normal values or reference ranges in neonates and infants are often different (designated N).
- The pattern of results or trend over time may be more useful than just the 'normal' versus 'abnormal' dichotomy.

Table 99.1 Clinical chemistry

Test	Measurement	Comment
Acid–base (arterial P)	pH 7.3–7.45; H$^+$ 35–48 nmol/l	
$PaCO_2$	4.5–6 kPa; 32–45 mmHg	
PaO_2	11–14 kPa; 80–100 mmHg	
Bicarbonate	18–26 mmol/l	
Base excess	–4 to +3	
Alanine transaminase (ALT) (P)	15–55 IU/l	Laboratories vary
Albumin (P, N)	30–55 g/l	
Alkaline phosphatase (ALP) (P, N)	250–1000 IU/l	Laboratories vary
Ammonia (NH$_3$) (P, N)	<50 micromol/l	
Amylase (P, N)	70–300 IU/l	Laboratories vary
Aspartate transaminase (AST) (P, N)	<50 IU/l	Laboratories vary
B$_{12}$ (S)	150–1000 ng/l	
Bicarbonate (P)	18–26 mmol/l	
Bilirubin (P, N):		
total	<17 micromol/l	
conjugated	<2 micromol/l	
Calcium (P, N) (total)	2.2–2.6 mmol/l	
Cholesterol (P, S, N):		
total:	3–5.8 mmol/l	Fasting
HDL	>0.9 mmol/l	Fasting
Creatine kinase (CK, CPK) (P, N)	60–300 IU/l (in dystrophies >5000 IU/l)	High with trauma
Creatinine (P, N)	25–120 micromol/l	Increases with age
C–reactive protein (CRP) (P)	<10 mg/l	
Erythrocyte sedimentation rate (ESR)	<10 mm/hr	Consult laboratory re bottle
Ferritin (S)	8–300 ng/mL	
Folate:		
serum (S)	3–20 ng/ml	
red cell (B)	100–640 ng/ml	
Iron (S)	5–34 micromol/l	
Lead (B)	<1.75 micromol/l	Consult laboratory re bottle
Lactate (P, flu ox)	0.6–2.4 mmol/l	
Magnesium (P)	0.6–1.0 mmol/l	

continued

Table 99.1   Clinical chemistry—cont'd

Test	Measurement	Comment
Potassium (P, N)	3.0–5.6 mmol/l	High if haemolysed
Phosphate (P, N)	0.7–1.8 mmol/l	
Glucose (P, flu ox, N)	3–6 mmol/l >2.5 mmol/l	Fasting, keep
Protein (P):		
total	60–80 g/l	
albumin	35–55 g/l	
Sodium (P)	133–145 mmol/l	
Thyroid-stimulating hormone (TSH) (P, N)	0.4–5 mIU/l	
Thyroxine (free T$_4$) (P, N)	6–26 pmol/l	Laboratories vary
Total iron binding capacity (TIBC) (P)	45–70 micromol/l	
Transferrin (S)	2.5–4.5 g/l	
Triglycerides	0.4–1.7 mmol/l	Fasting
Urate (P, N)	120–390 micromol/l	
Urea (P, N)	2.5–6.7 mmol/l	

B, whole blood; flu ox, fluoride oxalate; N, different in neonates; P, plasma; S, serum.

Table 99.2   Haematology indices (B in EDTA)

Age	Hb (g/l)	MCV (fl)	MCHC (%)	WBC (10^9/l)	(%)	Neutrophils (10^9/l)	(%)	Lympho-cytes (10^9/l)	Platelets (10^9/l)
Neonate	14–22	95–116	29–34	9–30	30–50	3–22	30–50	2–6	150–400
6 months	8.5–13	80–96	32–36	6–18	30–50	1–8	30–50	4–13	150–400
1–5 years	10–13	75–96	32–36	6–15	30–50	1.5–8.5	30–50	3–9	150–400
5–10 years	11–14	75–96	32–36	5–15	40–65	1.5–8	30–50	2–7	150–400
10–15 years	11–15	80–96	32–36	4–13	50–75	1.8–8	30–50	2–6	150–400

Expect: monocytes 2–10%, eosinophils 1–6%, basophils <1% of WBC.
Hb, haemoglobin; MCHC, mean corpuscular haemoglobin concentration; MCV, mean corpuscular volume; WBC, white blood count.

Table 99.3 Antiepileptic drug (AED) target range (TR)

Drug	mg/l (microgram/ml)	micromol/l	Comments
Carbamazepine	4–12	16–60	
Ethosuximide	40–100	300–750	
Lamotrigine	1.5–20	–	May be toxic >5 mg/l
Phenobarbital	10–50	45–200	
Phenytoin	10–25	40–100	May be toxic in TR or need higher level
Valproate	40–100	280–700	

Approximate concentrations (plasma, serum).

INFECTIOUS DISEASES – REFERENCE TABLES

Table 100.1

Infection	Incubation period	Period of infectiousness	Recommended exclusion period
Rashes			
Chicken pox (varicella)	11–20 days	–4 to +5 days	5 days from start of skin infection
fifth disease (erythema infectiosum, parvovirus, slapped cheek)	13–18 days	Not known	None because onset of disease occurs after transmission has occurred
Infectious mononucleosis	33–49 days	At least 2 months	None, there is a prolonged period of excretion which would not allow exclusion
Measles	6–19 days	Infectious 1–2 days before onset of rash	5 days from onset of rash
Roseola infantum (exanthema subitum)	10–15 days	Not known, maybe life-long	None
Rubella	15–20 days	Most infectious in prodrome	5 days from onset of rash
Scabies	7–27 days	If not treated, indefinite	Until treated
Scarlet fever	2–4 days	Not known	5 days from start of antibiotic treatment
Warts and verrucae	1–24 months	Some think could be duration of lesion	None

9

462

Table 100.2   Diseases notifiable (to local authority proper officers) under the Public Health (Infectious Diseases) Regulations 1988

Acute encephalitis
Acute poliomyelitis
Anthrax
Cholera
Diphtheria
Dysentery
Food poisoning
Leptospirosis
Malaria
Measles
Meningitis:
- meningococcal
- pneumococcal
- *Haemophilus influenzae*
- viral
- other specified
- unspecified

Meningococcal septicaemia (without meningitis)
Mumps
Ophthalmia neonatorum
Paratyphoid fever
Plague
Rabies
Relapsing fever
Rubella
Scarlet fever
Smallpox
Tetanus
Tuberculosis
Typhoid fever
Typhus fever
Viral haemorrhagic fever
Viral hepatitis:
- hepatitis A
- hepatitis B
- hepatitis C
- other

Whooping cough
Yellow fever
Leprosy is also notifiable, but to the Director, CDSC.

9

BASIC PAEDIATRIC LIFE SUPPORT

Flow charts outlining basic paediatric life support and advanced paediatric life support – based on the 2001 Resuscitation Council (UK) *Guidelines for Resuscitation* – are illustrated on the front and back covers, respectively, of this book.

DRUGS

Defibrillation:	2 joules/kg
then	2 joules/kg
then	4 joules/kg
Adrenaline:	0.1 ml/kg of 1:10,000 and repeat 3–5 minutes
Bicarbonate:	0.5 ml/kg of 4.2%
Fluids:	20 ml/kg (10 ml/kg for trauma)

Seizures

Midazolam:	0.5 mg/kg up to 10 mg, buccal or intranasal
Lorazepam:	0.1 mg/kg (maximum 4 mg)
Rectal diazepam:	0.5 mg/kg up to 10 mg IV solution

Hypoglycaemia

Glucose:	5 ml/kg of 10%

INDEX